D1206720

IMPROVING THE LONG-TERM MANAGEMENT OF OBESITY

WILEY SERIES ON
HEALTH PSYCHOLOGY/BEHAVIORAL MEDICINE

Thomas J. Boll, Series Editor

Improving the Long-Term Management of Obesity

Theory, Research, and Clinical Guidelines

Michael G. Perri
University of Florida

Arthur M. Nezu
Hahnemann University

Barbara J. Viegener
FDR V.A. Hospital

A Wiley-Interscience Publication

JOHN WILEY & SONS

New York / Chichester / Brisbane / Toronto / Singapore

RC628
.P465
1992

In recognition of the importance of preserving what has been written, it is a policy of John Wiley & Sons, Inc., to have books of enduring value published in the United States printed on acid-free paper, and we exert our best efforts to that end.

Copyright © 1992 by John Wiley & Sons, Inc.

All rights reserved. Published simultaneously in Canada.

Reproduction or translation of any part of this work beyond that permitted by Section 107 or 108 of the 1976 United States Copyright Act without the permission of the copyright owner is unlawful. Requests for permission or further information should be addressed to the Permissions Department, John Wiley & Sons, Inc.

This publication is designed to provide accurate and authoritative information in regard to the subject matter covered. It is sold with the understanding that the publisher is not engaged in rendering legal, accounting, or other professional service. If legal advice or other expert assistance is required, the services of a competent professional person should be sought. *From a Declaration of Principles jointly adopted by a Committee of the American Bar Association and a Committee of Publishers.*

Library of Congress Cataloging-in-Publication Data

Perri, Michael G.
  Improving the long-term management of obesity : theory, research, and clinical guidelines / Michael G. Perri, Arthur M. Nezu, Barbara J. Viegener.
     p.   cm.—(Wiley series on health psychology/behavioral medicine)
  Includes bibliographical references and indexes.
  ISBN 0-471-52899-4 (cloth : alk. paper)
  1. Obesity—Treatment. I. Nezu, Arthur M. II. Viegener, Barbara J. III. Title. IV. Series.
  [DNLM: 1. Behavior Therapy. 2. Models, Psychological.
  3. Obesity—psychology. 4. Obesity—therapy.   WD 210 P4561]
  RC628.P465   1992
  616.3'9806—dc20
  DNLM/DLC
  for Library of Congress   92-92
                                                                                CIP

Printed in the United States of America

10 9 8 7 6 5 4 3 2 1

For my parents
MGP

For Chris
AMN

For my parents and my children
BJV

JUL 1 6 1996

JUN 1 5 1936

Series Preface

This series is addressed to clinicians and scientists who are interested in human behavior relevant to the promotion and maintenance of health and the prevention and treatment of illness. *Health psychology* and *behavioral medicine* are terms that refer to both the scientific investigation and interdisciplinary integration of behavioral and biomedical knowledge and technology to prevention, diagnosis, treatment, and rehabilitation.

The major and purposely somewhat general areas of both health psychology and behavioral medicine which will receive greatest emphasis in this series are: theoretical issues of bio-psycho-social function, diagnosis, treatment, and maintenance; issues of organizational impact on human performance and an individual's impact on organizational functioning; development and implementation of technology for understanding, enhancing or remediating human behavior and its impact on health and function; and clinical considerations with children and adults, alone, in groups, or in families that contribute to the scientific and practical/clinical knowledge of those charged with the care of patients.

The series encompasses considerations as intellectually broad as psychology and as numerous as the multitude of areas of evaluation treatment and prevention and maintenance that make up the field of medicine. It is the aim of this series to provide a vehicle that will focus attention on both the breadth and the interrelated nature of the sciences and practices making up health psychology and behavioral medicine.

THOMAS J. BOLL

The University of Alabama at Birmingham
Birmingham, Alabama

Preface

In November of 1988, Oprah Winfrey announced to her talk show audience, and the rest of America, that she lost 67 pounds by using Optifast, a very-low-calorie formula diet. In the subsequent week, Sandoz Nutrition, the manufacturer of Optifast, reportedly received one million telephone inquiries from people interested in using their formula diet to lose weight (Foreyt, 1990).

In December of 1988, less than one month after Oprah's public disclosure, the *Journal of Consulting and Clinical Psychology* published a report by a well-respected group of obesity researchers (Wadden, Stunkard, & Liebschutz, 1988). The report described the long-term effectiveness of three treatments for obesity including a very-low-calorie diet similar to the one used by Ms. Winfrey. The results were disheartening. The large initial weight losses produced by the diet (M = 31.0 lb) were poorly maintained. At a one-year follow-up, patients regained two-thirds of their initial losses. Three years after treatment, the average subject was back to within 5 pounds of his or her original weight! The two alternative treatments in the study, behavior therapy and the combination of behavior therapy plus the very-low-calorie diet, fared no better. Participants in each of these treatments also showed significant relapses toward their pretreatment weights, albeit at a slightly slower rate. These findings foreshadowed the fate of Ms. Winfrey's 67-pound weight loss.

In November of 1990, two years after announcing her dieting success,

Oprah Winfrey publically acknowledged what the tabloids had heralded for months and what viewers of her show could plainly see, she had regained most if not all of her 67-pound weight loss. In a show called "The Pain of Regain," Oprah warned her audience "If you lose weight on a diet, sooner or later you'll gain it back."

Ms. Winfrey's unsuccessful effort at weight control dramatically illustrates the critical problem that confronts so many dieters, namely, the inability to maintain weight loss over the long run. Documenting the existence of a "maintenance problem" in the treatment of obesity will surprise few people. Most of us are well-acquainted with the commonly-cited estimate that 95% of those who diet regain all the weight that they have lost within one year. Yet several considerations make the problem of poor weight-loss maintenance increasingly disconcerting and ominous.

First of all, business is booming in the diet industry. Currently, Americans spend more than 30 billion dollars per year on weight-control products and treatments. Commercial weight-loss programs offering very-low-calorie diets continue to draw enormous numbers of people eager for rapid weight reductions. Consequently, more people are losing weight and losing greater amounts of weight than at anytime in U.S. history. However, the available research predicts that more obese people will be regaining weight and regaining larger amounts of weight that at any other time in U.S. history. Special cause for concern comes from recent epidemiological studies that indicate a significant health risk is associated with losing weight and regaining it (Lissner et al., 1991). Many obese people may be placing themselves in physical and psychological jeopardy by their patterns of dieting and regaining weight.

Finally, recent research, particularly studies directly targeted at the *long-term* management of obesity (e.g., Bjorvell & Rossner, 1985; Perri et al., 1988), indicate that something can be done to help obese individuals lose weight and maintain their losses. Unfortunately, the long-term maintenance of weight loss often remains a neglected area of clinical focus. Often, clinicians are so concerned about getting their patients to lose weight that they give inadequate attention to the problem of weight-loss maintenance. Unless the problem of poor maintenance of weight loss is successfully addressed, the treatment of obesity makes no sense.

We believe that health-care professionals must take a more careful look at the way they treat their obese patients. A responsible approach to the care of the obese person must include consideration of the following questions: Should this individual be treated at all? If so, which treatment is best suited to his or her needs? If treatment is initiated, what type of maintenance program will be employed? What procedures will be utilized to increase the chances of long-term success and diminish the possibility that initial weight loss will be followed by relapse and regaining of weight over the long run?

In writing this book, we attempt to address these questions and provide health-care professionals with a comprehensive guide to the long-term care of the obese patient. Our interest in the long-term management of obesity stems from our clinical and research experience. Over the past decade, we have worked with obese persons and have struggled to help them lose weight and keep it off. We have also conducted a programmatic series of studies addressing the problem of poor maintenance of weight loss. Our clinical and research experience suggests that successful long-term weight loss does not occur without long-term care. It is the rare case in which an obese individual loses a significant amount of weight in treatment, and then, on his or her own, maintains that loss over the long run.

Rather than lamenting the lack of long-term successes, we believe that health-care professionals ought to confront the problem of poor long-term outcome directly. In this book, we attempt to do just that. We argue that obesity is a chronic condition requiring continuous and possibly life-long care. Accordingly, we believe that in treating the obese patient the health-care professional's role is to serve as an active problem solver, one who systematically and continuously aids the patient in identifying effective strategies to sustain the behavioral changes needed for long-term success. Equipped with a variety of strategies designed to enhance the maintenance of weight loss, health-care professionals *may* be able to assist their patients in the long-term management of obesity. Without such assistance, the vast majority of patients are certain to relapse and regain most of their lost weight.

In PART I of this book, we provide a context for understanding obesity and appreciating why it is so difficult for obese persons to achieve long-term success in managing their weight. Our review is selective rather than exhaustive. We begin in Chapter 1 by defining the scope of the problem. We describe the prevalence of obesity, examine the physical and psychological consequences of this serious problem, and review both the substantial benefits and risks associated with dieting. In Chapter 2, we provide a biobehavioral perspective on the problem of obesity. We selectively review the pertinent literature on biological and behavioral contributions to the development and maintenance of obesity, and we discuss the implications of these factors for the treatment of obesity.

In Chapters 3, we consider the effectiveness of current treatments for obesity. We examine conservative approaches such as conventional diets, commercial weight-loss programs, self-help groups, and comprehensive behavioral treatments, and we also consider more aggressive interventions including pharmacotherapy, very-low-calorie diets, and bariatric surgery. Our review suggests a disturbing conclusion. At the present time, there is no safe and reliable means of producing large and lasting weight loss. Although many of the current treatments produce positive short-term results, long-term evaluations consistently show that weight reductions are poorly maintained, regardless of whether the weight loss was initially attained through dietary, behavioral or pharmacological means.

In Chapter 4, we describe a series of studies in which we tested the effectiveness of various weight-loss maintenance strategies including ongoing patient-therapist contacts, skills training, social support, exercise, and multicomponent programs. The most consistent finding in our research was that structured, long-term programs of continued contacts with health-care professionals successfully helped patients to maintain weight-loss progress. Consistent with a biobehavioral perspective on obesity, these findings suggest that obesity must be considered as a chronic condition similar to diseases such as diabetes or hypertension. The clinical implications of this perspective include the development of a continuous care model of obesity management, wherein a clinician who decides to treat obesity assumes responsibility for providing the obese person with long-term continuous care.

In PART II, we present a continuous care/problem solving model of obesity treatment. In Chapter 5, we delineate a problem-solving model consisting of five component processes: (1) problem orientation, (2) problem definition and formulation, (3) generation of alternatives, (4) decision making, and (5) solution implementation and verification. We describe how this framework can be used to guide the clinician's decision making in the long-term care of the obese patient. Within this model, we advocate adoption of a therapeutic orientation emphasizing: (a) that obesity is determined and maintained by multiple, varying biological and behavioral determinants; (b) that those factors that serve to maintain obesity, particularly the behavioral determinants, need to be idiographically assessed; (c) that interventions should be characterized as clinical strategies tailored to the individual problems of a particular person, rather than as a set of standard techniques uniformly applied to all patients; and (d) that treatment of obesity requires continuous implementation spanning long periods of time and involving different stages of care.

In Chapter 6, we describe the process of applying our continuous care/ problem solving model of obesity treatment. We characterize the management of obesity as consisting initially of a weight-loss treatment phase and a weight-loss maintenance phase. Within each of these phases, we identify four clinical tasks: (1) screening; (2) problem analysis; (3) treatment design; and (4) treatment implementation and evaluation. We illustrate how our problem-solving framework can be used to address the various clinical decisions encountered in each of these tasks. However, rather than describing *the* treatment program to use, we outline a methodology that the clinician can employ to idiographically design and evaluate such programs for a wide variety of patients.

In Part III, we present an array of clinical strategies that a health-care professional can use as a resource in developing an individualized approach to the long-term management of obesity. We begin in Chapter 7 by addressing several general clinical concerns regarding the implementation of our continuous care/problem solving model of long-term obesity treatment. These include suggestions and recommendations regarding assessment, the selection of treatment goals, the structure of treatment, and the client-therapist relationship. In Chapter 8, we presents a variety of skills training procedures that may be included in the long-term management of obesity. We describe how cognitive-behavioral therapy strategies can be used to help patients to cope with setbacks and to prevent relapse.

Chapter 9 summarizes the significant psychological and physical benefits of increased physical activity. Exercise is one of the few factors consistently associated with long-term weight-loss progress. Thus, we describe a variety of ways to incorporate exercise into the long-term care of the obese patient. Chapter 10 deals with dietary considerations in the management of obesity. In addition to providing an overview of what constitutes a nutritionally-sound approach to achieving weight loss, we also describe practical procedures that can help patients to modify those elements of their diet that are most likely to interfere with successful long-term management of their weight. Finally, in Chapter 11, we describe how social influence and social support strategies can be used to enhance weight-loss progress. Since effective long-term management of obesity often requires that the patient receive help from others, we present techniques that can be used in a group context, such as telephone networking, group contingency contracts, and competitions between members. We also examine the benefits and potential pitfalls of involving spouses, families, and peers in the maintenance process, and we describe how commercial weight-loss programs and self-help groups can be incorporated into a long-term plan for the management of obesity.

Thus, in this book, we present the problem of poor long-term maintenance of weight loss within the context of current theory and research regarding the causes of obesity and the effectiveness of its treatment. We provide a clinical guide to improving the long-term management of obesity, and we attempt to be as practical as possible in offering the reader ways of understanding and addressing obstacles to long-term success. We hope that the material that we present will stimulate further research, improve the clinical care of the obese patient, and contribute to higher rates of weight-loss maintenance.

Acknowledgments

Over the years, many individuals have contributed to our research on the treatment of obesity. We gratefully acknowledge their help and influence. Our sincere thanks go to Steve Richards, George McAdoo, Dave McAllister, Randy Jordan, Jim Gange, Peter Spevak, Rob Shapiro, Warren Ludwig, Craig Twentyman, Donna Yancey, Joan Lauer, David Newlin, Jim Rebeta, Charlie Wilson, Andy Eichmann, Mike Petronko, Karen McCann, Wendy McKelvey, Becky Schein, David Renjilian, and the late Peter Stalonas. We are particularly grateful to Chris Nezu, Jennifer Oglesby, and Shari Hatch, for suggestions that improved our manuscript, and to Nicole Engel, Melodye Gaskin, Sam Sears, and Jamie Temple for their technical assistance. We also express our appreciation to Herb Reich, our acquisitions editor at John Wiley & Sons, whose help made this book a reality. Finally, we thank those special people in our lives, Kathy and Katie Perri, Chris Nezu, and Jim Smith, who provided the support and encouragement that enabled us to complete this project.

Contents

PART I

THEORY AND RESEARCH

1

Obesity: Definition, Prevalence, and Consequences

Most health-care professionals would agree that obesity represents a common, serious, and difficult-to-treat clinical problem. The majority would also agree that obesity should be treated seriously. Yet few would admit to having confidence in the prospects for *long-term* success in the treatment of obesity. Such pessimism reflects the common belief that although many obese individuals may experience success in losing weight, most eventually regain much, if not all, of the weight they lost during treatment. The intriguing question of whether it is possible for an obese person to lose weight and keep it off permanently represents the heart of the "maintenance problem." Our aim in this book is to address this issue and to describe a therapeutic framework that can improve the long-term care of the obese person.

In this chapter, we provide a brief overview of the problem of obesity, including various definitions and classification schemes for obesity. We examine the prevalence of obesity in the United States, and we note the changes that have occurred over the past few decades. We also describe

3

the documented physical and psychological consequences of obesity, and we consider the impact of changes in weight on health and happiness.

DEFINING OBESITY

Obesity is defined by an excessive accumulation of body fat—excessive to the extent that it is thought to impair health. When body fat content equals or exceeds 30% in women or 25% in men, an individual is considered *obese; severe obesity* is characterized by a body fat content that exceeds 40% in women or 35% in men (Bray & Gray, 1988; Schlundt & Johnson, 1990). Unfortunately, body fat is difficult to measure. Aside from postmortem analyses of cadavers, there are no truly direct measures of body fat (Clarys, Martin, & Drinkwater, 1984). However, accurate estimates of percentage of body fat can be made indirectly through an assessment of body density. Because fat and fat-free mass have different specific densities, a comparison of a person's weight under water and then out of water allows a determination of the proportion of body weight that is fat. At present, this hydrostatic method of weighing represents the "gold standard" for assessing body fat. However, this cumbersome procedure requires an individual to be weighed while totally submerged under water and therefore is not practical for routine clinical purposes.

Alternative assessments of body fat, such as measurement of skinfold thickness, are less awkward; however, they suffer from problems related to the reliability of measurement. Newer technological developments (such as x-ray densitometry, bioelectrical impedance, infrared interactance, and computed tomography) have been developed for assessing body fat. However, these more sophisticated assessments have been developed from data derived from samples consisting primarily of normal-weight young adults; consequently, their current generalizability to obese populations is questionable (see Marshall, Hazlett, Spady, & Quinney, 1990).

Because of the difficulties inherent in measuring body fat, relative weight has become the most popular and convenient indicator of obesity. *Relative weight* is calculated by dividing a person's actual weight by the "ideal" weight for his or her height and sex. A relative weight of 1.20 or greater (i.e., 20% or more over ideal weight) is used as an operational definition of *obesity* (National Institutes of Health Consensus Development Panel on the Health Implications of Obesity, 1985).

There are several problems inherent in using either relative weight or percentage overweight as an indicator of obesity. First, a person may be overweight without being obese. The increased weight may reflect increased muscle mass rather than fat, as is often seen in athletes. Second, the degree of overweight at which an increased risk of disease develops remains an area of debate. The cutoff point of 20% overweight represents a value judgment rather than the precise starting point of a pathological state. Third, the ideal weights most commonly used—the 1983 Metropolitan height and weight tables (Metropolitan Life Insurance Company, 1984)—were derived from samples that were not representative of the U.S. population. The Metropolitan tables were based on findings from the 1979 Build Study (Society of Actuaries and Association of Life Insurance Medical Directors of America, 1980), in which weights associated with the lowest mortality were derived from 4.2 million life insurance policies issued between 1950 and 1971. The 1979 Build Study included a disproportionately larger number of males, whites, and individuals from middle and upper socioeconomic strata, and it omitted people over age 59 (cf. Foreyt, 1987a; Harrison, 1984). Finally, the ideal weights derived from the 1983 Metropolitan tables may require adjustment for age. Researchers have calculated the weights at which minimum mortality occurred for both men and women at each decade of life, based on the 1979 Build Study (Andres, Elahi, Tobin, Muller, & Brant, 1985). The results indicate that the so-called ideal weights are generally too high for younger adults and too low for older adults. Table 1.1 presents the age-specific weight-for-height recommendations calculated by Andres et al. (1985). Thus, although relative weight can be used as a simple and convenient indicator of obesity, clinicians should be aware of its limitations.

TABLE 1.1   AGE-SPECIFIC WEIGHT-FOR-HEIGHT RECOMMENDATIONS

Height (in.)	Weight (lb) range for men and women, by age (years)				
	25	35	45	55	65
58	84–111	92–119	99–127	107–135	115–142
59	87–115	95–123	103–131	111–139	119–147
60	90–119	98–127	106–135	114–143	123–152
61	93–123	101–131	110–140	118–148	127–157
62	96–127	105–136	113–144	122–153	131–163
63	99–131	108–140	117–149	126–158	135–168
64	102–135	112–145	121–154	130–163	140–173
65	106–140	115–149	125–159	134–168	144–179
66	109–144	119–154	129–164	138–174	148–184
67	112–148	122–159	133–169	143–179	153–190
68	116–153	126–163	137–174	147–184	158–196
69	119–157	130–168	141–179	151–190	162–201
70	122–162	134–173	145–184	156–195	167–207
71	126–167	137–178	149–190	160–201	172–213
72	129–171	141–183	153–195	165–207	177–219
73	133–176	145–188	157–200	169–213	182–225
74	137–181	149–194	162–206	174–219	187–232
75	141–186	153–199	166–212	179–225	192–238
76	144–191	157–205	171–218	184–231	197–244

Source: Reproduced, with permission, from Andres, R., Elahi, D., Tobin, J. D., Muller, D. C., & Brant, L. (1985). Impact of age on weight goals, *Annals of Internal Medicine* 1985; 103: 1030–1033.

The body-mass index (BMI) is an alternative weight/height ratio that offers several advantages over relative weight as an indicator of obesity. BMI is derived by dividing weight (in kilograms) by the square of height (in meters). The correlation between BMI and body fat measured from hydrostatic weighing ($rs = .70$ to $.80$) exceeds the correlations for percentage overweight and other height/weight ratios (Benn, 1970; Keys, Fidanza, Karvonen, Kimura, & Taylor, 1972). Because BMI is not encumbered by the problems of ideal weight, and because it corresponds more closely to percentage of body fat, it represents a preferable indicator of obesity, as compared to either relative weight or percentage overweight.

BMI values that correspond roughly to 20% above ideal weight, using the 1983 Metropolitan tables, are 27.2 for males and 26.9 for females. Table 1.2 presents body weights by height that correspond to BMI values of 20, 25, 30, 35, 40, and 45. The table can be used to quickly gauge an individual's approximate BMI values without having to resort to a calculator.

CLASSIFYING OBESITY

Because the overall category of obesity probably represents a heterogeneous group of disorders, the classification of types of obesity could serve

TABLE 1.2   BODY WEIGHTS CORRESPONDING TO HEIGHT AND BODY MASS INDEX (BMI)

| | Weight (lb), in relation to BMI | | | | | |
Height (in.)	20	25	30	35	40	45
58	96	119	143	167	191	214
59	99	124	148	173	198	223
60	102	128	153	179	204	229
61	106	132	158	185	211	238
62	109	136	164	191	218	245
63	113	141	169	197	225	254
64	116	145	174	204	232	262
65	120	150	180	210	240	270
66	124	155	186	216	247	279
67	127	159	191	223	255	286
68	131	164	197	230	263	296
69	135	169	203	237	270	304
70	139	174	209	243	278	313
71	143	179	215	250	286	321
72	147	184	221	258	294	331
73	151	189	227	265	303	340
74	155	194	233	272	311	350

an important organizational function for studying and treating obese individuals. Harrison (1984) noted that four different types of classification systems have been proposed in obesity research. Schemes have been based on (1) *etiology* (i.e., known cause), (2) *prognosis* (i.e., probability of improvement), (3) *functional consequences* (i.e., associated symptoms, such as hypertension), and (4) *therapeutic implications* (i.e., type of treatment required).

To date, etiological classifications have not been particularly productive because only a very small percentage of cases have known causes (e.g., endocrine or central nervous system disorders). Moreover, obesity is probably a multiply determined disorder without a single cause.

Prognostic classification schemes require reliable and accurate predictors of successful weight loss. For example, for a period of time, some researchers thought that childhood-onset obesity was more refractory to treatment than adult-onset obesity. Unfortunately, the childhood- versus adult-onset distinction has not proven to be a reliable predictor of response to treatment. At present, few indicators reliably predict who will lose weight and keep it off.

Functional classification schemes characterize individuals based on the physical or psychological consequences of their obesity (e.g., poor glucose tolerance or body-image disparagement). Functional classification may be useful in suggesting specific outcome measures, besides weight loss, that are relevant for particular obese individuals (e.g., improvements in glucose tolerance or reduction in body-image dissatisfaction).

Therapeutic classification schemes endeavor to match the type of obesity with the particular treatment that is likely to result in the best outcome. For example, Stunkard (1984) proposed that percentage over ideal weight can be used to classify obesity as "mild" (i.e., 20% to 39% over ideal weight), "moderate" (i.e., 40% to 99% over ideal body weight), or "severe" (i.e., 100% or more over ideal body weight). Stunkard suggested that this scheme holds clinical utility, in that the nature of treatment (i.e., behavioral, medical, or surgical) varies according to the severity of obesity. According to Stunkard, mild obesity, which accounts for 90% of the prevalence of obesity, is best suited to comprehensive behavioral intervention, which can be delivered by nonmedical personnel. Moderate obesity, which involves approximately 9% of the obese population, requires more aggressive treatment, such as a combination of behavioral treatment plus modified fasting and therefore necessitates medical management. Severe obesity, which accounts for approximately 0.5% of the cases of obesity, is the least responsive to behavioral intervention or severe caloric restriction and usually requires surgery for successful outcome.

Garrow (1981) has also proposed a therapeutic classification scheme for obesity based on severity. His system distinguishes three grades of obesity based on severity but defines obesity in terms of BMI rather than percentage over ideal body weight. In Garrow's system, Grade I (or "mild obesity") corresponds to a BMI in the range of 25.0–29.9, Grade II (or "moderate obesity") falls in the range of 30.0–40.0, and Grade III (or "severe obesity") is characterized by a BMI in excess of 40.0. The Panel on Energy, Obesity, and Body Weight Standards of the American Society of Clinical Nutrition has recently recommended adoption of Garrow's classification system (Jequier, 1987). Table 1.2 can be used to determine the grade of obesity based on BMI.

PREVALENCE OF OBESITY

In the United States, the National Center for Health Statistics (NCHS) has conducted three large-scale studies (1966, 1979, 1981) that included heights and weights on representative samples of Americans. These surveys included the National Health Examination Survey (NHES), from 1960 to 1962 (NCHS, 1966); the first National Health and Nutrition Examination Survey (NHANES-I), from 1971 to 1974 (NCHS, 1979); and the second National Health and Nutrition Examination Survey (NHANES-II), from 1976 to 1980 (NCHS, 1981).

In its surveys, the NCHS defined "overweight" as a BMI equal to or greater than the eighty-fifth percentile of men and women in their 20s and defined "severe overweight" as a BMI equal to or greater than the ninety-fifth percentile for the same group. In NHANES-II, the overweight and severe overweight categories for men corresponded to BMIs of 27.8 and 31.1, respectively. For women, the overweight and severe overweight categories corresponded to BMIs of 27.3 and 32.3. The values used in NHANES-II for defining overweight and severe overweight closely approximate the 20% and 40% over ideal weight cutoff points used by Stunkard to classify "mild" and "moderate" obesity (Stunkard, 1984).

The NHANES-II data (1976–1980) showed that 26% of American adults, about 34 million people, were considered to be overweight. Among these overweight people, approximately 12 million individuals were heavy enough to be classified as severely overweight. Moreover, a comparison with earlier surveys showed an ominous trend: the incidence of obesity in America was increasing, and particularly large increases in obesity were noted among children and adolescents (see Gortmaker, Dietz, Sobol, & Wehler, 1987).

The NHANES-II data also showed that gender, age, race, and poverty status influenced the prevalence of overweight. Fewer men than women were overweight, and among men, overweight increased up to 55 years of age and then declined. For women, the prevalence of overweight increased steadily up to 65 years of age and then leveled off. Furthermore, the prevalence of obesity at all ages was much higher among black women than white women; in fact, between the ages of 45 and 54 years, the prevalence of obesity among black women exceeded 60%, an amount double that of white women in the same age group.

The survey results also showed that the association between overweight and poverty status differed for men and women. Across all age groups, the prevalence of overweight was slightly higher for men above the poverty line than for those below it. For women, a much different picture was apparent: Independent of race, women below the poverty line showed a dramatically higher prevalence of obesity than those above it (Van Itallie, 1985).

CONSEQUENCES OF OBESITY

How does obesity affect physical health and psychological well-being? Over the past decade, the answer to this question has become increasingly clear. Obesity has a substantial adverse impact on health and well-being. Obesity is associated with a number of serious illnesses and with risk factors for diseases. Not only does obesity aggravate the onset and progression of some illnesses, but it also shortens life and decreases quality of life.

Obesity and Coronary Heart Disease

Obesity contributes to coronary heart disease primarily through its strong association with risk factors such as hypertension, hyperlipidemia, and impaired glucose tolerance. Cross-sectional studies have clearly documented the association between obesity and these risk factors. For example, NHANES-II results demonstrated that the prevalence of hypertension was almost three times higher in overweight versus nonoverweight individuals. Moreover, among persons in the 20- to 44-year-old age range, the prevalence of hypertension was more than five times higher for obese individuals than for their nonoverweight counterparts. Similarly, these young obese persons were more than twice as likely as their nonoverweight peers to have hyperlipidemia (i.e., blood cholesterol over 250 mg/dL).

Several large-scale prospective studies have explored the relationship of obesity to coronary artery disease. In a 1990 report from the Nurses' Health Study, Manson et al. examined the incidence of coronary heart disease in a prospective cohort over an 8-year period. The participants consisted of more than 115,000 female nurses who were 30 to 55 years old in 1976, and who were free of diagnosed coronary disease, stroke, and cancer at that time. In this sample, a higher BMI was positively associated with the occurrence during the study period of fatal and nonfatal coronary heart disease. Women in the heaviest weight category, those with BMIs ≥ 29, were more than *three* times as likely to develop coronary heart disease than those in the lightest group (BMI < 21). This finding has far-reaching significance because more than 25% of American women in the 35- to 64-year-old age group have a BMI greater than 29 and thus are at greater risk of coronary heart disease.

The Nurses' Health Study also assessed the *independent* contribution of obesity by statistically controlling for hypertension, diabetes, and hyperlipidemia. For women in the heaviest category, 70% of the instances of coronary heart disease were attributable to obesity. Across all weight categories, obesity accounted for 40% of coronary events. These findings dovetail with the results of the Framingham Heart Study, which also found that obesity is an independent risk factor for cardiovascular disease (Hubert, Feinleib, McNamara, & Castelli, 1983).

How overweight does one need to be before there is an adverse impact on health? Although the answer to this question is still a matter of debate, the data from the Nurses' Health Study showed that even *mild* amounts of overweight were associated with increased risk of coronary disease. For women with a BMI of 25 to 28.9 (mild obesity), the risk of heart disease was 80% greater than for those in the reference group. However, it is important to note that the reference group consisted of women with a BMI of 21 or less, who would generally be considered "underweight." Nonetheless, the authors of the Nurses' Health Study concluded that even mild amounts of overweight may result in substantial increases in coronary risk.

Obesity and Diabetes

Diabetes is the third most frequent cause of death in the United States, and obesity is a major risk factor for Type II or non-insulin-dependent diabetes mellitus (NIDDM). The NCHS (1986) indicated that there are almost 6 million Americans with a known diagnosis of diabetes, and the American Diabetes Association (Salans, Knittle, & Hirsch, 1983) estimates that there may be as many as 5 million individuals with *undiagnosed* diabetes. More than 80% of those with diabetes suffer from NIDDM, and *obesity is the single factor* most strongly associated with NIDDM. Estimates of the prevalence of obesity among NIDDM patients range from 60 to 90% (National Diabetes Data Group, 1979). Thus, the vast majority of Type II diabetic patients are obese.

The specific relationship between obesity and the development of NIDDM is complex and not completely understood. NIDDM involves an impairment in insulin secretion, resistance to the effects of insulin, or both (Kolterman, Olefsky, Kurahara, & Taylor, 1982). Obesity is associated with a decrease in the number and the binding of insulin receptors, thereby requiring greater amounts of insulin for the uptake of glucose. Family history, distribution of body fat, and degree of obesity seem to moderate the relationship between obesity and the development of NIDDM. Specifically, some people have a strong genetic predisposition for the development of NIDDM (NCHS, 1986; Rifkind, 1984); excess abdominal fat increases the potential for NIDDM (Hartz, Rupley, & Rimm, 1984; Kissebah et al., 1982; Ohlson, Larsson, Suardsudd, Welin, Eriksson, Wilhelmsen, et al., 1985); and the risk of developing NIDDM increases from twofold for the mildly obese, to fivefold for the moderately obese, and exceeds tenfold for the severely obese (Salans et al., 1983; Westlund & Nicholaysen, 1972).

Obesity and Cancer

Large-scale follow-up studies conducted by the American Cancer Society (e.g., Lew & Garfinkel, 1979) have shown that the risk of cancer increases with weight, particularly among those who are moderately or severely obese. For example, in the Lew and Garfinkel study, which included data from 750,000 subjects, the mortality from cancer was significantly higher for those who were 40% or more overweight, compared to a reference group of average-weight individuals. The mortality rate from cancer for men who were 40% or more overweight was one third higher than for men of average weight, with cancers of the colon and rectum contributing most to excess mortality. The mortality rate for cancer among women who were 40% or more overweight was 55% higher than for those of average weight, with cancers of the gallbladder, breast, cervix, endometrium, uterus, and ovary contributing most to increased mortality.

Obesity and Other Diseases

The association between obesity and gallbladder disease has also been well documented. Obese women of all ages are more likely to develop gallbladder disease than average-weight women (Bray, 1985; Friedman, Kannel, & Dawber, 1966; Sturdevant, Pearce, & Dayton, 1973). Moreover, some data suggest that one third of all obese women will have experienced gallbladder disease by the time they are 60 years old (Bernstein, Giefer, Vieira, Werner, & Rimm, 1977). Severely obese persons also suffer from higher rates of pulmonary dysfunction (Sharp, Barrocas, & Chokroverty, 1983) and sleep apnea (Block, 1985), and they are more likely to develop serious complications following surgery (Bray, 1985).

Body Fat Distribution and Health Risk

The health risks associated with obesity vary with the distribution of body fat (Bjorntorp, 1985; Lapidus et al., 1984). Individuals with body fat stored in the upper body (i.e., abdomen and flanks) are at greater risk for heart disease and diabetes than those with body fat stored in the lower body (i.e., buttocks and thighs). Upper-body (or android) obesity is more typically seen in men, whereas lower-body (gynoid) obesity is more characteristic of women (see Smith, 1985). The metabolism of *adipocytes* (i.e., fat cells) appears to vary with fat sites. Fat deposits in the abdomen and flank are more metabolically "active" (i.e., stored and utilized) than fat deposits in the thighs and buttocks, and upper-body obesity is more closely associated with abnormalities of blood pressure, glucose tolerance, and serum cholesterol levels than is lower-body obesity (Bjorntorp, 1985; Kissebah, Pieris, & Evans, 1986; Krotkiewski, Bjorntorp, Sjostrom, & Smith, 1983; Lapidus & Bengtsson, 1988).

The ratio of waist-to-hip circumferences has provided important information about body-fat distribution and its health consequences. In both men and women, *higher* waist-to-hip ratios (WHRs), which indicate upper body obesity, have been linked to increased risk of hypertension, diabetes, stroke, and death (Bjorntorp, 1985, 1986; Ducimetiere, Avons, Cambien, & Richard, 1983; Lapidus, Bengtsson, Larsson, Pennert, Rybo, & Sjostrom, 1984; Larrson, Svardsuud, Welin, Wilhelmsen, Bjorntorp, & Tibblin, 1984). For women, WHRs ratios that exceed 0.8 suggest a significantly increased health risk; for men, WHRs exceeding 1.0 fall in the high-risk category. Thus, upper body obesity, independent of the severity of obesity, may serve as an important clinical marker for increased risk of disease and death.

Obesity and Longevity

Given the many associations between obesity and illness, it is reasonable to expect that obesity reduces longevity. Indeed, several prospective investigations have documented that obesity is associated with a shortened life span. Several major studies have explored the effect of obesity on longevity.

The American Cancer Society Study (Lew & Garfinkel, 1979) followed 750,000 persons prospectively from 1959 to 1972 and determined the relation between weight and mortality from all causes. The reference group consisted of individuals who were within 90–109% of average weight (for the cohort); they were compared to subjects in six weight categories: < 80% of average, 80–89% of average, 110–119% of average, 120–129% of average, 130–139% of average, and ≥ 140% of average. The lowest mortality rates were observed in the reference group (average weight) and in the group that was 10–19% below average weight. For men and women who were 30–39% heavier than average, mortality was nearly 50% higher than for those of average weight. Moreover, for men and women in the heaviest weight category (i.e., 40% or more above average), mortality rates were nearly 90% higher than for those of average weight.

The effect of obesity on longevity varies according to degree of overweight. Findings from the 1979 Build Study (Society of Actuaries and Association of Life Insurance Medical Directors of America, 1980) demonstrated a curvilinear relationship between mortality and weight. Increased mortality was observed at both the lowest and highest levels of the weight spectrum. People in "average" weight and "slightly below average" weight categories had the lowest mortality rates. As weight increased beyond average, increases were also seen in the *mortality ratios* (i.e., the proportion of deaths observed, relative to the number of deaths expected). Thus, in the average weight category, mortality ratios of 95% and 97% were observed for men and women, respectively, whereas in the highest weight category reported (i.e., 55–65% over ideal body weight), the mortality ratios increased to 186% and 140% for men and women, respectively. Although the generalizability of the 1979 Build Study findings is limited because the sample is not representative of the U.S. population, the findings clearly indicate that increased weight is associated with a shortened life span.

The findings from the 1979 Build Study also showed that the increased mortality associated with being overweight was more pronounced in persons under age 50 than in older individuals. For an obese male (i.e., 30% overweight), the reduction in life expectancy is 3 years at age 30, and 2 years at age 60. For an obese woman (i.e., 30% overweight), the reductions in life expectancy are 2.2 years at age 30, and 1.6 years at age 60. These data support the argument that age-specific height–weight tables are necessary (Andres et al., 1985).

Obesity and Psychological Distress

Many obese people experience social discrimination and psychological distress as a direct consequence of their weight (Wadden & Stunkard, 1985). Our culture's emphasis on slimness and prejudice against obesity exacerbate the disdain that overweight people have for their own physical appearance (see Stunkard, 1976). Indeed, many obese people hate their bodies, and body-image disparagement serves as an ongoing source of distress that prompts many to seek professional help in losing weight.

Psychological or emotional disturbances have long been presumed to play a causative role in the development of obesity. According to this presumption, obese individuals overeat to compensate for feelings of inferiority, insecurity, and sexual inadequacy. Since the early 1980s, this perspective has changed significantly. Studies comparing obese persons with appropriate nonobese controls have failed to show clinically significant between-group differences in the rates of psychological disturbance, regardless of whether psychopathology was assessed by self-report in the general population (e.g., Stewart & Brook, 1983) or by psychiatric interviews in clinical samples (e.g., Halmi, Long, & Stunkard, 1980; Kaplan & Wadden, 1986; Wadden, Foster, Brownell, & Finley, 1984; for a review, see Wadden & Stunkard, 1985).

Although, as a group, the obese may not differ from the nonobese in terms of general psychological disturbance, many overweight *individuals* suffer from serious emotional difficulties, and some need professional help to cope with these problems (cf. McReynolds, 1982). Moreover, many obese persons suffer negative psychological consequences that are specific to being overweight. These range from a lack of self-confidence and a sense of frustration with repeated weight-loss failures, to severe body-image disparagement, accompanied by feelings of self-contempt and personal inadequacy.

Wadden and his colleagues (Wadden & Stunkard, 1985; Wadden, Stunkard, Rich, Rubin, Sweidel, & McKinney, 1990) have observed that the psychological consequences of obesity vary according to social context. For example, among lower-socioeconomic-status (SES) groups, in which obesity is highly prevalent, being overweight represents less of a social stigma than for higher-SES groups. As a consequence, obese individuals in this social context do not seem to experience a significant amount of weight-related distress. Also, there appear to be racial differences in preferred body types. Among African-Americans and some Hispanic-American groups, the preferred body type differs from the thin ideal that characterizes middle-class European-Americans.

Differences in sociocultural contexts may determine an individual's emotional response to being overweight (Wadden, Stunkard, et al., 1990). Consider the likely differences in the weight-related, emotional responses of two women: Each is 45 years old, 50 pounds overweight, and moderately obese; yet one is black and poor, the other white and wealthy. Among middle-aged black women below the poverty line, obesity is the norm rather than the exception, and among African-Americans, there is greater cultural acceptance of a heavier body type. Among upper-class white women, obesity is uncommon, and the European-American cultural standard dictates that "one can never be too rich or too thin." Thus, in the latter sociocultural context, obesity is likely to produce a greater adverse psychological impact. Based on her weight, the high-SES white woman is likely to judge herself quite harshly. Not only does her obesity mark her as pejoratively different from her peers, but she is also likely to see herself as "abnormal" and to experience adverse emotional consequences directly related to body-image disparagement (Moore, Stunkard, & Srole, 1962).

BENEFITS OF WEIGHT LOSS

The proposition that weight loss can reverse many of the disadvantages associated with obesity provides the rationale for the treatment of obesity. The data supporting the beneficial effects of weight loss have been derived from longitudinal studies of cohort groups from the general population and from intervention studies with clinical samples of obese subjects. In the following sections, we briefly examine a few examples of each type of study.

Cardiovascular Benefits

In the Framingham Heart Study, a cohort of 5209 adults has been followed since 1948, by means of biennial physical examinations and ongoing reviews of hospital admissions and death certificates. This longitudinal study has provided information about the long-term relationship between weight change and changes in the major risk factors for cardiovascular disease. The researchers have quantified the impact of weight change on risk factors for coronary heart disease. For example, Ashely and Kannel (1974) showed that a 10% change in relative weight is associated with clinically significant improvements in levels of systolic blood pressure (i.e., a decrease of 6.6 mm of mercury [mm Hg]) and serum cholesterol (i.e., 11.3 mg/dL).

The Framingham researchers have also calculated the risk of coronary heart disease corresponding to changes (increases or decreases) in relative weight of 10% and 20%. Their data suggest that dramatic increases in coronary risk are associated with weight gain. For example, among persons ages 35–44 years, an increase in relative weight of 20% corresponds to a 69% increase in coronary risk among women and an 86% increase among men. The data also show the corresponding benefits from weight loss. For a male between ages 45–54 years, a reduction of 10% in relative weight corresponds to a 20% reduction in the risk of coronary heart disease. For a younger man (age 25–44), there is an even greater reduction in risk (i.e., 24%). For women, the reduction in risk associated with a 10% loss in relative weight is less dramatic but noteworthy (i.e., 6% and 20% for those in the 45- to 54- and 35- to 44-year age groups, respectively).

The associations between weight change and risk for coronary disease observed in the Framingham Heart Study have significant implications for the prevention and treatment of obesity.

It is clear that weight gain leads to changes in levels of blood pressure, cholesterol, glucose tolerance, and uric acid. These changes significantly increase the risk of coronary disease. Weight reduction, on the other hand, leads to beneficial changes in atherogenic risk factors and thereby reduces the risk of coronary disease. For many health-care professionals, these data underscore the importance of preventing the development of obesity, even among older adults, and—when feasible—of encouraging weight loss among those who are obese.

Longevity Benefits

In addition to the findings from the Framingham Heart Study, insurance company data also indicate that weight loss has a beneficial impact on health. In the 1959 Build and Blood Pressure Study, for example, obese individuals who successfully lost weight had mortality ratios comparable to persons who were never overweight (Society of Actuaries, 1980). More specifically, a group was identified that consisted of individuals who were initially 25% or more overweight but subsequently reduced their weight to within normal limits. Their mortality ratios declined from 128% to 109%. Similarly, another group whose members were initially 35–40% overweight successfully reduced their weights to the average range. For this group, a corresponding reduction emerged in their mortality ratios, which dropped from 151% down to 96%. These longitudinal findings clearly highlight the beneficial impact of weight loss on longevity. Indeed, these data suggest that successful weight reduction can *undo* the decrease in life expectancy that is associated with obesity.

Other Physiological Benefits

Numerous intervention studies using clinical samples have also documented the benefits of weight loss. Weight loss produces beneficial effects on hypertension, glucose tolerance, and hyperlipidemia. We now examine two studies with clinical samples that demonstrate some of the health benefits of weight reduction.

In a randomized, controlled trial, MacMahon, Wilcken, and Macdonald (1986) evaluated the effects of a weight-reduction program versus medication (beta-blocker) versus a placebo in obese patients with essential hypertension. At the conclusion of a 21-week treatment period, patients in the weight-reduction group showed significantly greater decreases in weight and in diastolic blood pressure than subjects in either the medication or the placebo conditions (see Table 1.3). Furthermore, the researchers used echocardiograms to determine the impact of treatment on ventricular hypertrophy, a serious complication of hypertension. The results indicated that patients in the weight-reduction group, compared to subjects in the other two conditions, demonstrated a significant decrease in left ventricular mass. More specifically, the thickness of the walls of the left ventricle was significantly reduced as a result of weight loss. The findings in this study, although limited by the absence of follow-up data,

TABLE 1.3   CHANGES IN WEIGHT, BMI, BLOOD PRESSURE, AND LEFT VENTRICULAR MASS IN THREE TREATMENT GROUPS

	Treatment condition		
	Weight Reduction	Medication	Placebo
Dependent Measure			
Weight (lb)	−18.3**	+5.5	+1.1
BMI	−2.8**	+0.8	+0.1
Blood pressure			
Systolic	−14.2	−12.4	−8.9
Diastolic	−12.7*	−7.5	−4.4
Left ventricular mass (g)	−37.8*	+0.7	−3.3

Source. Adapted from information appearing in *NEJM*. MacMahon et al. (1986). The effect of weight reduction on left ventricular mass. *New England Journal of Medicine, 314,* 334–339.

*$p < .05$, compared to medication and placebo conditions.

**$p < .001$, compared to medication and placebo conditions.

suggest that weight loss exerts beneficial effects in the treatment of high blood pressure, and weight loss may prevent or attenuate left ventricular hypertrophy.

Wing and her colleagues (Wing, Koeske, Epstein, Nowalk, Gooding, & Becker, 1987) have documented the health benefits of weight loss in diabetic patients. One hundred and fourteen adults with Type II diabetes (NIDDM) underwent behavioral treatment of obesity and were followed for 1 year. Wing et al. divided patients into five weight categories, based on their weight change from pretreatment to 1-year follow-up: lost 30 or more pounds, lost 15 to 29.9 pounds, lost 5 to 14.9 pounds, lost 0 to 4.9 pounds, or gained weight. Table 1.4 presents the number of patients in each category and the average changes in glucose, insulin, and lipid levels observed 1 year after treatment.

Table 1.4 shows that at the 1-year follow-up, six patients (5% of the sample) had weight losses that exceeded 30 pounds. These individuals showed dramatic improvements on measures of blood-glucose control

TABLE 1.4   WEIGHT, GLUCOSE, AND LIPID LEVELS AT PRETREATMENT AND 1-YEAR FOLLOW-UP

	Weight-change category (lb)				
Dependent measure	15–29.9 ≥30 lost	5–14.9 lost	0–4.9 lost	Gained lost	weight
N	6	21	42	22	23
Weight (lb)					
Pre	215	214	214	214	215
1 Year	156*	192*	201*	211*	221*
Hemoglobin A_1 (%)					
Pre	9.7	9.8	9.8	9.8	9.8
1 Year	7.1*	8.7*	9.8	10.4	10.6*
Fasting blood glucose (mg/dL)					
Pre	186	191	191	191	187
1 Year	109*	162*	185	197	217*
Insulin (picomoles [pmol]/L)					
Pre	151	131	131	131	136
1 Year	21*	75*	85*	105	107
Triglycerides (mg/dL)					
Pre	194	194	191	202	193
1 Year	87*	155*	166*	176	204
HDL-cholesterol (mg/dL)					
Pre	38.2	38.8	38.4	38.4	38.6
1 Year	48.8*	41.3*	40.3	38.4	39.7

Source. Adapted from Wing et al., (1987). Long-term effects of modest weight loss in Type II diabetic patients. *Archives of Internal Medicine, 147,* 1749–1753. Copyright 1987, American Medical Association. Adapted with permission.

*Indicates significant within-group change over time (p's < .05).

(i.e., hemoglobin A_1, fasting blood glucose, and insulin), and they also experienced significant improvements in blood lipid levels (i.e., triglyceride and high-density lipoprotein [HDL] cholesterol). Despite average weight losses of almost 60 pounds, these patients were still more than 20% above ideal weight at the end of the study. Twenty-one patients (18.4% of the sample) had weight losses in the 15- to 29.9-pound range (mean = 21.8 pounds). At the 1-year follow-up, these individuals remained on average 42% above their ideal body weight. Nevertheless, they too demonstrated significant improvements in all measures. Those patients who lost more than 5 but fewer than 15 pounds (36.8% of the sample) showed significant improvements in insulin and triglyceride levels but did not experience benefits in their hemoglobin A_1, fasting blood-glucose, or HDL-cholesterol levels. Finally, subjects who lost fewer than five pounds (19.3%) failed to demonstrate significant improvements on any of the clinical measures, and those who gained weight (20.2%) experienced a significant worsening of blood-glucose control.

Although previous research had reported that weight loss can produce short-term benefits for diabetic patients (e.g., Rifkind, 1984), the study by Wing and her colleagues showed that the benefits of weight loss for obese diabetic patients persist even 1 year after treatment. Furthermore, the Wing et al. study also demonstrated that it is not necessary for the obese person to achieve ideal body weight in order to reap the benefits of weight loss. *Modest* reductions (e.g., 15 pounds) produced clinically significant improvements in both blood-glucose control and levels of blood lipids. These findings are particularly noteworthy because it is quite rare for moderately obese persons to attain ideal body weight (let alone to maintain such a loss). Based on these findings, moderately obese patients can be reassured that weight losses of 15–30 pounds are achievable and do indeed produce clinically significant benefits.

Psychological Changes

The impact of weight loss on psychological functioning represents an area of some debate. Studies from the 1950s and 1960s routinely showed that weight reduction was accompanied by adverse psychological reactions, including depression, nervousness, weakness, and irritability (e.g., Stunkard, 1957). If weight reduction does indeed produce a negative psychological state, these adverse emotional consequences may help precipitate relapse. Indeed, some have speculated that such negative emotional states are directly attributable to reductions in body weight below a biological set-point. Thus, for the obese person, the lower body weight induced by dieting may represent an apparently "unnatural" physiological state because it deviates from an elevated, but natural, biological set-point for weight.

What is the evidence that weight loss does produce adverse emotional consequences in people who are obese? Findings of an adverse impact typically come from studies that (a) employed psychodynamic treatment; (b) used idiographic assessments, such as open-ended, interview-based judgments of emotional sequelae; and (c) conducted frequent assessments during the course of treatment (see Smoller, Wadden, & Stunkard, 1987, for a review). In strong contrast to these results, benign or even beneficial emotional consequences have been observed in studies in which (a) behavior therapy was the treatment mode, (b) standardized objective tests were used to assess mood, and (c) change from baseline was assessed following the completion of treatment (Wing, Epstein, Marcus, & Kupfer, 1984). Some authors (e.g., Stunkard, 1984; Stunkard & Rush, 1974) have speculated that the negative emotional complications may not arise until weight loss exceeds a particular threshold (i.e., 15–20 pounds). When the threshold is exceeded, adverse emotional consequences may be precipitated by metabolic processes operating in defense of a biological set-point for weight (Stunkard, 1984). Thus, the question arises whether the benign emotional effects observed in behavior therapy for obesity are a function of the specific type of treatment versus the modest effects of treatment (i.e., mean weight loss of 20 pounds or less). A recent study may help to answer such questions about the effects of weight reduction on emotional well-being.

In a well-controlled study, Wadden and Stunkard (1986) tested the effects of three conditions: (1) a very low-calorie diet (VLCD; i.e., 400–500 kcal/day), (2) behavior therapy, and (3) the combination of VLCD and behavior therapy. Subjects in all three conditions demonstrated substantial weight losses of 30 pounds or greater. In addition to assessing the effects of the treatments on weight loss, the researchers also examined the impact of the three conditions on mood. Thus, the participants each completed the Beck Depression Inventory at four intervals: pretreatment, after 3 months, at posttreatment, and at a 1-year follow-up. These results are summarized in Table 1.5.

At posttreatment, the mean weight losses were substantial (i.e., 31.0, 31.5, and 42.5 pounds for the diet, behavior therapy, and combination treatments, respectively). Furthermore, these weight losses were certainly large enough to exceed the presumed threshold for emotional complication associated with significant weight reduction. As Table 1.5 shows, however, there were *no* significant *increases* in depression in any group, whether during treatment, at its conclusion, or at follow-up. Moreover, participants in both the behavior-therapy-alone and the combined-treatment conditions demonstrated significant *decreases* in depression during treatment, and these improvements were maintained at the 1-year follow-up assessment. Subjects in the diet-only condition did not show improvements in depression despite accomplishing posttreatment weight losses equivalent to those in the behavior-therapy-only condition.

The results of the Wadden and Stunkard (1986) study are important

TABLE 1.5   MEAN BECK DEPRESSION INVENTORY SCORES AT FOUR INTERVALS,
ACCORDING TO TREATMENT CONDITIONS

	Condition		
Assessment	VLCD	BT	BT + VLCD
Pretreatment	9.3	11.8	12.4
3 Months	8.9	7.6	4.2
Posttreatment	7.1	5.4	3.3
1-Year follow-up	8.4	6.6	3.9

Source. Adapted from Wadden and Stunkard, (1986). Controlled trial of very-low-calorie diet, behavior therapy, and their combination in the treatment of obesity. *Journal of Consulting and Clinical Psychology, 54,* 482–488. Copyright 1986 by the American Psychological Association. Adapted by permission.

Note. VCLD = very-low-calorie diet; BT = behavior therapy

because they dispel the myth that weight loss in general, and large losses in particular, are routinely accompanied by depression. Indeed, the findings from an array of studies indicate that behavioral treatment of obesity is associated with a significant *improvement* in mood (see Wing et al., 1984). As Wadden and Stunkard (1986) noted, many of the skills taught in the behavioral programs may enable participants to cope effectively with emotional stresses that arise during the course of weight reduction.

The literature on surgical interventions for severe obesity provides additional support for the beneficial psychological effects of weight loss. Dramatic improvements in mood, self-esteem, body image, and social functioning have been documented following the now-outdated jejunoileal (intestinal) bypass surgery (Solow, Silberfarb, & Swift, 1974) and the newer forms of gastric-restriction surgery (Gentry, Halverson, & Heisler, 1984; Halmi, Stunkard, & Mason, 1980; Stunkard, Stinnett, & Smoller, 1986). Overall, then, the impact of weight loss on psychological functioning appears to be at least benign, and many obese patients who undergo behavioral treatment or surgery often experience beneficial psychological changes as a result of weight loss.

EFFECTS OF WEIGHT FLUCTUATIONS ON HEALTH

Many obese people successfully lose large amounts of weight only to experience over time a substantial regaining of weight. Therefore, it is very important to know whether cyclical patterns of gaining and losing have a negative impact on health. Hamm, Shekelle, and Stamler (1989) addressed this question, using data from a 25-year longitudinal investigation, to determine whether large fluctuations in weight are associated with increased risks for coronary disease and cancer.

The investigators examined the mortality rates due to heart disease in a cohort of 2107 men who participated in the Western Electric Study from 1957 through 1983. The researchers identified subjects who showed one of three distinctly different patterns of weight change from ages 20 to 40. The first group contained 98 men who experienced large weight fluctuations, as evidenced by both *gain and loss* in body weight of 10% or more. The second group included 133 individuals whose weight histories showed steady *gain* in body weight. The third group consisted of 178 men whose body weight from age 20 to age 40 years showed *no change* except for fluctuations of 5% or less. Finally, the majority of subjects (n = 1550) formed an additional group whose members did not meet the weight-change criteria for inclusion in any of the other three groups.

The results demonstrated that a history of large fluctuations in body weight was associated with an increased risk of death due to coronary disease. The men who had both large gains and losses in body weight had a significantly higher risk of coronary death than men with all other patterns of weight change, including those with large gains and no losses. The researchers found that this increased risk was present even after adjusting for potential confounds, including age, cholesterol level, blood pressure, alcohol intake, smoking history, and BMI. It should be noted, however, that these results are limited by the use of male subjects only, by the reliance on subjects' self-reported weight histories, and by examination of a single cycle of weight gain and loss.

Hamm et al. (1989) speculated that when a large weight loss is followed by a rapid regaining of weight, cholesterol levels can become extremely elevated. These high concentrations of serum cholesterol may increase the rate of atherogenesis and, thus, of heart disease (see Keys, 1979). In addition, Rodin, Radke-Sharpe, Rebuffe-Scrive, and Greenwood (1990) have recently shown that repeated cycles of weight gain and loss contribute to increased abdominal obesity. The hormonal changes associated with greater upper body obesity may be partly responsible for the negative health impact of body-weight fluctuations.

Other studies that have examined the association between body-weight variability and mortality have produced mixed results. Two studies (Lissner, Andres, Muller, & Shimokata, 1990; Stevens & Lissner, 1990) did not find a significant relationship, but two other investigations (Lissner, Bengtsson, Lapidus, Bengtsson, & Brownell, 1989; Lissner et al., 1991) found that fluctuations in body weight were a significant risk factor for coronary heart disease and excess mortality.

In the most methodologically sophisticated of these studies, Lissner et al. (1991) employed a large sample that included women as well as men, examined the influence of *multiple* cycles of gain and loss, and controlled for a host of potential confounding variables. The subjects in this study were 1804 women and 1367 men who participated in the Framingham Heart Study. The pattern of subjects' weight fluctuations was based on nine measurements (i.e., the participant's self-reported weight at age 25 and body weight measured during the first eight biennial examinations of the Framingham Heart Study). The first health outcome measures used were those taken 4 years after the last measurement of weight (to control for the influence of preexisting illnesses). In addition, the researchers employed a statistical model that controlled for age, obesity, trends in weight over time, smoking status, cholesterol level, blood pressure, glucose tolerance, and level of physical activity.

Lissner et al. (1991) found that variability in body weight was significantly associated with increased mortality and with increased morbidity and mortality due to coronary heart disease in both men and women (all p's $\leq$ .01). Moreover, the strong association between weight fluctuations and poor health outcome was independent of obesity, the rate of change in body weight, and other risk factors for coronary heart disease. The researchers also calculated the relative risks of adverse health outcomes among subjects whose weights were most variable (upper third) versus those whose weights varied the least (lower third). Table 1.6 presents the relative risk of each outcome for the subjects with the highest degree of weight variability, compared to those with the least variable weights. As Table 1.6 shows, the relative risk estimates for total mortality for men and women with greatest variability in weight were 1.65 and 1.27, respectively. These findings indicate that compared to individuals with relatively stable body weights, people with frequent or large fluctuations in body weight have a significantly higher risk of coronary heart disease and death!

TABLE 1.6   AGE-ADJUSTED RELATIVE RISK OF EACH OUTCOME FOR SUBJECTS WITH THE HIGHEST DEGREE OF VARIABILITY OF WEIGHT, AS COMPARED WITH THOSE WITH THE LEAST VARIABLE WEIGHTS

Outcome	Relative risk
Men	
Total mortality	1.65
Morbidity due to coronary heart disease	1.78
Mortality from coronary heart disease	1.93
Morbidity due to cancer	1.33
Women	
Total mortality	1.27
Morbidity due to coronary heart disease	1.38
Mortality from coronary heart disease	1.55
Morbidity due to cancer	1.05

Source. Adapted from information appearing in *NEJM.* Lissner, Odell, D'Agostino, Stokes, Kreger, Belanger, and Brownell (1991). Variability of body weight and health outcomes in the Framingham population. *New England Journal of Medicine, 324,* 1839–1844.

Note. The group of subjects was divided into thirds, according to weight variability.

The available research on weight cycling is not yet consistent enough to allow *definitive* conclusions. Nonetheless, there appears to be sufficient cause for concern about the negative impact of body-weight fluctuations on health. At any given time, approximately 50% of American women and 25% of American men are dieting to lose weight (National Research Council, 1989), and dieting patterns represent the single factor most likely to account for cycles of weight loss and regain in healthy adults. The results from the studies of the Western Electric and the Framingham cohorts suggest that dieting may contribute significantly to the development of chronic diseases and decreased longevity. Diets that produce initial losses followed by a regaining of weight may actually pose a greater risk to an individual's health than no treatment at all.

This sobering thought should cause the general public and health-care professionals alike to consider carefully the potential negative consequences of initiating weight-loss treatment. Efforts at weight reduction must be taken *seriously*. Clinicians must inform patients seeking obesity treatment about the potential risks associated with cyclical patterns of weight loss and regain, and if the patient and therapist decide to proceed with obesity treatment, it is imperative that they collaboratively plan a course of treatment that includes a strong component designed to enhance the long-term *maintenance* of weight loss.

SUMMARY

Obesity is defined as an excess accumulation of body fat. Reliable and convenient measures of body fat are not yet widely available. Consequently, percentage over so-called ideal weight (for height and gender) has become a popular and practical indicator of obesity; 20% over ideal weight is commonly used as an operational definition of obesity. Percentage overweight should be interpreted with a degree of caution, however, because ideal weights have been derived from insurance company samples that were not representative of U.S. adults. The BMI (i.e., the ratio of weight in kilograms to height in meters squared) correlates highly with reliable measures of body fat and may be a preferable indicator of obesity.

It is quite likely that obesity represents not just a single condition, but rather a heterogeneous group of disorders. At present, researchers have not developed a widely accepted system for classifying types or subtypes of obesity. Categorization based on degree of overweight has been recommended for use in matching obese individuals to the type of treatment that is most likely to produce a favorable outcome. *Mild obesity*, defined as 20–39.9% over ideal weight or a BMI of 25.0–29.9, represents 90% of the prevalence of obesity and responds best to behavioral interventions. *Moderate obesity*, defined as 40–99% overweight or a BMI of 30.0–40.0, involves 9% of the prevalence and often requires behavioral treatment plus medical management. Finally, *severe obesity*, defined as 100% or more over ideal weight or a BMI greater than 40.0, accounts for less than 0.5% of the prevalence and frequently necessitates surgical intervention for successful outcome.

National surveys indicate that more than one out of every four adults in the United States is overweight, and the prevalence of obesity in America appears to be increasing. A variety of factors (including gender, age, race, and poverty) are associated with obesity. More women than men are obese; overweight is associated with increased age in both sexes but tapers off at an earlier age (i.e., 55 years) in men than in women. Obesity is more common among black women than among white women, and it is much more prevalent among women below the poverty line than among those above it.

Obesity has a substantial adverse impact on health and well-being. It is associated with important risk factors for disease, such as hypertension, hyperlipidemia, and impaired glucose tolerance. In addition, obesity is directly related to a variety of serious illnesses, including coronary artery disease, cancer, and diabetes. The health risks of obesity vary according to the distribution of body fat. Individuals with body fat stored in the upper body appear to have a greater risk for heart disease and diabetes than those with body fat stored in the lower body. The impact of obesity on life expectancy varies according to degree of overweight, with mortality ratios rising as body weight increases above average. In addition to its negative impact on health and longevity, obesity also diminishes the quality of life. Many obese people experience social discrimination and psychological distress as a direct consequence of their obesity.

Weight loss can reverse many of the disadvantages associated with obesity. Reductions in body weight, even if modest (i.e., 15 pounds), produce beneficial effects on hypertension, glucose tolerance, and hyperlipidemia. Moreover, treatment of obesity often results in significant improvements in mood. Although weight loss is often accompanied by beneficial changes in health and well-being, recent research has indicated that cyclical patterns of gaining and losing weight may pose a special risk to health. Therefore, it is extremely important to develop interventions for obesity that enhance the *long-term* maintenance of weight loss.

2

A Biobehavioral Perspective on the Development and Maintenance of Obesity

A complex interaction of genetic, physiological, and life-style variables produces and maintains obesity. The relative contributions of various biological and behavioral factors varies from person to person, and people become overweight through multiple pathways. In this chapter, we consider some of the major contributors to obesity. We examine biological and physiological factors, including genetic susceptibility to obesity, metabolic regulation of energy expenditure, fat-cell size and number, and set-point regulation of body weight. We also consider factors that represent behavioral or life-style contributions to obesity, including the influences of culture, personality, eating and exercise habits, nutritional composition of diet, and the effects of dieting itself on obesity.

BIOLOGICAL CONTRIBUTORS TO OBESITY

Genetic Susceptibility

Since the early 1980s, research into the influence of genetics on obesity has increased dramatically. However, calculating the degree to which hereditary factors determine obesity is a complex research endeavor. Different methods employed to address the question have yielded varying, if not contradictory, results.

Studies with adoptees and twins have indicated that obesity is highly determined by genetic control. For example, in an often-cited study (Stunkard, Sorensen, et al., 1986), the weights of 540 Danish adoptees were compared with the weights of both their biological and adoptive parents. The adoptees were classified as "thin," "median," "overweight," or "obese," and the parents' degree of overweight was based on BMI. The researchers found a strong positive linear relationship between the weight category of the adoptees and the BMIs of their biological mothers ($p <$ .0001) and their biological fathers ($p <$ .02). Moreover, no relation existed between the weight category of the adoptees and the BMIs of their adoptive parents. These findings did indeed suggest that shared genes rather than shared environment were responsible for the development of obesity. Furthermore, two other recent adoption studies (Price, Cadoret, Stunkard, & Troughton, 1987; Sorensen, Price, Stunkard, & Schulsinger, 1989) also provided data indicating that genetic factors strongly influence the development of obesity.

In a 1990 study of twins, Stunkard and his associates (Stunkard, Harris, Pedersen, & McClearn) examined the adult weights of 93 monozygotic (MZ) twins reared apart and found further evidence for a strong genetic contribution to the development of obesity. The researchers calculated a heritability estimate and found that genetic factors accounted for 66% of the variance in weight. Collectively, the data from these recent studies of adoptees and twins seem to indicate that (a) the development of obesity is largely under genetic control, and (b) environmental factors play a relatively minor role in determining whether an individual becomes obese.

However, comprehensive reviews of the research on the genetics of obesity have painted a cloudier picture (e.g., Bouchard, 1989; Price, 1987). A puzzling pattern of results has emerged, with reported heritability estimates ranging from 0 to 0.90. One researcher (Bouchard, 1991) has suggested that methodological limitations may help to explain the wide disparity in findings. Bouchard (1991) argues that an examination of the correlations between only one or two types of relatives, as is typically done in studies of adoptees and twins, does not allow an accurate assessment of either the simple (additive) genetic effect or the *interaction* of genetic and environmental factors. Bouchard contends that a large-scale, complex data base is necessary in order to determine the relative contributions of genetic, cultural, and nontransmissible factors in the development of obesity. Crucial sources of information include both within-generation and second-generation relatives, including parent–child, adoptive parent–child, siblings, siblings by adoption, MZ and dizygotic (DZ) twins.

Bouchard and his colleagues (Bouchard, Perusse, Leblanc, Tremblay, & Theriault, 1988) have conducted such a study by examining the correlations of BMI among *nine* different types of relatives, using 1698 individual members of 409 families. Table 2.1 presents the correlations (adjusted for age and gender) of BMIs for the nine pairs of relatives. As expected, the highest correlation occurred in pairs of MZ twins; lower-order but significant correlations were also observed in pairs of DZ twins, in nontwin siblings, in children and their biological parents, *and* in children and their adoptive parents. The researchers used a path analysis to determine the relative contributions of the (additive) genetic and cultural transmission components to BMI. The calculated genetic effect was only 5%, whereas the cultural transmission effect was 30%.

Most studies of the genetics of human obesity have *not* measured obesity directly. Researchers have relied instead on the BMI, which indirectly assesses body fat. From a research perspective, the use of the BMI can be problematic. Even though the correlation between BMI and percentage of fat is relatively high (i.e., 0.6 to 0.8), any indirect assessment of body fat introduces a significant degree of error variance, particularly when the BMI is below 30 (Garn, Leonard, & Hawthorne, 1986). Moreover, BMI is a weight–height ratio, which cannot account for the degree to which body fat contributes to weight. Thus, the genetic effects observed for BMI are influenced to a certain, but unknown, extent by variations in the

TABLE 2.1   INTERCLASS CORRELATION FOR THE BMI IN VARIOUS PAIRS OF RELATIVES

Pairs of relatives	N (pairs)	Correlation
Spouses	348	0.10
Foster parent–adopted child	322	0.22*
Siblings by adoption	120	0.08
First-degree cousins	95	0.14
Uncle/aunt–nephew/niece	88	0.14
Parent–child	1239	0.23*
Brothers and sisters	370	0.26*
Dizygotic (DZ) twins	69	0.34*
Monozygotic (MZ) twins	87	0.88*

Source. Bouchard, C., Perusse, L., Leblanc, C., Tremblay, A., & Theriault, G. (1988). Inheritance of the amount and distribution of human body fat. *International Journal of Obesity, 12,* 205–215. Adapted with permission.

Note. Scores were adjusted for age and gender effects and normalized by generation.

*$p \leq .01$.

amounts of muscle tissue and bone mass that affect BMI but not percentage of body fat.

In a subsequent project, Bouchard and his colleagues (Bouchard et al., 1988) addressed the limitations inherent in using BMI as an indicator of obesity (a) by utilizing hydrostatic weighing to assess fat mass and percentage of body fat, and (b) by using skinfold measures to assess subcutaneous body fat. The researchers employed these direct measures of body fat in a large sample of nine types of relatives (as in their previous study). For percentage of body fat and body mass, they found that cultural and genetic transmission together accounted for 55% of the variance, with 25% of the variance observed as an additive genetic effect and 30% as a culturally transmitted effect. For subcutaneous fat, they found a cultural transmission effect of about 30% and a simple genetic effect of only 5%. Consequently, they reasoned that if the simple genetic effect for subcutaneous body fat was only 5%, whereas the effect for total fat mass was 25%, then it is reasonable to conclude that the genetic effect observed for fat mass is determined primarily by the visceral or deep fat component of fat mass. These methodologically sophisticated studies suggest that the simple genetic effect on BMI may be quite small, and that the genetic impact on the development of body fat, although significant, is modest. Thus, the research by Bouchard and his colleagues serves as a counterpoint to the studies by Stunkard and associates, which show a very strong genetic contribution to obesity.

Energy Expenditure

The way in which the body expends energy (or *thermogenesis*) represents one specific mechanism through which inherited characteristics may influence the development of obesity. Are obese people more energy efficient than lean individuals? Do they require fewer calories to maintain their body weight? Since the early 1970s, scientists have speculated that a defect in thermogenesis may be responsible for the development of obesity. The three major components of energy expenditure are (a) resting metabolic rate (RMR), (b) the thermic effect of food (TEF), and (c) the thermic effect of exercise (TEE). Each of these components may play a role in the development or maintenance of obesity.

Resting Metabolic Rate (RMR).   RMR is responsible for approximately 60 to 80% of daily energy expenditure and is proportional to the amount of lean or muscle tissue that an individual has (Ravussin, Lillioja, Anderson, Christin, & Bogardus, 1986). Because obese individuals generally have more muscle mass than their nonobese counterparts, their RMR is higher. This does not mean, however, that obese people necessarily expend more energy than average-weight individuals: Differences in other components of energy expenditure, such as TEF, may offset higher RMR. Also, because women have a lower proportion of lean body mass than men, their RMR is lower. Furthermore, a loss of lean tissue accompanies aging, and therefore, a decline in RMR and caloric expenditure occurs as people age. Thus, if older people do not decrease their caloric intake, over time, they will gain weight.

Members of the same family have highly similar RMRs (Bogardus et al., 1986), and studies of MZ and DZ twins suggest that genetic factors partly determine RMR (Fontaine, Savard, Tremblay, Despres, Poehlman, & Bouchard, 1985). Several studies have demonstrated that RMR affects weight gain and are directly relevant to understanding obesity.

A recent *prospective* study was carried out with the specific objective of determining whether people with a lower RMR are more likely to gain weight than those with higher RMR. Ravussin et al. (1988) calculated RMR in a sample of southwestern Native Americans, a group that is known to be prone to the development of obesity. The researchers found that baseline energy expenditure correlated significantly with weight change over a 2-year period ($r = -0.39$; $p < .001$). Ravussin et al. (1988) divided subjects into *tertiles* (i.e., into three groups), based on their RMR at baseline. Subjects in the middle and highest tertiles of RMR had mean weight changes of 0.51 and –0.15 pounds per year, whereas those in the lowest tertile showed a mean weight gain of 6.05 pounds per year ($p < .01$). The researchers also compared the characteristics of subjects who gained more than 22 pounds with those who did not gain weight. At baseline, no between-group differences existed for age, height, weight, or percentage of body fat; however, the group that later gained weight had a mean RMR that was lower by 70 calories per day than that of the group that did not gain weight ($p < .03$). At follow-up, the RMRs of the two groups were equivalent, but those who gained weight showed mean increases of 34.5 pounds of body weight, including a gain of 21.6 pounds of fat mass.

This longitudinal study is significant because it clearly demonstrated that low RMR predicts weight gain in a population prone to obesity. These results indicate that enhanced metabolic efficiency may indeed be a significant contributor to the development of obesity. Moreover, other studies show that, following weight loss, increased metabolic efficiency may make it very difficult for obese people to maintain their weight reductions. For example, Geissler, Miller, and Shah (1987) found that 16 formerly obese subjects had metabolic rates that were 15% lower than a matched control group of lean individuals. Furthermore, Leibel and Hirsch (1984) showed that, in order to stay at their reduced weight, formerly obese individuals required 24% fewer calories (per unit of body surface area) than control subjects. Collectively, the results from these studies suggest that lowered RMR may contribute to *both* the development *and* the maintenance of obesity.

Thermic Effect of Exercise (TEE). The second largest component of energy expenditure is the TEE. TEE represents the cost of physical activity beyond resting and generally accounts for 15–20% of the energy that the average person expends. In terms of TEE and obesity, two questions arise: (1) Is there a reduced TEE in obese versus lean individuals? and (2) Are the obese more energy efficient because of decreased physical activity?

Segal and colleagues (Segal, Gutin, Albu, & Pi-Sunyer, 1987; Segal, Gutin, Nyman, & Pi-Sunyer, 1985) conducted two studies to determine whether TEE is lower in obese than in lean individuals. In the first study, Segal et al. (1985) compared a group of obese men (mean = 30% body fat) with a group of lean men (mean = 10% body fat). Although the two groups differed in fat percentage, they were equivalent in total body weight (means = 212 vs. 209 pounds, respectively). Therefore, the researchers could determine whether differences in TEE were caused specifically by adiposity rather than by body weight. The data revealed that energy expenditure in exercise did not differ for the obese versus the lean individuals. In their second study, Segal et al. (1987) compared a group of obese men (mean = 29.6% body fat) with a group of lean men (mean = 12.8% body fat). This time, however, the groups were matched with respect to lean body mass (means = 141 versus 143 pounds of lean body mass for the obese and lean groups, respectively). Again, the results failed to show differences in TEE for the obese versus the lean individuals. The findings of these two studies indicate that energy expenditure during physical activity is neither diminished nor increased in obesity.

If reduced energy expenditure during exercise is not a source of impaired energy metabolism in obesity, could it be that obese people are simply less active than lean individuals? Studies of physical activity routinely reveal that obese adults are indeed less active than their nonobese counterparts; moreover, as the percentage of overweight increases, physical activity decreases (e.g., Brownell, 1982; Brownell & Stunkard, 1980; Perusse, Tremblay, Leblanc, & Bouchard, 1989). Thus, a decreased TEE in obese individual is attributable to a lower amount of regular physical activity rather than to a specific metabolic defect (Segal & Pi-Sunyer, 1989). Differences in amounts of energy expended in physical activity may also explain how an obese person with a high RMR expends fewer total calories per day than a lean person with a lower RMR.

The lower level of physical activity observed in the obese may well be a consequence rather than a cause of their obesity: The more obese an individual is, the more aversive physical activity may become. It would be ideal to assess the contribution of decreased physical activity to the development of obesity; this requires a prospective investigation of the relationship between overweight and physical activity in very young subjects who had not yet become obese. Roberts and her colleagues (Roberts, Savage, Coward, Chew, & Lucas, 1988) conducted such a study by examining energy intake and expenditure during the first year of life. The subjects were infants born to 6 lean and 12 overweight mothers. Total energy expenditure and energy intake at 3 months of age were related to the infants' weight at 12 months of age. Over 1 year, none of the infants born to lean mothers became overweight, whereas 6 of the 12 infants born to overweight mothers exceeded the ninetieth percentile for weight and were classified as "overweight." At 12 months, the overweight infants had significantly higher BMIs and significantly greater skinfold thicknesses, showing that they were fatter, as well as heavier than the nonoverweight babies.

A comparison of the total energy intake and expenditure at 3 months of age for infants who later became overweight versus those who did not revealed an interesting pattern. Energy intake was equivalent for the two groups, but the infants who became overweight had a total energy expenditure that was 20.7% lower than the expenditure for the other infants ($p < .05$). This difference could account for the differences in weight gain. Furthermore, by determining that no between-group difference in the RMR or TEF existed, the researchers concluded that *reduced energy expenditure from physical activity* was the primary reason for the lower level of total energy expenditure in the infants who became obese.

This study by Roberts and associates has several important implications. First, the development of obesity may result from low energy expenditure rather than from an excessive energy intake. Second, a reduced level of physical activity may be the major cause of the low energy expenditure. These findings dovetail with the literature showing lower rates of habitual physical activity in obese adults (Perusse et al. 1989). Furthermore, because the results for energy intake/expenditure were obtained prospectively and before the infants actually became overweight, the study provides evidence that a low level of physical activity may play a significant *etiological* role in the development of obesity.

Thermic Effect of Food (TEF). Eating an average meal results in an increase in energy expenditure (above baseline RMR) that is roughly equivalent to 7–10% of the caloric content of the meal. The energy expended is utilized for digestion and for the synthesis of nutrients. The increase in metabolic rate varies according to the nutrient consumed, with a 5% rise in response to fat, a 10% increase in response to carbohydrate, and a 20% rise in response to protein. Some research has suggested that obese people may have a TEF that is 1–2% lower than the response of lean individuals. Over a long period of time, the cumulative impact of this slightly lower energy expenditure may be a substantial increase in weight. The decreased TEF appears to be mediated by insulin resistance or glucose intolerance (Ravussin, Acheson, Vernet, Danforth, & Jequier, 1985). Specifically, an inverse relationship exists between TEF and degree of insulin resistance. Overeating and weight gain appear to exacerbate this problem, whereas weight loss and decreased caloric intake appear to improve it. Thus, lowered TEF may contribute significantly to lowered energy expenditure in a subset of obese individuals. Such findings may be particularly salient to understanding the nature of obesity in Type II diabetic patients.

Adaptive Thermogenesis (AT).   The TEF is the body's short-term or acute response to food. Adaptive thermogenesis (AT), on the other hand, represents the longer-term or chronic response to caloric intake. Individual variations in AT help explain both the propensity to gain weight and the difficulty in weight loss for many obese individuals. AT affects the tendency to gain weight and the difficulty in reducing weight because it adjusts the metabolic response to periods of caloric excess and caloric deficits, as described in the following paragraphs.

When an excess caloric intake (of 1000 calories or more per day) persists for 10 days or longer, there is an increase in hormonal response, which in turn results in an increase in RMR of 7–10% (Katzeff, O'Connell, Horton, Danforth, Young, & Lansberg, 1986). Because this increase in thermogenesis is not proportional to a change in lean body mass, it is attributed to AT. Some research has suggested that excess caloric intake may result in smaller increases in RMR for individuals who are prone to the development of obesity than for lean individuals. Therefore, compared to lean individuals, people prone to obesity have more calories in excess of their energy needs and are thus more likely to convert those calories into fat and therefore to gain weight.

In a 1990 study, Bouchard and his colleagues (Bouchard et al.) examined the response to overfeeding in 12 pairs of MZ twins. Each of the 24 subjects consumed 1000 calories above his normal intake, for 6 days per week, during a period of 100 days. The caloric surplus was 84,000 calories. Without an AT effect, subjects would gain 1 pound for every 3500 calories consumed above their normal intake. At the end of 100 days, the expected weight gain would be 24 pounds. The actual mean weight gain observed was 17.8 pounds, which is 26% less than anticipated. Moreover, weight gains varied considerably, ranging from 8.8 to 28.6 pounds! Similarly, an examination of changes in body mass indicated that the increases in body fat and fat-free mass accounted for only 63% of the excess energy consumed. Because subjects maintained a sedentary mode of activity, the differences between the observed and the expected changes in weight and body mass could only result from adaptations in thermogenesis. In fact, RMR increased significantly in response to the excess caloric intake, and TEF increased marginally, with marked variability.

The results from the Bouchard et al. (1990) study also revealed two other instructive findings. First, in response to overfeeding, more than three times as much variability occurred *between* pairs of twins than within pairs, indicating a substantial genetic influence on the amount of weight gained or fat accumulated. Second, the researchers observed considerable individual differences in amounts of fat and muscle tissue gained. The average ratio of fat to fat-free tissue gained was 2:1, but the variability ranged from 1:2 in one person to 4:1 in several others. Moreover, a high correlation existed between the amount of weight gain and the proportion of weight gained as fat ($r = .61$, $p < .01$). This phenomenon, known as *nutrient partitioning*, is quite relevant to understanding the plight of the obese individual. Some individuals may have a genetic predisposition such that, when faced with a surplus of calories, they show less of an AT effect and instead demonstrate a propensity to gain weight and fat mass.

During prolonged periods of caloric restriction, AT produces a slowing of weight loss. Prolonged caloric restriction results in decreases of insulin and catecholamines. In turn, RMR declines to the point that it is no longer proportional to changes in lean body weight. From an evolutionary perspective, these changes are adaptive and protect the organism from excessive weight loss during periods when food is scarce. However, for the person who is trying to lose weight through dieting, this formerly adaptive change in energy expenditure leads to a progressive slowing of weight loss and can make the dieting effort seem frustrating and futile.

Katzeff (1988) has lucidly described the effect of AT on the weight loss effort of a moderately obese woman.

At the start of her weight loss effort, our hypothetical patient (we call her Martha) weighs 176 pounds and has a sedentary life-style. An energy intake of 1900 calories per day maintains her weight, with the energy expenditure allocated in the following manner: RMR, 1250 calories; TEE, 500 calories, and TEF 150 calories. Martha decides that she would like to lose weight, so she places herself on a diet of 1000 calories per day. After 1 month of dieting, she loses 13.2 pounds (an unusually large amount!). A breakdown of this weight loss shows that only 50% of the change is due to fat loss; 33% is due to the loss of lean tissue, and the remaining 17% is a result of the loss of water and salt. After just 1 month of dieting, however, Martha's RMR has dropped 15.4% (i.e., the equivalent of 203 calories per day), and her TEF and TEE decreased because she ate and exercised less than usual. Thus, her total energy expenditure declines from 1900 to 1547 calories per day, for a decrease of 18.6% from baseline.

During the second month of her diet, Martha's RMR and TEF decline a bit further, and her total energy expenditure drops below 1500 calories per day. Although Martha is working just as hard on her diet during the second month, she is losing weight at a much slower rate (i.e., less than 1 pound per week). Feeling frustrated at this slow weight loss, and uncertain whether all her hard work is really worth the effort, Martha abandons her diet and reverts to her former caloric intake of 1900 calories per day. As a consequence, her levels of insulin, catecholamine, and sodium increase, and Martha experiences an immediate weight gain from water retention. Her lean body mass and her body weight are now lower than when she first began restricting her caloric intake. Her RMR and TEE are also lower, and her daily energy requirement for maintenance of body weight is now 8% less than when she began the diet (i.e., 1763 vs. 1900 calories per day)! Therefore, it is quite easy to see that Martha will regain weight quickly and end up feeling like a failure at dieting.

Fat Cells: Size and Number

Although the debate continues regarding the extent to which defects in energy expenditure contribute to obesity, it is an accepted fact that, regardless of etiology, obesity involves the storage of an excessive amount of fat. In recent years, many researchers have explored the role that fat-cell size and number may play in the development of obesity and in its resistance to treatment. The average adult's body contains about 30 billion *adipocytes* (fat cells) (Leibel, Berry, & Hirsch, 1983). Although each individual cell contains only a tiny amount of triglyceride (i.e., 0.5 micrograms [μg]), the total amount of energy stored as fat can sustain an individual for 40 days (Hirsch, Fried, Edens, & Leibel, 1989).

An intricate process regulates the synthesis of dietary fats into the storage of lipid as an adipocyte. The enzyme lipoprotein lipase (LPL) mediates this process and appears to serve a gatekeeper function in the development of fat cells. A key issue currently under study is whether adipose tissue merely serves as a passive site for the storage of energy or whether it plays an active role in the regulation of energy. For example, according to some animal models of obesity, fat-cell size plays a regulatory role in food consumption, such that when existing fat cells are filled to capacity, a signal is transmitted that results in lowered intake (Faust, Johnson, Stern, & Hirsch, 1978). Therefore, when exposed to a palatable diet, an individual with an excessive number of fat cells would be less likely to reach the threshold signal for decreased consumption than would a person with fewer fat cells.

In humans, fat-cell proliferation occurs primarily during infancy and puberty, and the number of fat cells present in childhood and adolescence appears to be associated with whether the individual later develops obesity. Increased numbers of fat cells (i.e., hyperplastic obesity) have been observed in cases of childhood-onset obesity (Knittle, Timmens, Ginsberg-Fellner, Brown, & Katz, 1979) and in individuals who are 70% or more over ideal body weight (Hirsch & Batchelor, 1976). More common, however, is adult-onset obesity, which is associated with normal cell number but increased cell size (i.e., hypertrophy).

Excess caloric intake generally results in increased fat-cell size; however, periods of extreme weight gain can produce increases in fat cell number when existing cells exceed their capacity for triglyceride storage (Sjostrom, 1980). Weight loss typically produces a decrease in cell size, but not cell number. Obese persons who have both excessive numbers of fat cells and enlarged fat-cell size have particular difficulty in their weight-reduction efforts. In these individuals, plateaus in weight loss appear to occur, despite minimal caloric intake, when their previously enlarged fat cells reach average size. If fat-cell size plays a role in the regulation of energy metabolism, such persons may find it hard to lose additional weight after their fat cells have been reduced to a normal size; that is, they may remain obese because they have excessive numbers of fat cells. Furthermore, the reduction of fat-cell size may trigger a physiological process that stimulates food consumption, enhances the storage of fat, and hinders the long-term maintenance of weight loss.

When fat-cell size is reduced through weight loss, a signal may be transmitted from adipose tissue to the central nervous system. As previously noted, animal research has suggested that LPL functions as a gatekeeper enzyme. Following weight loss, increases in LPL may signal the brain to replenish fat stores by increasing food consumption. Recent research in humans has supported this hypothesis. Kern, Ong, Saffari, and Carty (1990) studied LPL in the adipose tissue of very obese individuals both before and after the subjects had achieved large weight losses. Following weight loss, the release of LPL dramatically increased, accompanied by a rise in the level of LPL messenger-RNA. Moreover, Kern et al. (1990) observed a strong positive correlation between subjects' degree of obesity at pretreatment and the amount of LPL activity detected following weight loss. These findings suggest that in very obese people, LPL may act as the messenger between adipose tissue and the central nervous system. In such individuals, the excessive production of LPL that follows weight loss may stimulate hunger and facilitate the conversion of food into storage fat. The clinical implications of this process are indeed significant. For some obese people, LPL activity may be a key physiological mechanism contributing to poor maintenance of weight loss.

Set-Point Theory

Keesey (1989) has proposed that "at any particular point in time, there is but one body weight for each individual at which he or she expends energy at the normal rate. It is proposed that this weight be regarded as the set-point for that individual" (p. 19). Keesey (1980, 1986, 1989) has theorized that, just as a thermostat regulates the temperature of a room, physiological mechanisms operate to maintain body weight at a constant level, or "set-point." Within this framework, obesity is a "normal" condition, insofar as the obese person's natural pattern of energy intake and expenditure simply maintains a constant level of body weight and adipose tissue, which happens to be higher than the cultural or statistical norm. Thus, Keesey does not view obesity as a consequence of defective energy regulation resulting from excessive food intake or lowered energy expenditure. In short, the obese person may neither eat too much nor exercise too little. Rather, the natural weight and adiposity level for the obese person is apparently set at a high level, and the body responds to attempts to modify weight with compensatory resistance.

Research has demonstrated that the body does appear to defend its set-point weight in response to efforts to either increase or lower body weight. When set-point weight is challenged, adjustments occur in both food intake and energy expenditure in order to maintain body weight at a constant level. For example, research with animals indicates that weight gain from forced feeding results in decreased eating, whereas weight loss from caloric restriction produces increased eating (Cohn & Joseph, 1962; Levitsky, 1970). Similarly, corresponding accommodations in energy expenditure also serve to defend against weight gain and weight loss. Research with humans has demonstrated that basal metabolic rate declines during periods of decreased intake, resulting in a slowing of weight loss and a preservation of body fat. Conversely, periods of excessive intake produce increases in basal metabolic rate that lessen the degree of weight gain and fat accumulation. Such findings explain how the defense of body weight occurs and help provide an understanding of the obstacles to producing long-term weight changes in humans through dietary manipulations (e.g., Keys, Brozek, Henschel, Mickelsen, & Taylor, 1950; Sims, 1974).

Genetic factors may determine a person's initial set-point for body weight. Some individuals may inherit a low RMR that disposes them to become obese when consuming the same diet on which peers of the same height and sex maintain a normal weight (Ravussin et al., 1988). For such individuals, their natural set-point may be higher than the cultural or statistical norm and may be significantly higher than the weight desired by the individual. Environmental factors can also contribute to raising the set-point. A high-calorie, high-fat diet may result in weight gain and an upward resetting of the set-point. As a consequence, the individual may experience difficulty reducing weight below the new set-point.

Keesey has proposed two broad categories of obesity: one type regulated by homeostatic mechanisms that defend set-point weight; the other type without apparent homeostatic regulation. For example, when animals become obese through prolonged exposure to a high-fat diet, regulatory defense of set-point weight occurs. On the other hand, when a lesion of the ventromedial hypothalamus produces obesity, regulatory defense of set-point weight does *not* develop. Keesey (1989) suggests that such findings may have implications for the assessment and treatment of human obesity.

In order to determine whether an individual displays what he calls "regulatory" obesity, he recommends an assessment of the individual's RMR both before and after a period of dieting. If the person shows a drop in RMR that is proportional to weight loss, their obesity may *not* be under the regulatory control of homeostatic mechanisms, and they may be good candidates for conventional methods of weight reduction. If, on the other hand, the individual displays a disproportionately larger drop in resting energy than in weight, their obesity is probably under regulatory control and they are probably below their natural set-point for body weight. For such individuals, conventional approaches to treatment such as dieting or behavior therapy will be minimally effective due to defensive changes in RMR. Furthermore, for such individuals to achieve long-term success, treatment of obesity will require a significant degree of cognitive and behavioral control to override the compensatory mechanisms of the relentless set-point. Successful long-term weight loss will involve a *lifelong* commitment to sustain a daily caloric intake that may be less than needed to satisfy hunger and will almost certainly be lower than the intake of an average person of similar weight.

PSYCHOLOGICAL AND BEHAVIORAL CONTRIBUTORS TO OBESITY

Traditionally, most researchers and clinicians have viewed obesity as a consequence of an unbalanced energy equation: Body fat accumulates because an individual consumes more energy than he or she expends. This section examines the sociocultural, psychological, and behavioral factors that affect food intake and energy expenditure and thereby contribute to the development or maintenance of obesity.

Sociocultural Influences on Obesity

Throughout human history, periodic shortages of food have plagued most societies, and obesity has rarely been a common health problem. From an evolutionary perspective, the scarcity of food acted as an agent of natural selection. Because body fat in humans serves primarily as a reserve source of energy, genetic traits and cultural patterns that contribute to the accumulation of adipose tissue would serve an adaptive role by enhancing the chances of survival in times of scarcity. In societies with constant and abundant supplies of food, inherited traits and cultural characteristics that contribute to adiposity no longer serve an adaptive function. Thus, as preindustrial societies undergo the transition to modernization (i.e., Westernization), a dramatic increase in the prevalence of obesity typically occurs. For example, in a naturalistic study of the association between obesity and modernization in Polynesia, Prior (1971) found that the prevalence of obesity in the highly Westernized region of Maori was more than double the rate of obesity observed on the more traditional island of Pakupaku (i.e., 35% versus 15%, respectively). Because of similar findings across a number of societies undergoing Westernization, some authors (Trowell & Burkitt, 1981) have described obesity as the "first disease of modernization."

Several factors may contribute to the association between modernization and obesity. In preindustrial populations, periodic food shortages required the expenditure of the energy reserves stored as body fat. In modern societies, on the other hand, the constant and abundant supply of food, combined with decreased energy expenditure in physical activity, frequently results in excess accumulation of adipose tissue. Moreover, modern diets include less dietary fiber and significantly more sugar and fats than the diets observed in preindustrial societies. Indeed, fats comprise less than 30% of caloric intake in most preindustrial diets (Eaton & Konner, 1985; Whiting, 1958). By contrast, more than 40% of calories consumed in the contemporary American diet consists of fats. Thus, the combination of a constant, high-fat diet plus diminished energy expenditure may interact with the formerly adaptive biological tendency to accumulate fat stores and thereby result in the high prevalence of obesity in modern societies.

The Obese Personality

In affluent societies, virtually all members of the population participate in a life-style requiring minimal physical activity and offering an endless cornucopia of fattening foods. Because an abundant food supply is available to all members of a population, why do only certain individuals become obese? Some theorists have attributed individual differences in the development of obesity to personality factors. Psychodynamic writers (e.g., Bruch, 1981) have proposed that overeating represents a psychological process wherein the obese individual uses food to cope with feelings of personal inadequacy. This perspective views the obese person as a passive and dependent individual who has not learned appropriate ways of dealing with the problems of living. The overweight person overeats to ameliorate feelings of anxiety or depression resulting from personal ineffectiveness. Food serves as a substitute for maternal nurturance and thereby provides temporary relief from distress.

Over a period of years, the pattern of overeating leads to overweight, and the socially unattractive appearance of the obese person reduces opportunities for interpersonal contact, particularly with members of the opposite sex. Consequently, the psychological significance of eating becomes further enhanced. For the obese person, food becomes a "best friend," a soothing companion who is always available in times of trouble. Although overeating may momentarily diminish feelings of dysphoria, it inevitably results in a heightened sense of personal ineffectiveness and social isolation. Thus, the obese person's psychological need for nurturance increases in intensity, and the individual develops a dependency on food to cope with the distress of personal inadequacy.

The psychodynamic portrayal of the overweight individual as an ineffective and dependent person suggests that obese people in general experience greater amounts of distress and maladjustment than normal-weight individuals. As noted previously, however, studies with samples from the general population and from clinical settings generally have failed to detect higher levels of psychiatric disturbance, emotional distress, or psychological maladjustment in obese versus nonobese individuals. On the other hand, several studies have suggested that obese people eat more than normal-weight subjects when confronted with anxiety-arousing circumstances (e.g., Abramson & Wunderlich, 1972; McKenna, 1972; Ruderman, 1983a), and obese patients in psychotherapy often report problems with depression and describe themselves as overeating in response to negative emotions (McReynolds, 1982; Wadden & Stunkard, 1987). Rodin, Schank, and Striegel-Moore (1989) have observed that obese persons who are experiencing subjective distress are more likely than other obese individuals to seek psychological treatment. For such individuals, anxiety or depression related to obesity, not obesity itself, probably prompts them to seek clinical attention.

Thus, many of the psychological features suggested as causes of overeating may in fact be consequences of obesity and of the pervasive social discrimination experienced by the obese person. Rodin and her colleagues (1989) suggest, for example, that the social rejection experienced by overweight individuals often damages their sense of self-esteem, thereby leaving them vulnerable to depression. Furthermore, chronic dieting itself, particularly if caloric restriction is severe, may produce irritability, anxiety, and depression in the obese individual, and repeated dieting failures may further reduce the obese person's sense of self-esteem.

Behavioral Characteristics of the Obese

Behavioral theorists, like their psychodynamic counterparts, have proposed psychological mechanisms to explain the development and maintenance of obesity. They have invoked the principles of operant and classical conditioning to explain how learned patterns of overeating and underexercising produce a positive energy balance and result in the excess accumulation of adipose tissue. The behavioral perspective suggests that obese individuals are distinguishable from normal-weight individuals based on four sets of behaviors: (1) excessive caloric intake; (2) a heightened responsiveness to stimuli associated with food; (3) a characteristic eating style typified by a rapid pace and large bites; and (4) a diminished rate of physical activity.

In their classic paper, Ferster, Nurnberger, and Levitt (1962) described how learning principles could explain overeating and the development of obesity. From an operant-conditioning perspective, they postulated that overeating is a behavior largely controlled by immediate positive consequences. The taste of food serves as a powerful positive reinforcer, and the removal of the unpleasant sensation of hunger acts as a negative reinforcer. This combination of reinforcing properties strengthens the eating habit. In terms of classical conditioning, an association develops between the environmental circumstances that precede eating (e.g., mealtimes, the sight of food) and internal stimuli that are perceived as hunger (e.g., predigestive response of stomach motility). The act of eating further strengthens the association between environmental stimuli and the sensation of hunger via operant conditioning, and a variety of noneating stimuli (e.g., negative emotional states) may elicit the perception of hunger and in turn may prompt eating. Thus, for some individuals, the combination of operant and classical conditioning can produce inappropriate stimulus control over eating, thereby resulting in faulty eating patterns, excessive food consumption, and eventually obesity.

Both the behavioral and psychodynamic models of obesity assume that overeating is largely responsible for the development and maintenance of obesity. However, over the years, a set of research literature has challenged the assumption that obesity is simply the result of overeating. Reviewers of the research comparing the eating behavior of obese and nonobese individuals (e.g., Garrow, 1974; Wooley, Wooley, & Dyrenforth, 1979) have found that, in general, mildly or moderately obese individuals do not consume more calories than their average-weight counterparts. For example, the authors of a recent review (Rodin et al., 1989) noted that 20 laboratory studies have failed to demonstrate between-group eating differences, compared to only 8 studies that showed that obese individuals consumed more than normal-weight subjects.

Rodin et al. (1989) have cautioned, however, that obese people may be more self-conscious about their eating, and thus may eat less in the laboratory setting than average-weight individuals. Several investigators have sought to overcome this problem by studying the eating behavior of obese and nonobese people in the natural environment. Trained raters have observed and recorded the amounts eaten by obese and nonobese individuals in public settings, such as restaurants and cafeterias. Rodin et al. (1989) reviewed eight of these naturalistic studies and found that five showed that the obese ate more than nonobese individuals, and three found no differences in total consumption. Obviously, the validity of such naturalistic studies is questionable because the raters are not blind to the subjects' weight status. Consequently, subjects' size and appearance may have exerted a subtle but consistent bias in the raters' estimates of subjects' food consumption.

Most of the studies that have failed to show differences in consumption for obese versus average-weight people have examined eating behavior during a single meal. It is possible that obese individuals may consume more than average-weight people, either between meals or cumulatively (e.g., day, week, month). Nevertheless, the majority of available research has failed to show greater energy intake in obese individuals. Such findings indicate that overeating may not be responsible for the *maintenance* of obesity: once obese, overweight individuals may not require excessive caloric intake to remain obese.

However, overeating may be crucial to the development of obesity.

Overconsumption during certain critical periods such as the first year of life seems to lead to excess adiposity. Over time, however, adaptive physiological mechanisms may diminish the need for a higher-than-average caloric intake for obesity to be maintained. The literature on energy intake in children has generally failed to demonstrate differences between obese and nonobese children. Of course, it is conceivable that available research has simply not adequately examined caloric consumption during the developmental periods (i.e., infancy or puberty) critical to excess accumulation of fat cells.

Also, it may be that not all individuals who become obese do so via the same mechanism. If obesity is determined by multiple factors, then people may become obese by different routes. Overeating may be only one of several contributors that independently or in combination with other factors leads to the development of obesity. Any given sample of obese people may include people with the same endpoint (obesity) but different causes for their excess adiposity. The etiological significance of any single factor such as overeating may be important for only a specific subgroup of obese individuals rather than for all obese persons in general.

Clearly, then, the relationship between caloric consumption and fat accumulation is neither simple nor straightforward. A complex constellation of variables determines whether calories will be stored as fat, and individuals vary widely in their proneness to gain weight in response to similar caloric intake. For example, the previously described study by Bouchard and colleagues (1990) found that, in response to the same amount of overeating, some people gained very little weight, whereas others gained large amounts of weight. Such results are especially important to keep in mind when considering the contribution of overeating to obesity.

Eating Habits and Sensitivity to Food Cues

During the 1960s and 1970s, several researchers proposed that obese individuals displayed a unique and distinctive pattern of eating habits (Ferster et al., 1962; Mahoney, 1975; Schachter, Goldman, & Gordon, 1979; Schachter & Rodin, 1974). This "obese eating style" was characterized as a heightened responsiveness to external cues for eating and a rapid pace of food consumption. This perspective was consistent with the view of obese people as overeaters whose eating behavior was inappropriately controlled by a wide variety of external stimuli. The eating of the obese person was conceptualized as being highly "stimulus bound." In other words, this viewpoint considers obese people, regardless of their internal state of hunger, to be especially vulnerable to minimal "external" cues, such as particular times of the day (e.g., mealtime) or the mere sight of food. Moreover, the obese person was thought to eat at a rapid pace, taking large bites at frequent intervals. The speed of food consumption was seen as contributing to overeating. Rapid eating was thought to allow greater amounts of food to be consumed before internal cues signaling fullness or satiety could be recognized. Thus, stimulus-control procedures to limit external cues for eating and techniques to slow the pace of eating became standard components of behavioral treatment programs for obesity.

Although some early research studies were supportive of the externality hypothesis, the accumulated evidence suggests that average-weight individuals are just as sensitive as obese persons to external cues for eating (Rodin, 1981; Rodin et al., 1989). Similarly, the bulk of recent research findings indicate that if rate of eating is measured across an entire meal, eating pace does not differentiate obese from nonobese individuals (e.g., Kisseleff, Klingsberg, & Van Itallie, 1980). Assessing eating rate during only part of a meal may have influenced some of the early findings, which suggested that obese people ate more rapidly than the nonobese (Lebow, Goldberg, & Collins, 1977).

In one area, the eating style of obese persons appears to vary consistently from that of average-weight individuals. A variety of studies have indicated that obese people may be highly sensitive to particular types of foods. Specifically, obese individuals appear to prefer highly palatable, calorically dense foods and eat more of them than average-weight individuals (e.g., Hill & McCutcheon, 1975; Nisbett, 1968). It is conceivable that dieting patterns involving significant caloric restriction may be responsible for the greater responsiveness to good-tasting, high-fat foods observed in obese individuals (Polivy & Herman, 1985). If the preference for such foods results in the consumption of a high proportion of fat in the overall diet, it could contribute significantly to the maintenance of obesity (Miller, 1991).

Physical Activity

Studies of physical activity routinely show that obese adults are less active than their nonobese counterparts; furthermore, as the percentage of overweight increases, physical activity decreases. Researchers have replicated such findings using a variety of methods to assess physical activity, including self-reports, pedometer readings, and naturalistic observations (see Brownell, 1982; Brownell & Stunkard, 1980; Perusse et al., 1989). Studies with children have revealed a mixed pattern of results. Some studies suggest that obese children are less physically active than their average-weight peers (e.g., Gortmaker, Dietz, & Cheung, 1990), whereas others indicate that overweight children expend equivalent or even greater amounts of energy in exercise than nonobese children (Brownell, 1982; Waxman & Stunkard, 1980).

The behavioral perspective on obesity provides a reasonable explanation for the findings of lower levels of physical activity for obese persons, compared to average-weight individuals. Increases in physical activity typically entail negative short-term consequences, including shortness of breath and muscle soreness. For obese individuals, physical activity is particularly aversive because they must expend greater amounts of energy in order to move larger amounts of weight. Thus, the negative short-term effects of physical activity may serve as aversive consequences (or punishers) that decrease the likelihood that an obese individual's life-style will involve a high level of exercise. Moreover, obese individuals are often highly sensitive to the aversive social aspects of working up a sweat, out of fear that they will be perceived according to a pejorative stereotype that portrays obese people as fat and sweaty. By avoiding opportunities for sustained exercise or increased physical activity, the overweight person will expend less energy and will not achieve the long-term reinforcing consequences associated with physical activity, including improvements in physical fitness and enhancements in self-esteem. Moreover, in the treatment of obesity, long-term success is unlikely without substantial increases in physical activity (Kayman, Bruvold, & Stern, 1990).

Dietary Composition

Some research has suggested that the nutritional composition of a person's diet may be more crucial to the development and maintenance of obesity than total energy consumed. Recently, Miller and his colleagues (Miller, Lindeman, Wallace, & Niederpruem, 1990) examined the relationships among energy intake, diet composition, and obesity in a study of 216 men and women, ranging in age from 18 to 71. Rather than relying on indirect indicators of obesity, such as percentage overweight or BMI, the researchers directly assessed the participants' body fat content through hydrostatic weighings. The researchers determined both diet composition (percentages of protein, carbohydrates, and fats) and total energy intake through 3-day dietary recall and a food-frequency questionnaire.

Miller and his colleagues failed to find a significant relationship between daily energy intake and percentage of body fat for either men or women. Moreover, when energy intake was expressed in terms of calories consumed per pound of lean body weight, the researchers observed significant *negative* correlations between caloric intake and body fat for both women ($r = -.37$) and men ($r = -.42$). Thus, the more obese the individual, the *fewer* calories he or she consumed (per pound of lean body weight). A further comparison of groups of lean subjects (i.e., body fat $\leq 15\%$ for men and 20% for women) versus obese participants (i.e., body fat $\geq 25\%$ for men and 35% for women) revealed that the daily energy intake of the two groups was virtually identical when expressed as calories per pound of lean body weight. These findings are consistent with the results of other researchers (Dreon et al., 1988; Romieu et al., 1988) and with large-scale population studies (e.g., Braitman, Adlin, & Stanton, 1985), which have failed to find a relationship between overeating and obesity.

Miller et al. (1990) also evaluated the relationship between diet composition and adiposity. Some research has demonstrated that animals on high-fat and high-sugar diets can become extremely overweight without an increase in total energy consumption (e.g., Oscai, Miller, & Arnall, 1987). Miller et al. (1990) examined the relationship of dietary composition and percentage of body fat, to determine whether the intake of dietary fats and/or carbohydrates is associated with adiposity in humans.

The authors found that dietary-fat intake was positively and significantly related to body fatness in both women ($r = .37$; $p < .001$) and men ($r = .38$; $p < .001$). In other words, the more obese the individual, the more dietary fat they consumed. In addition to this correlational analysis, the researchers compared the fat intake of subgroups consisting of lean versus obese individuals. This between-group analysis revealed a striking differences: The obese men and women consumed significantly greater proportions of fat in their diets than the lean men and women (see Table 2.2). Other researchers (Dreon et al., 1988; Romieu et al., 1988) have also found a significant association between dietary fat content (particularly saturated fats) and adiposity. Such findings suggest that although the relative total energy intake of obese individuals may be equivalent to average-weight persons, the obese may derive a significantly greater amount of their energy in the form of dietary fat.

Collectively, these findings regarding fat intake have important implications, particularly because the intake of fat produces a lower TEF than either protein or carbohydrate. Foods consumed in the form of fat require less energy expenditure to be stored as fat than foods consumed in the form of carbohydrate or protein. The synthesis of fat from carbohydrate requires an energy expenditure of equivalent to 23% of the original calories from the carbohydrate, whereas the cost of storing dietary fat as adipose tissue is only 3% of the original calories (Flatt, 1987). Thus, if an

TABLE 2.2   PERCENTAGES OF TOTAL ENERGY CONSUMED AS FAT AND CARBOHYDRATES IN LEAN AND OBESE SUBJECTS

	Subject classification			
Nutrients	Lean females	Lean males	Obese females	Obese males
Fats				
Mean	28.6%	28.7%	36.3%	33.1%
SD	2.25	1.00	2.25	1.00
Carbohydrates				
Mean	52.9%	52.6%	44.3%	48.0%
SD	2.25	1.69	2.89	1.21

Source: Miller, W. C., Lindeman, A. K., Wallace, J., & Niederpruem, M. (1990). Diet composition, energy intake, and exercise in relation to body fatness in men and women. American Journal of Clinical Nutrition, 52, 426–430. © Am. J. Clin. Nutr. American Society for Clinical Nutrition. Adapted with permission.

individual consumes a high-fat diet on a continuous basis, he or she may readily accumulate excess adipose tissue without consuming excess calories.

Miller et al. also found a significant negative relationship between carbohydrate intake and adiposity in both females ($r = -.39$; $p < .001$) and males ($r = -.30$; $p < .001$). Comparing the diet composition of lean and obese subjects, they found that the obese individuals derived significantly smaller percentages of their energy intake from carbohydrates than did the lean subjects (see Table 2.2). Other researchers (e.g., Dreon et al., 1988) have also demonstrated a negative relationship between carbohydrate consumption and adiposity. These findings dovetail with the observed association between dietary fat intake and adiposity. Collectively, these research studies indicate that diet composition may influence the balance between energy intake and expenditure and may lead to the accumulation of body fat (Jen, 1988; Levin, Triscari, & Sullivan, 1986; Oscai, Brown, & Miller, 1984; Oscai et al., 1987). Furthermore, the findings suggest that a high-fat, low-carbohydrate diet may play a significant role in the development and maintenance of obesity.

Effects of Dieting on Obesity

In our weight-conscious society, dieting is a common way for people to respond to being overweight or "feeling fat." Dieting itself, however, contributes to a variety of psychological and physiological changes that may further perpetuate or exacerbate obesity. Let us consider how some of the methods people use in their attempts to control their weight may actually contribute to the development and maintenance of obesity.

Herman and Polivy (1980) have suggested that people who are chronic dieters or "restrained eaters" rely heavily on cognitive-control methods to keep themselves from eating as much as they would like. "Nonrestrained eaters," on the other hand, are people who appear to eat as much as they would like without preoccupation about dieting or fear of weight gain. Dieters often display an all-or-none approach to eating. Periods of strict control over eating are punctuated with bouts of binge eating, wherein the individuals consume a great deal, with little apparent control over their eating.

The binge eating of dieters (described by Herman and Polivy as "disinhibited" or "counter-regulatory" eating) has been observed consistently under specific laboratory conditions. Following the consumption of a small amount of food or no food at all (i.e., a small preload or no preload), the ad lib eating behavior of dieters appears controlled and consistent with their efforts to limit caloric intake. However, after consuming a large preload (i.e., a significant amount of a high-calorie food), dieters subsequently eat a great amount of food ad lib and exhibit little control over their consumption (see McCann, Perri, Nezu, & Lowe, 1992). In contrast, nondieters show a normal pattern of regulation in their eating. Like their dieter counterparts, after initially eating little or no food, their subsequent ad lib intake shows a large amount of eating; however, unlike dieters, following a high preload, they reduce their subsequent ad lib consumption and eat very little (Herman & Polivy, 1975, 1980; Polivy & Herman, 1985). Thus, when forced to eat an initial high-calorie snack, dieters respond by breaking their diet and overeating. Their eating behavior suggests that they are saying to themselves: "Because I've already blown my diet, I may as well go ahead and eat as much as I would like." A wide variety of experiences may cause dieters to break their restraint and engage in disinhibited or binge eating. In the laboratory setting, negative emotional states (Baucom & Aiken, 1981; Herman & Polivy, 1975), alcohol intake (Polivy & Herman, 1976), and the mere *perception* of having eaten a high-calorie snack (Polivy, 1976) trigger binge eating in dieters.

Patients with bulimia nervosa often compensate for episodes of binge eating by vomiting after eating or by engaging in vigorous exercise; consequently, their body weight may not be affected. In individuals who do not engage in compensatory behaviors, binge eating may lead to weight gain. Moreover, because many obese people may have a biological predisposition to store excess calories as fat, episodes of binge eating without purging may contribute significantly to increased weight and adiposity. Recent studies have indicated that binge eating is a common problem among obese individuals, with estimates of its prevalence ranging from 20% to 46% (Marcus & Wing, 1987). Some research has shown that obese binge eaters have increased psychopathology, are more obese, and have higher rates of relapse than obese non-binge eaters (Marcus, Wing, & Hopkins, 1988; Telch, Agras, & Rossiter, 1988).

Recently, Spitzer et al. (in press) conducted a multisite field trial of diagnostic criteria for "binge-eating disorder" (BED) for possible inclusion in the fourth edition of the American Psychiatric Association's *Diagnostic and Statistical Manual of Mental Disorders (DSM-IV)*. The major goal of the research was to gather information about people who have a serious problem with binge eating but do not engage in the purging behaviors of bulimia nervosa. The study included self-report data from 1984 subjects. The researchers compared episodes of binge eating in obese patients attending hospital-based weight-control programs with subjects from community samples, including a group of college students. Frequent episodes of overeating were most common in the weight-control sample (59.5%), were relatively high among the college students (38.7%), and were lowest, but not uncommon, in the community sample (19.3%). When the authors applied the proposed diagnostic criteria for binge-eating disorder (which are similar to those for bulimia nervosa but exclude compensatory behaviors such as purging), they found that 30.1% of the individuals from the weight-control sample met the BED criteria, compared to only 2.0% of the subjects from the community sample. In both samples, the presence of

BED was strongly associated with marked obesity (i.e., BMI ≥ 35) and with a history of weight cycling (i.e., losing and gaining back 20 pounds or more at least five times). By definition, subjects who met the criteria for BED had an average of two or more eating binges per week. When asked to provide information about the duration of a typical binge and the amount of calories consumed, the obese binge eaters reported that an average binge lasted more than 2 hours (mean = 138 minutes) and involved the consumption of more than 2000 calories (mean = 2231 calories). Although based solely on self-reports of patients in weight-loss treatment, the findings suggest that for many obese people, binge eating contributes significantly to the development or exacerbation of their obesity.

Polivy and Herman (1985) have argued that dieting causes binge eating. They reason that dieting, when successful, may result in a decrease in body weight to a level below the set-point weight that is physiologically defended. Consequently, the dieter may be faced with a chronic state of deprivation and hunger. Binge eating may constitute a physiologically adaptive means of restoring intake to a more biologically appropriate level.

Several mechanisms may be responsible for overeating when body weight drops below the set-point. Because of their state of relative food deprivation, the response of dieters to salient food cues may be more intense than it is for other individuals. For example, when presented with the attractive sight and aroma of freshly baked cookies or pizza, dieters salivated more than nondieters (Klajner, Herman, Polivy, & Chhabra, 1981). The heightened responsiveness of dieters to external food cues, particularly to highly palatable foods, may trigger metabolic processes (e.g., higher insulin levels) that lead to increased hunger and food consumption, and eventually lead to weight gain (Rodin, 1985; Rodin, Wack, Ferrannini, & DeFronzo, 1985).

Cognitive factors further exacerbate the plight of the dieter. Caloric restriction and weight loss often produce thoughts of food and eating that preoccupy the dieter's thinking. In order to sustain their weight-loss efforts, dieters frequently develop dichotomous rules that distinguish "good" foods from "bad" foods and "good amounts" of food from "bad amounts." The "good" categories are those foods or amounts that they perceive to be consistent with their efforts at weight loss: Anything else is "bad." The dieter marshals willpower and cognitive control to eat the so-called good foods in good amounts, and thereby consumes an amount that is less than the physiological demands for return to set-point weight. In this chronic state of hunger, any minor disruptions in the dieter's cognitive restraint will produce overeating because the dieter's cognitive set dictates that if they are not on their diet and being good, then they must be off their diet and being bad. Being bad often means the binge eating of forbidden foods. The binge eating produces guilt and self-blame and results in either a total abandonment of the diet or in a renewed commitment to being good through a return to rigorous dieting. Thus, the cognitive set of the dieter interacts with the body's physiological response to decreased caloric intake to produce a cyclical pattern of dieting and binging.

Cycles of weight loss and regain (i.e., "yo-yo" dieting) may have an adverse impact on the management of obesity and the health of the dieter. Preliminary research with animals (Brownell, Greenwood, Stellar, & Shrager, 1986) revealed that, over the long run, repeated cycles of weight loss followed by weight gain had made it harder to lose weight and easier to regain weight. Some studies in humans have demonstrated a similar effect for weight cycling.

For example, Blackburn and his colleagues (Blackburn et al., 1989) examined the weight-loss patterns of a group of obese people who were treated initially with a VLCD (very-low-calorie diet) on either an inpatient or an outpatient basis. The subjects subsequently regained weight and returned for a second period of treatment, again with the same VLCD. The researchers found that during the second dieting period, the subjects showed a lower rate of weight loss than during the first dieting period. For the inpatients, the mean rate of weight loss dropped significantly, from 1.03 pounds per day during the first dieting cycle to 0.81 pounds per day during the second diet ($p < .05$). For the outpatients, the pattern was similar; they lost 0.42 pounds per day during the first diet and 0.33 pounds per day on the second cycle ($p < .004$).

It is possible that decreased behavioral adherence during the second dieting period was at least partly responsible for the subjects' reduced rate of weight loss. A 1991 study (Smith & Wing) replicated the findings that obese individuals lost less weight during a second period of VLCD, and demonstrated that decreased compliance strongly contributed to their smaller losses. The findings from these studies suggest that periods of weight loss and regain may make subsequent weight loss more difficult to achieve (for whatever reason) and may also leave the dieter more susceptible to weight gain. Thus, an extensive history of dieting may represent an unfavorable prognosis for future success in weight loss.

Steen, Opplinger, and Brownell (1988) have suggested that the adverse effects of weight cycling on subsequent weight loss may be the result of increased metabolic efficiency. These researchers found that high school wrestlers who routinely used fasting or drastic diets to cut down their weight had RMRs that were on average 14% lower than the RMRs of their teammates who did not diet. Steen et al. (1988) postulated that a significant decline in RMR results from the combined effects of decreased caloric intake and the loss of muscle tissue that results from dieting (see Bray, 1969). The reduced RMR may persist beyond the dieting period and may predispose the individual to weight gain (Bjorntorp & Yang, 1982; Jen, 1988). When yo-yo dieters regain weight, the majority of their gain is fat tissue, thereby increasing their overall adiposity. Moreover, the regained weight is likely to be stored as abdominal fat and therefore may increase the risks of cardiovascular disease and diabetes mellitus (Rodin et al., 1990).

Empirical support for weight-cycling theory has been mixed. Studies with both animals (e.g., Cleary, 1986; Gray, Fisler, & Bray, 1988) and humans (e.g., Melby, Schmidt, & Corrigan, 1990; Van Dale & Saris, 1989) have failed to demonstrate increased metabolic efficiency following weight cycling. Moreover, recent research with obese humans has not supported the hypothesis that an extensive history of dieting represents a poor prognosis for successful weight loss. In a well-controlled study, Wadden and his colleagues (Wadden et al., in press) examined the impact of weight cycling on RMR, body composition, and weight loss. The researchers identified a sample of 50 obese women who were able to provide reliable information about their histories of dieting and weight loss. RMRs and hydrostatic weighings were obtained on each subject. The researchers found that a history of weight cycling was *not* associated with reduced RMR; however, the total amount of weight that an individual lost during her lifetime was associated with greater body weight, increased body fat, and earlier onset of obesity. These correlational findings raise an intriguing "chicken or egg" question: Did the subjects' history of dieting and weight loss cause their increased obesity, or did their increased obesity precipitate cycles of dieting, weight loss, and regain?

Wadden et al. (in press) also conducted a prospective clinical trial and compared the weight losses of individuals with a marked history of weight cycling (i.e., mean of 7.1 diets and a lifetime loss of 173.3 pounds) versus those with only a mild history (i.e., a mean of 2.8 diets and a lifetime weight loss of 58.1 pounds). The results showed that the "high cyclers" were just as successful in losing weight as the "low cyclers." However, Wadden et al. did not include a group of obese people with *no* history of weight cycling, and they did not assess whether high cyclers subsequently regained more weight or regained weight more rapidly than the low cyclers.

Although Wadden et al. did not find an association between weight cycling and either diminished RMR or decreased success in weight loss, additional research is necessary to clarify what role, if any, weight cycling plays as a contributor to obesity. Furthermore, there may be cause for concern about the effects of weight cycling, independent of its impact on the development of obesity. As noted in Chapter 1, recent epidemiological research (e.g., Lissner et al., 1991) has indicated that a cyclical pattern of fluctuations in body weight increases the risks of coronary heart disease.

SUMMARY

A complex interaction of biological and behavioral factors produces and maintains obesity. Moreover, obesity can develop through a wide variety of individual pathways. For many people, an inherited susceptibility interacts with environmental conditions to produce excess adiposity. Determining the degree to which heredity determines obesity represents a complex research endeavor, and the different methods employed to address the question have yielded varying results. Studies of adoptees and twins suggest that shared genes rather than shared environments are largely responsible for the development of obesity. On the other hand, studies that simultaneously examine several types of familial relatedness show that cultural influences exert a greater impact than genetic factors on the development of obesity.

Defects in energy expenditure may contribute to both the development and maintenance of obesity. Recent longitudinal research has demonstrated that low RMR is associated with weight gain in populations prone to obesity. Furthermore, following weight loss, increased metabolic efficiency makes it very difficult for obese people to maintain weight reductions. Although energy expenditure *during* exercise does not appear to be a source of impaired energy metabolism in obesity, studies of physical activity routinely reveal that obese adults are less active than their nonobese counterparts, and, as percentage overweight increases, physical activity decreases. Moreover, a recent prospective study of infants who later became obese showed that reduced energy expenditure from physical activity was the major predictor of the development of obesity during the first year of life. Finally, investigations of AT suggest that some obese individuals have a genetic predisposition such that, when faced with a surplus of calories, they do not show an adaptive thermogenic effect but instead demonstrate a propensity to gain both weight and fat mass.

Fat-cell number and size may play a key role in the maintenance of obesity. Weight loss typically produces a decrease in cell size but not in cell number. In obese persons who have both excessive numbers of fat cells and enlarged fat-cell size, plateaus in weight loss occur when their fat cells reach a normal size. Thus, despite rigorous dieting, some individuals remain obese because they have excessive numbers of cells. In addition, the reduction of fat-cell size may trigger the production of adipose tissue enzyme LPL, which stimulates food consumption, enhances the storage of fat, and thus hinders the long-term maintenance of weight loss.

Collectively, the effects of AT, fat-cell number, and LPL activity may maintain body weight at a constant level or set-point. Within this framework, obesity may be viewed as a "normal" condition in which the obese person's natural pattern of energy intake and expenditure simply maintains a constant level of body weight and adipose tissue that is higher than the cultural norm. Attempts to modify body weight are met with compensatory physiological resistance that makes the maintenance of changes in body weight exceedingly difficult to achieve.

Both environmental and biological factors contribute significantly to obesity. Genetic traits that contribute to the accumulation of adipose tissue served an adaptive evolutionary role by enhancing the chances of survival in times of scarcity. Such traits no longer serve an adaptive function in modern societies, which provide constant and abundant supplies of food. Continuous exposure to a diet of highly palatable foods, rich in fats and sugars, combined with decreased opportunities for physical activity, are largely responsible for the high prevalence of obesity in Westernized countries.

A variety of psychological formulations have been proposed to account for the development of obesity. Psychodynamic theorists have hypothesized that obesity is the manifestation of poor emotional adjustment; however, empirical studies demonstrate that the psychological features suggested as causes of overeating may in fact be consequences of obesity and the social discrimination experienced by the obese person. Behavioral theorists have proposed that learned patterns of overeating and underexercising produce the positive energy balance responsible for the development of obesity. The behavioral perspective suggests that obese individuals are distinguishable from normal-weight individuals based on their excessive caloric intake, a characteristic eating style typified by a rapid pace and large bites, a heightened responsiveness to food-related stimuli, and a diminished rate of physical activity. The majority of research studies have failed to show that obese persons either consume more or eat differently than average-weight individuals; however, there is evidence that obese people are less physically active than nonobese individuals.

Some research has indicated that obese people may be particularly sensitive to highly palatable, calorically dense foods. Moreover, the nutritional composition of a person's diet may be more crucial to the accumulation of adipose tissue than is the total energy consumed. Recent findings suggest that a high-fat, low-carbohydrate diet may play a significant role in the development and maintenance of obesity.

Dieting itself may contribute to a variety of psychological and physiological changes that perpetuate or exacerbate obesity. Periods of restricted caloric intake may dispose an individual to subsequent binge eating. Self-reports of patients in weight-loss treatment suggest that for many obese people, binge eating contributes significantly to the development and maintenance of their obesity. Finally, weight-cycling theory has suggested that repeated bouts of weight loss and regain might result in increased metabolic efficiency, thereby making subsequent weight loss more difficult to achieve. Empirical support for the weight-cycling hypothesis has been mixed; additional research is needed to clarify the impact of losing and regaining weight on subsequent efforts to reduce weight.

This selective overview of the major variables that contribute to the development and maintenance of obesity provides a context for understanding why obesity is such a difficult problem to treat. In the next chapter, we review the effectiveness of the major modalities currently available for the treatment of obesity.

3

The Effectiveness of
Treatments for Obesity

How effective are treatments for obesity? Is there evidence that
current treatments produce weight losses that are maintained over the
long run? In this chapter, we consider these questions by reviewing the
major modalities currently available for the treatment of obesity. We examine conservative approaches, such as conventional diets, commercial
weight loss programs, self-help groups, and comprehensive behavioral
treatments, and we also consider more aggressive interventions, including
pharmacotherapy, VLCDs, and bariatric surgery.

CONSERVATIVE APPROACHES TO TREATMENT

Conservative approaches to treating obesity generally involve modest
restrictions in caloric intake and entail low risk for negative side effects
(Bray & Gray, 1988; Stunkard, 1987). In a stepped-care approach to treating
obesity wherein low-cost/low-risk treatments are attempted before interventions of higher cost and risk are implemented, conservative treatments represent first-line therapy for obesity (Black & Threlfall, 1986;
Brownell & Wadden, 1991; Perri, 1989). Conservative treatments include
(a) conventional diets, which may be self-administered or directed by a

health-care professional; (b) commercial weight-loss programs and self-help groups; and (c) comprehensive behavioral treatment for obesity.

Conventional Low-Calorie Diets

Conventional low-calorie diets are characterized by moderate reductions in food intake that supply the individual with at least 800 calories per day and more than 40% of the energy needed to maintain body weight (Bray & Gray, 1988; Stunkard, 1987). Numerous studies (e.g., Kinsell, Gunning, Michaels, Richardson, Cox, & Lemon, 1964) have demonstrated that when energy intake is reduced below energy expenditure, weight loss follows. It is indeed quite clear that "calories do count." Moreover, studies of weight loss conducted on metabolic wards (i.e., closed environments where food intake is precisely measured and continuously monitored) show that obese patients placed on a fixed low-calorie diet lose weight in a relatively predictable manner.

We now look at an example. Recently, Webster and Garrow (1989) admitted 108 obese women to a metabolic ward and examined weight changes produced by an 800-calorie-per-day diet over a 21-day period. The mean weight loss during this interval was 11 pounds, but individual weight losses ranged from a low of 2.0 pounds to a high of 27.9 pounds. At first glance, the vast individual differences in weight loss produced by the same low-calorie diet seemed remarkable. The researchers found, however, that during the second and third weeks of the study, the rate of weight loss was constant and predictable. Subjects had a mean daily loss of 0.46 pounds and the variability was relatively small ($SEM = 0.18$ pounds). Moreover, individuals' RMR at admission predicted their rate of weight loss during Weeks 2 and 3 quite well ($r = .66$, $p < .0001$). On the other hand, average daily weight losses during the first week were large (mean $= 0.73$ pounds) and highly variable (i.e., 21 subjects gained weight). In addition, these initial losses were not well predicted by RMR ($r = .20$, $p < .05$). Webster and Garrow attributed the "labile" weight changes of the first week to high variability in the loss or retention of fluids. The first-week weight fluctuations due to water retention obscured the overall rate of weight loss, such that it took almost 2 *weeks* for some patients to experience a net weight loss. Imagine how frustrating an experience it must be for an obese person to eat just 800 calories per day and not see a downward turn in the scales for 2 weeks! Such an experience could indeed convince an individual that it is impossible to lose weight on a conventional diet.

The findings from the Webster and Garrow (1989) study have important clinical implications. Despite considerable variability in response to the 800-calorie-per-day diet, particularly during the first week, *all* subjects lost weight by the end of the study. Some obese patients believe that they have such highly efficient metabolisms that it is impossible for them to lose weight on a conventional diet; many believe that they must reduce their daily intake to 400 or 500 calories to achieve a weight reduction. The findings of Webster and Garrow (1989) contradict such beliefs and yet provide an understanding of how some individuals might draw such faulty conclusions. Moreover, Bray and Gray (1988) have noted that no adult studied in a metabolic chamber has ever required fewer than 1200 calories per day to maintain body weight. Clinicians can use such information to help their patients understand that any dietary intervention needs to be judged on its long-term effectiveness, and that over time, moderate caloric restrictions will produce weight loss in the vast majority of obese individuals.

The nutrient composition of a low-calorie diet appears to have a significant impact on weight loss during the first and second week of dieting (Van Itallie, 1980). Reductions in the intake of carbohydrates produce a diuretic effect, and low-calorie, low-carbohydrate diets, such as the Scarsdale Diet (Tarnower & Baker, 1978) and the Stillman Diet (Stillman & Baker, 1977), produce large initial weight reductions that are attributable for the most part to a loss of fluids rather than to an actual reduction in body fat (Nicholas & Dwyer, 1986). Over the long run, such losses have a negligible impact on the treatment of obesity. Nonetheless, short-term weight changes may affect the obese person's interpretation of the efficacy of a particular dietary regimen. Some individuals become convinced that they lose weight best when eliminating carbohydrates from their diet. By following a regimen that is low in carbohydrates, they often end up consuming a *high-fat*, high-protein diet. As we described in the previous chapter, consumption of a high-fat diet will actually *decrease* their chances of successfully losing weight and reducing body fat (Miller et al., 1990). Thus, a prudent low-calorie regimen should include a nutritionally balanced diet with energy intake derived from nutrients in a manner that approximates the Recommended Daily Allowances (National Research Council, 1989): 15% from proteins, 55% from carbohydrates (i.e., 40% complex carbohydrates and 15% refined sugars), and 30% from fats (i.e., 20% unsaturated and 10% saturated fats).

Weight losses produced by low-calorie diets vary according to the context in which treatment is delivered. Hard data about weight reductions that people accomplish on their own are scarce (see Perri, 1985; Perri & Richards, 1977; Schachter, 1982). Schachter (1982) interviewed two nonrepresentative samples of adults and found that a remarkably high proportion (62.5%) of once-obese individuals retrospectively reported "self-cures" of their obesity (i.e., a reduction of 10% or more in body weight and a current weight within 10% of ideal). The people in Schachter's samples reported that through their own dieting efforts, they had achieved mean weight losses of 25.9 pounds, which were maintained on average for more than 8 years.

Orme and Binik (1987) attempted to replicate Schachter's findings by using a design that allowed a check on the accuracy of patients' recollections about weight change. The researchers studied so-called self-cures of obesity in a sample of diabetic patients that included a subgroup of individuals for whom 5 to 10 years of documented weights were available through hospital records. Orme and Binik found that when the results were based solely on the patients' retrospective self-reports, about one third of the sample could be classified as cured of their obesity. When *documented* weight changes were used to determine success, however, only 8.7% of the patients met the criteria for self-cure of obesity. The documented findings did show that 20.6% of the subjects had achieved a 10% reduction in their predieting weight.

The participants in the Orme and Binik study differed from those in Schachter's investigation in several important ways: they were older, had diabetes, and were under medical care. Nonetheless, Orme and Binik's findings suggest that the actual percentage of obese people who lose weight through their own dieting efforts and the degree of success that they achieve is far less than the very optimistic figures reported by Schachter (1982).

How successful are low-calorie diets when provided by health-care professionals? Here again, success appears to depend on the context of treatment. For example, Bray and his colleagues (Bray, Glennon, Ruedi, Cheifetz, & Cassidy, 1969) admitted obese individuals (mean pretreatment weight = 240 pounds) to a metabolic ward and studied their response to a conventional diet of 1300 calories per day. The researchers prescribed the identical diet on an outpatient basis to an equivalent group of obese individuals. Over the course of a 4-week period, the same diet produced twice as much weight loss when used on an inpatient versus an outpatient basis. Patients on the metabolic ward, on average, lost 9.7 pounds, whereas those seen on an outpatient basis had a mean weight loss of 4.8 pounds.

These results testify to the impact of environmental control on adherence to dietary prescriptions. The findings also imply that individual differences in weight losses produced by conventional diets are due in large measure to how precisely patients follow the diet. On an outpatient basis, errors in the amount of food or the distribution of nutrients, together with decisions not to follow the diet on a given day or particular time, lead to substantially less weight loss than is produced by the equivalent diet in the precisely controlled environment of a metabolic ward. Awareness of the beneficial effects of a controlled environment on weight loss leads some obese individuals to seek treatment through residential programs (see Miller & Sims, 1981; Van Itallie & Hadley, 1988). For most obese individuals, however, inpatient or residential treatment is not a feasible or practical option.

We now examine in greater detail the effectiveness of conventional diets administered on an outpatient basis. Over the past decade, few studies have investigated the effectiveness of low-calorie diets as the *sole* component of treatment. Instead, studies using conservative treatment typically have combined a conventional diet with a program of behavioral treatment procedures, thereby making it difficult to isolate the specific impact of the diet alone. (We discuss the effectiveness of comprehensive behavioral treatments in the next section of this chapter.)

In 1979, Wing and Jeffery reviewed the results of outpatient treatments for obesity published between 1966 and 1977. Their review included nine studies that used dietary interventions as the primary mode of treatment. The dietary interventions in these studies entailed low-calorie diets and weekly treatment sessions but varied in the nutritional composition of the diet used. On average, the interventions produced a mean weight loss of 18.3 pounds during the course of treatment, which were generally carried out over a 10-week period. Very little information was available about how well these losses were maintained. Seven of the nine studies failed to include follow-up data. Two studies reported follow-ups showing that subjects subsequently regained an average 4.0 pounds during the 32 weeks following treatment.

Wing and Jeffery (1979) also identified 43 studies in which low-calorie diets (i.e., 1000–1500 calories per day) were combined with a placebo which they used as a comparison treatment or control group in relation to studies that evaluated drug treatments for obesity. These studies presented a less favorable impression than the investigations of dietary treatments alone. Over the course of treatment periods of 10–12 weeks, the combination of low-calorie diet plus placebo were used by a total of 1043 subjects. The average weight losses were a meager 4.6 pounds. It is conceivable, of course, that subjects expected dramatic effects from the use of a drug and therefore adhered poorly to the dietary component of treatment. Nonetheless, the findings observed across 43 studies and more than 1000 subjects suggests that prescribing a low-calorie diet for obese patients often results in minimal weight loss.

In a study conducted by our research group (Perri, Shapiro, Ludwig, Twentyman, & McAdoo, 1984), we compared a treatment group undergoing a conventional low-calorie diet in conjunction with nonbehavioral group sessions to a group undergoing behavior therapy for obesity. An examination of the weight losses accomplished by participants in the former of the two interventions may provide an indication of the short- and long-term effects of conventional diets. Over the course of 15 weekly treatment sessions, participants achieved a mean weight loss of 17.8 pounds, a posttreatment finding quite similar to the average weight loss of 18.3 pounds reported for dietary interventions in the Wing and Jeffery (1979) review. Over the course of a 12-month follow-up period, however, the subjects regained on average 11.0 pounds and maintained a mean weight loss of 7.0 pounds. Thus, the participants regained more than 61% of the weight that they had initially lost during treatment. If the findings in this study accurately reflect the longer-term results of low-calorie diets, it would appear that poor maintenance of weight loss represents a significant problem.

Commercial and Self-Help Programs

Each year, Americans spend more that $30 billion on commercial weight-loss programs. How effective are conventional diets when provided as part of a commercial weight-loss program? In evaluating the effectiveness of such programs, it is important to consider the impact of attrition. Volkmar, Stunkard, Woolston, and Bailey (1981) prospectively studied 108 women who enrolled in a commercial weight-loss organization that utilized weekly group meetings and a conventional low-calorie diet. These investigators found that during the first 6 weeks, fully half of the subjects dropped out of treatment. At 12 weeks, the dropout rate reached 70%. Clearly, such high attrition rates diminish the significance of weight losses reported for those who remained in the program. Participants who stayed in the commercial program for 24 weeks (and who did not receive additional treatment from the investigators) lost on average 11.9 pounds, an amount representing approximately 7.3% of their pretreatment weight.

In a prospective study of 187 participants who joined a commercial weight-loss program, Nash (1977) also found that the rate of attrition over 24 weeks exceeded 80%. In Great Britain, Ashwell and Garrow (1975) conducted a random sample of 600 participants in three commercial weight-loss programs. The researchers contacted subjects exactly 1 year after the participants had first joined their weight-loss groups. A total of 341 subjects (56.8%) completed the researchers' survey. Ashwell and Garrow found that the 1-year attrition rates for the three programs approached or exceeded 80% and that the mean initial weight loss reported by subjects was 20.5 pounds. The researchers sent out follow-up questionnaires to determine how well these weight losses were maintained. They contacted those individuals ($n = 136$) who had achieved initial weight losses of 14 pounds or more. Sixty-eight percent of the subjects responded to the follow-up survey. The results showed that only 13.1% of the participants had maintained their initial weight loss, 63% had regained part of their lost weight, and 23.9% had regained all of their lost weight.

Collectively, the research reviewed herein indicates that modest weight losses of 11 to 22 pounds are typically achieved in commercial programs that use conventional low-calorie diets. The significance of these weight losses is severely limited, however, by the dual problems of high attrition and poor maintenance of weight loss.

Do individuals who join self-help groups fare any better than those who enter commercial weight-loss programs? Overeaters Anonymous (OA) and Take-Off Pounds Sensibly (TOPS) represent the two most common self-help programs for weight loss. The TOPS program, which was begun in 1948 by a housewife from Milwaukee, typically involves weekly group meetings led by a nonpaid volunteer. Meetings are opened with a song, followed by a weigh-in of each group member. Weight changes are announced publicly. Often, a token reward (e.g., designation as "queen of the week") goes to the member with the largest weight loss, and occasionally a symbolic punishment (e.g., designation as "pig of the week") befalls the individual who gained the most weight. The heart of the meeting centers on a group discussion of the way individuals engage in what is called "game-playing," through less-than-sincere efforts at dieting. Competition among members is often encouraged, and special ceremonies are used as rewards whenever an individual accomplishes a milestone in weight reduction (e.g., each 10-pound loss). A special diet is not required, but members are expected to decrease their caloric intake and to follow their physician's dietary advice.

Two surveys of the effectiveness of TOPS have been conducted by Stunkard and his colleagues (Garb & Stunkard, 1974; Stunkard, Levine, & Fox, 1970). The results showed that attrition rates were 47% at 1 year and 70% at 2 years. Although these figures are high, they are superior to the dropout rates observed in commercial weight-loss programs (Ashwell, 1978; Volkmar et al., 1981). In terms of weight reduction, an average net weight loss of approximately 14.5 pounds was observed (subjects had been in TOPS for an average of 19 months at the time of the survey). This degree of weight loss represented a mean reduction of 7.8% in subjects' pretreatment weight.

Perhaps the most prominent of the self-help groups for weight control is OA. OA entails a 12-step program based a model identical to Alcoholics Anonymous (AA). The 12 steps of OA have been adapted from those of AA and differ only in their reference to food rather than alcohol as the substance of abuse. OA seeks to help its members recover from what they call the "disease" of compulsive overeating. The approach entails a strong network of social support, referred to as a "fellowship," which includes frequent group meetings and the availability of a sponsor to provide advice and support. OA meetings are typically held several times per week, and an individual's sponsor often provides daily contact. OA does not include a program of diets or exercise, and there are no weigh-ins at group meetings. Rather the focus of OA is to promote "physical, emotional, and spiritual healing" through contact with "recovering" compulsive overeaters and adherence to OA's 12-step program. At this time, there are no published empirical studies of the effectiveness of OA as a treatment for obesity. In Chapter 11, we discuss the utility of this particular self-help approach in greater detail.

Comprehensive Behavioral Treatment

In behavioral treatment of obesity, participants are taught to modify their eating and exercise habits so as to produce a negative energy balance and weight loss. The presumed process of change is straightforward. The clinician suggests a series of changes in eating and exercise behaviors. The obese patient's adherence to these recommended changes results in a negative energy balance, and consequently, weight loss ensues. As we are aware from research presented in Chapter 2, this model represents an oversimplification of the complex biobehavioral interactions involved in weight loss. Nonetheless, the scheme presents in a straightforward manner the rationale of the behavioral approach to treating obesity.

In its earliest form, behavior therapy for obesity generally involved four sets of strategies: (1) self-monitoring of eating, (2) control of the stimuli that elicit eating, (3) modification of the topography of eating, and (4) reinforcement of appropriate behavioral changes. Since the mid-1980s, adjunctive strategies, such as cognitive restructuring, exercise, and nutritional training, have commonly been added by many clinicians (see Stunkard, 1987).

Self-monitoring. Daily completion of an eating diary has served as the foundation of behavioral treatments for obesity. Participants in behavioral treatment are required to keep daily written records of the quantity and content of the foods they eat and the specific circumstances of their eating, such as the time, place, and presence of others. Self-monitoring is often viewed by participants and therapists alike as the single most effective technique in behavioral treatment (see Brownell & Foreyt, 1985). Recording food consumption vastly increases participants' awareness both of how much they eat and of the environmental cues or "triggers" that elicit their eating. When combined with a specific goal of decreased intake, self-monitoring provides feedback that facilitates reduced consumption. In addition to tracking food intake, self-monitoring is also used to record increases in physical activity and decreases in weight.

Stimulus Control. Self-monitoring of eating behaviors often reveals that a variety of circumstances prompt eating. The aroma of food, the sight of others eating, or feelings of emotional upset—all of these may trigger eating or overeating. Stimulus-control techniques are used to set specific limits on the types of circumstances that will be appropriate antecedents for eating. Eating is generally restricted to particular places (e.g., kitchen, restaurant) and specific times of the day (e.g., mealtimes, planned snack).

Modifying the Topography of Eating. A variety of changes are often introduced to engender a sense of control over eating, to slow the speed of eating, and to enhance the enjoyment of eating. Individuals are encouraged to put down their utensils between mouthfuls, to chew their food thoroughly, to pause during the middle of the meal, and to make eating a "pure experience" by not reading or watching television during mealtimes (Johnson & Stalonas, 1981). This combination of changes purportedly allows greater awareness of internal signals of satiety, as well as greater opportunity to enjoy the taste and texture of foods while eating smaller quantities (Spiegel, Wadden, & Foster, 1991).

Reinforcement of Program Behaviors. A formal system of positive reinforcement is employed to enhance adherence to behavioral changes prescribed by the treatment program. A monetary refund contingency is often established, such that at the start of treatment, patients deposit money (e.g., $100) that is returned to them on a contingency basis. Attendance at treatment sessions, completion of self-monitoring records, and adherence to other behavioral changes earn specific financial rewards. In addition, point systems based on adherence to changes in eating and exercise behaviors are often used as the basis of a *self*-reinforcement system. Patients are taught to use tangible or covert rewards to reinforce their progress in the program.

Adjunctive Behavioral Strategies. In addition to these basic four strategies, a variety of other techniques and procedures are sometimes included in behavioral treatments. These include social supports in the form of spouse involvement in treatment, relaxation exercises for dealing with stress-related episodes of eating, and assertiveness training to teach participants how to say "no" to friends bearing food. Brownell (1990) has recently catalogued 86 specific techniques that are now commonly utilized in behavior therapy programs for obesity. Although many incidental procedures are sometimes used, three *major* elements have become standard components of comprehensive behavioral programs: cognitive restructuring, increased physical activity, and nutritional training.

Cognitive Restructuring. Many obese people engage in negative or self-defeating monologues about themselves and their ability to lose weight. Maladaptive cognitions often result in emotional distress and poor adherence (Mahoney & Mahoney, 1976). For example, after having a high-calorie dessert, a dieter may say to him- or herself "This proves that I'm a failure and that I will never lose weight." Consequently, the individual is likely to experience distressful feelings of guilt or depression. These negative emotions may lead to an abandonment of the weight-loss effort and to additional episodes of inappropriate eating. In current behavioral programs, cognitive restructuring techniques are employed to teach participants to identify negative monologues and to challenge negative thinking with constructive counterarguments. Thus, in the situation just described, a rational counterargument—such as "I'm not happy that I overate in this situation, but I'm not going to let this minor setback get in the way of my long-term goal of losing weight"—is likely to result in a positive motivational state and a resumption of constructive behavioral changes.

Increased Physical Activity. Since the early 1980s, research regarding the contribution of exercise to the management of obesity (see Stern & Lowney, 1986) has led to its regular inclusion in behavioral treatment programs. In addition to increasing caloric expenditure, exercise limits the amount of muscle tissue that is lost during weight reduction and produces psychological benefits, including improvements in mood and self-concept (Folkins & Sime, 1981; Thompson, Jarvie, Lahey, & Cureton, 1982). Moreover, regular exercise has been linked to the long-term maintenance of weight loss (Kayman et al., 1990; Perri, McAdoo, McAllister, Lauer, & Yancey, 1986; Perri et al., 1988). In current behavioral programs, participants are encouraged to incorporate routine changes into their life-style as a means of increasing their physical activity. For example, a person could choose routinely to use stairs rather than elevators and to park somewhat farther from the destination than is customary; these two examples show how life-style changes can be used to increase energy expenditure on a regular basis. In addition, many behavioral programs also include aerobic exercise. For most obese persons, a brisk walk of 20–40 minutes per day constitutes a sensible and beneficial aerobic workout and one that can contribute to improved weight loss (Craighead & Blum, 1989; Perri et al., 1986, 1988; Wing et al., 1988).

Nutritional Training. In the early days of behavioral treatment, participants were encouraged to reduce their overall caloric intake, but little attention was paid to dietary counseling. In recent years, the recognition that high-fat diets (independent of their overall caloric value) can contribute to obesity (e.g., Miller et al., 1990) and can increase the risk of disease has resulted in nutritional education becoming a regular component of behavioral treatment. Patients are provided with information about the significant role that the composition of diet plays in health and weight loss. Moderate reductions in overall caloric intake are encouraged, and daily goals are commonly set at 1200 calories for women and 1500 calories for men. Some programs utilize food-exchange lists (e.g., American Diabetes Association, 1986) to provide participants with a means of calculating the nutritional makeup of their diet. Most programs recommend increased consumption of complex carbohydrates, coupled with a reduction in dietary fats. Rather than going on a "diet," however, participants are encouraged to gradually increase their consumption of fruits, vegetables, and high-fiber cereals, and to limit their intake of red meats and other foods that are high in saturated fats. It is now common for patients in behavioral programs to monitor their consumption of fats and to limit their intake to 30% or less of total calories consumed (see Viegener, Perri, Nezu, Renjilian, McKelvey, & Schein, 1990).

Effectiveness of Behavior Therapy. More than 100 studies have evaluated the effectiveness of behavior therapy for obesity, and numerous reviews of the literature are available (e.g., Brownell & Wadden, 1986; Jeffery, 1987). Wadden and Bell (1990) recently summarized the data from 13 controlled trials of behavior therapy conducted during the years 1985 to 1987. Their findings provide a perspective on the short-term effects of current behavioral treatments. The 13 studies included 931 subjects who, on average, received 15 or 16 weeks of behavior therapy. The average participant, who initially weighed 191.8 pounds, lost 18.5 pounds during the course of treatment. Subjects reduced their total body weight by 9.6% and decreased their percentage over ideal weight by 27.1%. The rate of weight loss observed during treatment was relatively slow (i.e., 1.1 pound per week) but consistent with the findings in other reviews of the behavioral literature. Thus, Wadden and Bell's (1990) review indicates that moderately obese people who undergo behavioral treatment generally can expect short-term benefits that include a 10% reduction in body weight and a 25% decrease in their amount overweight. This seemingly modest degree of weight loss is of sufficient magnitude to represent potentially significant improvements in physical health and psychological well-being (see Chapter 1). The clinical significance of a 10% reduction in body weight is determined, however, by whether the weight loss is maintained over the long run. Ten of the 13 studies reviewed by Wadden and Bell (1990) included follow-up assessments that provide a glimpse at what happens to participants' weights following behavior therapy. The follow-up evaluations showed that within 48 weeks of completing behavioral treatment, subjects regained an average of 38% of their posttreatment losses. This disturbing trend diminishes the luster of behavior therapy for obesity. Modest weight losses are beneficial only if they are maintained.

Follow-up evaluations of 1-year or less provide only a partial view of how well weight reductions are maintained. Brownell and Jeffery (1987) summarized the net weight losses in behavioral studies with follow-ups of more than 1 year. They found a consistent trend of weight gain over time such that at 5-year follow-up the average net weight loss maintained by subjects was 7.5 pounds. Brownell and Jeffery (1987) noted that a fair evaluation of the long-term effects of behavioral treatment requires an appropriate yardstick for comparison. They point out that extrapolations from population studies suggest that weight gains of at least 1 to 2 pounds per year are the norm for middle-aged Americans. Thus, it is reasonable to assume that equivalent increases would be expected in adults in seeking treatment for obesity (Hartz & Rimm, 1980). If this population norm is used as a comparison group, Brownell and Jeffery (1987) suggest that the 5-year follow-up results of behavioral treatment would be more favorable than a net loss of 7.5 pounds appears to suggest; that is, 5–10 pounds *not gained* could be added to the 7.5 pounds lost, for a net effect of 12.5–17.5 pounds.

The *cross-sectional* mean weight losses such as those summarized by Brownell and Jeffery (1987) provide a limited perspective on the long-term benefits of behavioral treatment. Group means do not show the proportion of individuals who benefited from treatment, and cross-sectional data may obscure particular patterns of weight gain within individuals. In order to better describe patterns of weight change and the proportion of patients benefiting from behavioral treatment, Kramer, Jeffery, Forster, and Snell (1989) presented both cumulative and cross-sectional data on 114 men and 38 women who received behavioral treatment and were seen for annual follow-ups over a 4-year period. The men in this study had a mean posttreatment weight loss of 28.6 pounds, an amount representing a 12.9% decrease in body weight and a 44.0% reduction in excess weight. The women had a mean posttreatment weight loss of 18.9 pounds, reflecting a 10.3% decrease in body weight and a 37.2% reduction in excess weight.

Table 3.1 presents the cumulative and cross-sectional data on the percentage of posttreatment weight loss maintained at the four-year follow-up. Cumulative data indicate the proportion of individuals who maintained a specific percentage of their posttreatment weight losses at *all* four annual follow-ups. The cross-sectional values indicate status at the 4-year point only. Table 3.1 shows that for men, the cumulative and cross-sectional data were quite similar. This finding indicates that in men, weight gains during follow-up were not typically followed by subsequent weight losses. For the women, however, a different pattern emerged. At the 4-year follow-up, the cumulative data indicated that only 5.3 % of the women had maintained their entire posttreatment weight loss through *all* four follow-up evaluations. On the other hand, the cross-sectional data indicated that 28.9% of the women weighed the same or less than they did at the end of treatment. This result shows that during follow-up, a substantial propor-

TABLE 3.1　PERCENTAGE OF MEN AND WOMEN MAINTAINING DIFFERENT AMOUNTS OF INITIAL WEIGHT LOSS CUMULATIVELY AND AT THE 4-YEAR FOLLOW-UP

Percentage of initial loss maintained		Men	Women
100+	Cumulative	0.9	5.3
	Cross-sectional	2.6	28.9
75–100	Cumulative	3.5	7.9
	Cross-sectional	3.5	2.6
50–75	Cumulative	10.5	13.2
	Cross-sectional	19.3	18.4
25–50	Cumulative	18.4	7.9
	Cross-sectional	18.4	13.2
0–25	Cumulative	29.8	26.3
	Cross-sectional	26.6	13.2
<0	Cumulative	36.9	39.5
	Cross-sectional	29.8	23.7

Source: Kramer, F. M., Jeffery, R. W., Forster, J. L., & Snell, M. K. (1989). Long-term follow-up of behavioral treatment for obesity: Patterns of weight gain among men and women. *International Journal of Obesity, 13,* 123–136. Adapted with permission.

tion of women experienced relapses but subsequently reduced their weights to posttreatment levels. The sex differences in the cross-sectional data may reflect the greater social pressure on women to lose weight. The findings reported by Kramer et al. are consistent with other long-term studies (e.g., Stalonas, Perri, & Kerzner, 1984) and show an invariant pattern of substantial weight gain following behavioral treatment. Fewer than 3% of the participants maintained their posttreatment weight losses throughout the entire 4 years of follow-up. Moreover, during the follow-up period, almost 40% of the subjects regained the total amount that they lost in treatment. A degree of partial success was evident, in that 18.5% of the subjects maintained at least half of their posttreatment losses throughout follow-up, and one third of the sample maintained 25% or more of their posttreatment weight reductions.

AGGRESSIVE TREATMENTS OF OBESITY

Some writers (e.g., Mason et al., 1987) have argued that aggressive approaches to the treatment of obesity are warranted because (a) moderate and severe forms of obesity are closely associated with serious medical consequences, and (b) conservative interventions have been shown to have little effectiveness in the treatment of moderate and severe obesity. Pharmacotherapy, VLCDs, and surgery represent three aggressive approaches to treating obesity. These approaches generally entail a greater degree of risk for negative side effects than conservative treatments for obesity. In this section, we consider the near- and far-term effects of aggressive therapies for obesity.

Pharmacotherapy

Drugs have been used to treat of obesity since the 1930s, when the anorectic effects of amphetamine were first observed. During the 1950s and 1960s, amphetamines were commonly used for weight control, but their negative side effects, especially the strong potential for abuse, severely tarnished the image of drug therapy for obesity (Silverstone, 1987). Table 3.2 summarizes the anorectic drugs currently available by prescription in the United States. The table shows the Controlled Substance Act (CSA) classification of each drug's potential for abuse. Of those listed in the table, Schedule II drugs are most likely to be abused, whereas drugs in Schedule IV have little or no risk of abuse.

Anorectic drugs that act on the central nervous system (CNS) can be categorized into two major types based on whether or not they have stimulant properties. The phenylethylamines (which include amphetamine, phenmetrazine, phentermine, chlorphentermine, and diethylpropion) constitute the largest group of anorectic agents with

TABLE 3.2   ANORECTIC DRUGS CURRENTLY AVAILABLE BY PRESCRIPTION IN
THE UNITED STATES

Generic name	Trade name	CSA schedule
Amphetamine	Dexedrine, Obetrol	II
Methamphetamine	Desoxyn	II
Phenmetrazine	Preludin	II
Benzphetamine	Didrex	III
Phendimetrazine	Plegine, Statobex	III
Diethylpropion	Tenuate, Tepanil	IV
Fenfluramine	Pondimin	IV
Mazindol	Sanorex, Mazanor	IV
Phentermine	Fastin, Ionamin	IV

Note. Drugs in Controlled Substances Act (CSA) schedule II are most likely to be abused, whereas those in Schedule IV have little or no risk of abuse.

stimulant properties. These drugs stimulate the CNS mainly through the release of dopamine and noradrenalin. Mazindol, which is chemically different from the phenylethylamines, produces stimulation by inhibiting the uptake of noradrenalin. The CNS stimulation decreases appetite and fatigue and elevates mood, motor activity, and mental alertness. The anorectic effects of stimulant drugs appears to be due in part to a decrease in the frequency of eating. Schedule II stimulants have significant negative short-term side effects, including insomnia, restlessness, palpitations, and tachycardia, and if taken on a long-term basis, these potent stimulants can lead to addiction. Consequently, most experts strongly recommend against the use of Schedule II drugs for the treatment of obesity (Gotestam & Hauge, 1987). Diethylpropion (Tenuate) and phentermine (Fastin), which are Schedule IV stimulants with mild side effects (e.g., insomnia, dry mouth), have much less potential for abuse and are appropriate alternatives.

The second category of anorectic agents are those that do not have stimulant properties. These drugs act predominantly on the serotonin system. Fenfluramine and D-fenfluramine block the uptake of serotonin, and fluoxetine (Prozac), which is not yet approved by the Food and Drug Administration (FDA) for weight control, selectively inhibits the reuptake of serotonin. The anorectic effects of drugs that act on the serotonin system appear to result from decreased meal size and decreased consumption of carbohydrates.

Fenfluramine has a depressant rather than a stimulant effect on the CNS. Its side effects include drowsiness, sedation, and diarrhea, and depression sometimes occurs after its withdrawal. Clearly, fenfluramine is not a drug to be used with patients who are prone to depression. Fluoxetine, on the other hand, is an antidepressant medication. Observations of its anorectic effect have led to its consideration as a treatment for obesity. The side effects of fluoxetine include nausea, nervousness, insomnia, and drowsiness (Zerbe, 1987).

Dozens of double-blind studies have demonstrated that anorectic drugs produce greater weight losses than treatment with placebo. Although the between-group differences in weight loss for drug versus placebo have been statistically significant, the key question that often arises is whether such differences are clinically meaningful. Bray and Gray (1988) presented data from 41 studies that compared drug treatment (with or without diet) versus placebo (with or without diet). Studies that include a diet more closely approximate delivery of treatment in the clinical setting, and they allow for an assessment of the incremental advantage of drug therapy over conservative treatment.

The data summarized by Bray and Gray (1988) showed that, during an average treatment phase of 14 weeks, the combination treatments of drug plus diet produced a mean weight loss of 13.7 pounds compared to 6.34 pounds for placebo plus diet. The total incremental benefit for drug plus diet treatment versus placebo plus diet was a net loss of 7.4 pounds. Thus, over the course of treatment, the use of an appetite-suppressing drug enhanced the rate of weight loss by 0.5 pounds per week. The short-term effects of drug treatment in this selected group of studies are comparable to the findings summarized in larger-scale reviews of the drug-therapy literature (Scoville, 1975; Sullivan & Comai, 1978; Weintraub & Bray, 1989).

The studies reviewed by Bray and Gray did not include treatment with fluoxetine. Two 8-week trials with nondepressed, obese patients (Ferguson & Feighner, 1987; Levine, Rosenblatt, & Bosomworth, 1987) showed that fluoxetine plus diet increased the weekly rate of weight loss by 0.86 pounds, compared to placebo plus diet. In addition, one of the studies (Ferguson & Feighner, 1987) suggested that fluoxetine may be particularly effective for patients who experience cravings for carbohydrates.

What happens when patients stop using anorectic medications? Reviews of the longer-term effects of drug treatments consistently show that weight lost during drug treatment is almost completely regained following withdrawal of the drug (Munro & Ford, 1982). This disappointing result has led researchers to speculate that the efficacy of drug therapy could be enhanced by combining it with other treatments for obesity. Behavior therapy appeared to be a logical choice, because behavioral programs incorporate habit-change strategies with the potential to improve the long-term effects of treatment.

In an important study, Craighead, Stunkard, and O'Brien (1981) compared the short- and long-term effects of pharmacotherapy (fenfluramine), behavior therapy, and the combination of pharmacotherapy plus behavior therapy. At the conclusion of the 6-month treatment phase of this study, weight losses in the pharmacotherapy (31.9 pounds) and combined treatment groups (33.0 pounds) were significantly greater than results obtained with behavior therapy alone (25.1 pounds). The magnitude of weight loss in all three conditions was impressive, and the results showed that the addition of fenfluramine to behavior therapy improved the short-term effects of treatment. At a 12-month follow-up, however, a surprising reversal occurred. Patients who received pharmacotherapy or combination treatment showed dramatic relapses; they experienced weight gains of 18.0 and 22.9 pounds, respectively. The behavior therapy participants, on the other hand, had a minor increase of only 4.2 pounds.

The most surprising aspect of these results was poor maintenance of weight loss by the combination treatment. In 12 months, subjects who received pharmacotherapy plus behavior therapy regained almost 70% of their initial weight loss. Two explanations have been offered for these findings. Craighead (1987) has offered a psychological interpretation suggesting that *attributions* regarding success account for the differential long-term effects. Craighead suggests that subjects in the combined treatment attributed their initial success to an *external* agent—their medication. Thus, when the drug was withdrawn, they did not have sufficient self-confidence in their own abilities to sustain the behavior changes required to maintain weight loss. On the other hand, Stunkard (1989) has offered a physiological interpretation of the results. Stunkard suggests that the effect of an anorectic agent is to lower the set-point for body weight. Withdrawal of the drug, in turn, results in a return of set-point to the pretreatment level, and consequently, a regaining of weight occurs. Accordingly, Stunkard (1989) has recommended that drug therapy should be used on a continuous rather than a short-term basis.

A large-scale trial of the *long-term* use of drug therapy for obesity has recently been reported (Guy-Grand et al., 1989). A total of 822 obese patients received a *yearlong* treatment consisting of either drug plus diet or placebo plus diet. The drug used was dexfenfluramine, which is similar to fenfluramine but has fewer side effects. Over the course of the 12-month study period, a substantial proportion of participants dropped out of the study (45% in the placebo-plus-diet group and 37% in the drug-plus-diet condition). The mean weight losses at 1 year were 21.6 pounds for the drug-plus-diet condition versus 15.73 pounds for the placebo-plus-diet condition. These losses represented reductions in initial weight of 10.26% versus 7.18% and decreases in amount overweight of 31.78% versus 20.98% (for drug vs. placebo, respectively). In both groups, virtually all weight lost was accomplished during the first 6 months of treatment. During the second 6 months, the placebo-plus-diet group gained a small but significant amount of weight, whereas the drug-plus-diet group did not experience a significant change in weight. Thus, the researchers suggested that continuous drug therapy for obesity may enhance maintenance of weight loss without harmful side effects.

Very-Low-Calorie Diets (VLCDs)

Fasting represents the most aggressive approach to dietary treatment of obesity. Although fasting produces large, rapid weight losses (e.g., 49.7

pounds in 51 days; Drenick & Smith, 1964), it exposes the patient to an undue risk of physical danger. Weight losses from fasting entail severe reductions in muscle mass that can damage the vital lean tissues of the heart and can result in death (Garnett, Bernard, Ford, Goodbody, & Woodhouse, 1969; Spencer, 1968).

As an alternative to fasting, VLCDs were developed to preserve lean body mass while maximizing weight loss. To accomplish this objective, researchers formulated diets that were very low in calories (i.e., 400–800 calories per day) but included sufficient amounts of protein (i.e., 30–100 grams per day) to minimize the loss of lean tissue. Some VLCDs, such as the protein-sparing modified fast (Blackburn, Bistrian, & Flatt, 1975), rely on conventional foods (e.g., lean meats, fish, and fowl) as a source of protein, whereas other VLCDs consist of a liquid diet with protein derived from a milk- or egg-based powdered formula (e.g., Optifast 70, the commercially prepared product of Sandoz Nutrition Co. of Minneapolis, Minnesota). VLCDs also differ as to whether carbohydrate is included. The protein-sparing modified fast provides 1.5 grams of protein per kilogram of ideal body weight, and no carbohydrate is included. Most commercially available products contain some carbohydrate (e.g., Optifast 70 includes a daily total of 70 grams of protein, 30 grams of carbohydrate, and 2 grams of fat). According to Blackburn, Phinney, and Moldawer (1981), the exclusion of carbohydrates produces a high degree of ketosis and a low level of plasma insulin, thereby resulting in enhanced protein-sparing and increased fat mobilization. Other researchers (Howard, Grant, Edwards, Littlewood, & McLean Baird, 1978) have favored the inclusion of small amounts of carbohydrate in VLCDs so as to minimize the severity of diuresis, the loss of electrolytes, and the occurrence of orthostatic hypotension. Both types of VLCDs entail vitamin and mineral supplements. Equivalent weight losses have been obtained in each approach (Wadden, Stunkard, Brownell, & Day, 1985).

The use of a VLCD requires close medical supervision. During 1976–1977, a liquid-protein diet (Linn & Stuart, 1976) was associated with more than 60 fatalities. These deaths were subsequently attributed to cardiac dysfunction resulting from insufficient amounts or poor quality of protein consumed, prolonged periods of dieting, and severe vitamin and mineral deficiencies (Lantingua, Amatruda, Biddle, Forbes, & Lockwood, 1980; Van Itallie, 1978). Current VLCDs include protein of high biological quality and appropriate supplements of vitamins and minerals, and VLCD use is generally limited to 12 weeks. This aggressive form of treatment is recommended only for moderately or severely obese individuals. Contraindications include a history of heart disease, stroke, cancer, Type I diabetes, liver or renal failure, and serious psychiatric disorder (Atkinson, 1989). A complete medical evaluation is essential prior to treatment, and ongoing medical monitoring and testing is required throughout treatment.

Administration of VLCDs is usually conducted in three phases. A preliminary phase of 2–4 weeks involving a 1200-calorie per day balanced diet allows for gradual physiological and psychological accommodation to caloric restriction. In the middle phase, the VLCD itself is used. During this interval, close medical monitoring is required, including brief physical exams to check vital signs and side effects, routine blood tests to evaluate electrolyte balance, and occasional electrocardiograms (ECGs) to assess cardiac functioning. A refeeding phase of 2–4 weeks follows the period of VLCD use. During refeeding, the patient gradually is reintroduced to ordinary foods. Starches and refined sugars are the last items to be reinstated, to minimize the rapid gain in fluid weight that is associated with carbohydrate consumption. Following the refeeding phase, patients are often encouraged to participate in an aftercare program to enhance maintenance of weight loss.

VLCDs appear to be a safe form of treatment when used appropriately (Doherty, Wadden, Zuk, Letizia, Foster, & Day, 1991; Wadden, Stunkard, & Brownell, 1983). Proper use entails (a) close medical supervision throughout treatment; (b) the exclusion of patients who are not moderately or severely obese or who have contraindicated physical conditions; (c) the use of high-quality sources of protein, with appropriate vitamin and mineral supplementation; and (d) a limit of 12 weeks on the VLCD phase of treatment. Side effects of VLCDs include headaches, fatigue, postural hypotension, constipation, exacerbation of gallbladder disease, and menstrual irregularity (Atkinson, 1989).

VLCDs have become a very popular means of treating obesity. In the week following Oprah Winfrey's disclosure on nationwide television that she lost 67 pounds using Optifast, 1 million people telephoned Sandoz Nutrition for information about VLCD treatment (reported in Foreyt, 1990). Public interest in VLCDs remains quite high, and in any given week, tens of thousands of obese individuals are on a VLCD. How effective is this aggressive approach to treating obesity?

The short-term effects of VLCD treatment are quite impressive. Wadden, Stunkard, and Brownell (1983) summarized weight losses in eight major studies of VLCDs conducted prior to 1982. Treatments ranged in duration from 4 weeks to 24 weeks, and the resulting mean weight losses, which were highly correlated with the duration of treatment, ranged from 20.5 pounds to 90.4 pounds. Across studies, the mean duration of treatment was 14.7 weeks, and the mean weight loss was 47.3 pounds. These remarkable short-term results have been replicated in recent studies showing that VLCDs routinely produce initial weight losses of 33 to 44 pounds (Pavlou, Krey, & Steffee, 1989; Sikand, Kondo, Foreyt, Jones, & Gotto, 1988; Wadden & Stunkard, 1986; Wadden, Stunkard, Brownell, & Day, 1985).

Standing in stark contrast to the positive short-term effects of VLCDs are findings of *poor maintenance* of weight loss. The large weight reductions achieved by VLCDs are rarely sustained over the long run. Wadden and his colleagues (Wadden, Sternberg, Letizia, Stunkard, & Foster, 1989) have carefully documented the pattern of weight change over 5 years in a sample of 76 moderately and severely obese women who were initially treated by VLCD, behavior therapy, or the combination of VLCD plus behavior therapy. An examination of the findings in this study provides a sobering view of the long-term effects of VLCD treatments and of other therapies for obesity, as well.

In the Wadden et al. study, participants in the VLCD condition received 4 months of dietary treatment, including an initial month on a 1200-calorie-per-day diet, 2 months on a 400- to 500-calorie-per-day protein-sparing modified fast, and a final month of a 1200-calorie-per-day diet. Subjects in the behavior therapy condition received a 6-month program that included training in behavioral weight-control methods and instructions to follow a 1200-calorie-per-day diet throughout the course of therapy. Participants in the combined treatment also received a 6-month program that included behavioral training and 2-month use of a protein-sparing modified fast. At the end of treatment, the combination of VLCD and behavior therapy resulted in significantly greater reductions in weight than either of the VLCD-alone or the behavior-therapy single-modality conditions. The combined treatment produced a mean weight loss of 37.0 pounds, compared to 28.8 pounds in the VLCD-alone condition and 28.6 pounds in the behavior-therapy-alone condition.

The 1-year follow-up evaluation showed that *all* groups regained substantial proportions of their posttreatment losses, with 64% of lost weight regained in the VCLD-alone condition, 49% in the behavior therapy group, and 37% in the combined treatment. Net weight loss from baseline was significantly greater in the combined treatment group than in the VLCD-alone condition. In addition, only 5% of the VCLD-alone subjects maintained their end-of-treatment weight loss, as compared with 36% of the behavior-therapy subjects and 32% of the combined-treatment subjects. Thus, the 1-year follow-up evaluation showed that regaining of weight occurred in all conditions, but it was most common and most severe in the group treated by VLCD alone.

The findings from the 5-year follow-up evaluation were even more discouraging. After correcting for the effects of any subsequent therapy for obesity that subjects received, the researchers found that the *majority* of participants in *all three* conditions had regained the *entire* amounts that they lost during treatment! Only 11.1% of the VCLD-alone subjects, 13.3% of the behavior-therapy subjects, and 27.3% of the combined-treatment subjects had maintained weight losses of 11 pounds or more at the 5-year follow-up. Furthermore, just three participants (one in each condition) had maintained their entire end-of-treatment weight losses.

Findings of very poor maintenance of weight loss following VLCD treatment have been reported in a number of recent studies. For example,

Sikand and colleagues (Sikand, Kondo, Foreyt, Jones, & Gotto, 1988) evaluated the effects of VLCD with and without structured exercise training during treatment. At a 2-year follow-up, the investigators found that patients in the VLCD-plus-exercise group had regained 58% of their posttreatment losses and those in the VLCD-alone condition regained 96% of their end of treatment losses. Hovell et al. (1988) examined the results for 400 health-maintenance organization (HMO) patients who were treated with VLCD plus behavior therapy. The investigators found that although patients initially lost 84% of their excess weight, they regained an average of 59–82% of their initial excess weight by the time of a 30-month follow-up evaluation. Finally, Andersen and associates (Andersen, Stockholm, Backer, & Quaade, 1988) conducted a 5-year follow-up of subjects treated with VLCD and found that only 17% of their patients maintained 22 pounds or more of their original average 48.4-pound weight losses.

Surgical Treatment

Gastroplasty and gastric bypass are the two major types of bariatric surgery currently available. Gastroplasty entails a severe reduction of the volume of the stomach so as to restrict the amount of food that can be eaten. Gastric bypass involves circumventing a portion of the stomach, to decrease the absorption of foods that have been eaten. At present, gastroplasty is the more common surgical treatment for obesity.

In gastroplasty, the size of the stomach is surgically reduced. Typically, a small vertical pouch is created, to limit the amount of solid food that can be ingested during a single eating. A ring or "collar" with a circumference of 4.5 to 5.5 cm is placed at the outlet of the pouch, to slow the rate at which food passes through the remainder of the stomach and into the small intestine. Gastroplasty exerts a regulatory effect on eating behavior through aversive conditioning. Ingestion of more than the small amount of solid food that the stomach pouch can accommodate typically results in regurgitation. Fear of vomiting provides a powerful disincentive for overeating, and the perception of fullness associated with distention of the stomach serves as a discriminative stimulus to control consumption. Thus, when surgery is successful, the gastroplasty patient will feel full after eating a small amount of food and will discontinue eating to avoid the aversive consequences associated with regurgitation.

Prior to the 1980s, intestinal (i.e., jejunoileal) bypass procedures constituted the standard surgical treatments for obesity. In this procedure, a portion of the small intestine was removed, so that a significant amount of nutrients ingested by the obese person would not be absorbed in the intestine but would be expelled in stools. The jejunoileal bypass procedure produced dramatic weight losses. Unfortunately, numerous complications from this surgery led to an unacceptably high mortality rate (Halverson,

Wise, Wazna, & Ballinger, 1978), and it was eventually abandoned in favor of safer procedures.

Gastric bypass surgery, also based on the principle of malabsorption, entails bypassing part of the stomach rather than the small intestine. In this procedure, the size of the stomach is reduced (usually through horizontal stapling), and the resulting pouch is attached to a loop of small intestine. Ingested food passes through only a portion of the stomach before entering the intestine. In addition to the decreased absorption that results from gastric bypass, there is also an aversive consequence experienced by the patient. The dumping of nutrients directly from the stomach into the upper intestine often produces a variety of unpleasant symptoms, such as light-headedness, sweating, and palpitations. The combination of these aversive consequences and the malabsorption of nutrients may be responsible for the greater weight losses reported for gastric bypass than for gastroplasty (Kral, 1989; Sugerman, Starkey, & Birkenhauer, 1987; Sugerman et al., 1989).

What characteristics make an obese person an appropriate candidate for bariatric surgery? In 1985, a Task Force of the American Society of Clinical Nutrition described guidelines for patient selection suggesting that surgery be reserved for *refractory* cases of *morbid* obesity. The guidelines include an actual body weight that is either 100 pounds or 100 percent over ideal weight, coupled with the presence of an obesity-related, serious medical condition and a history of substantial obesity despite repeated attempts at weight reduction. Some bariatric surgeons consider a body weight that is 60% or more over the ideal to be "morbid obesity" due to its statistical association with poor health and decreased longevity. Moreover, some (e.g., Mason et al., 1987) argue that because the efficacy of surgery is superior to that of alternative treatments, surgery may be an appropriate intervention for obese individuals who are less than 100% overweight *and* who are yet to experience other medical illnesses.

Mason and colleagues (Mason et al., 1987) have summarized the results of surgical treatments of obesity in a very large sample of patients. The authors described findings for two major types of surgery: vertical-banded gastroplasty and Roux-en-Y gastric bypass. In addition, they compared the results for patients with what they called "morbid" obesity (i.e., 60–125% over ideal weight) versus those with their category of "super" obesity (i.e., greater than 125% over ideal weight). Data were reviewed from a total of 1073 surgeries, including 1000 gastroplasties and 73 gastric bypasses. The authors found that gastric-bypass surgeries took longer (an average of 2 1/2 to 3 hours) and resulted in a higher infection rate (15%) than the gastroplasty procedures, which averaged less than 2 hours and had an infection rate of about 2%. Both types of surgery were longer and had higher infection rates for patients with super versus morbid obesity. The overall mortality rate was 0.4%, and there were no significant differences by type of surgery or patient. Weight loss achieved with the gastroplasty was described as "slightly less" than that obtained with gastric bypass.

Mason et al. (1987) have summarized mean weight losses for groups of patients seen 2 and 5 years after gastroplasty (using a 5-cm collar). The 2-year data showed that 120 patients with morbid obesity had a mean weight reduction of 79.2 pounds, a loss representing more than 60% of their excess body. The corresponding mean weight loss for 159 superobese patients was 114 pounds, an amount representing slightly more than half of their excess body weight. Mason et al. also presented weight-loss results for 80 patients who were 5 years postsurgery. These data were similar to the 2-year findings. A group of 58 morbidly obese patients had a mean weight reduction of 74.8 pounds, whereas 22 superobese persons had a mean loss of 105.6 pounds.

Collectively, the findings from Mason et al. demonstrate the impressive magnitude of weight losses that can be accomplished through bariatric surgery. Nonetheless, several considerations are worth noting. First, the aforementioned data are the results for the most successful of three variations of gastroplasty performed by the Mason et al. group (i.e., use of 5.0-cm collar); the alternative procedures (i.e., using collars of 4.5 or 5.5 cm) produced less weight loss at 5 years. Second, a significant portion of the patients required a second surgery, often because the stapling came undone or their stomach pouch was stretched, presumably as a result of overeating. The percentages of patients who underwent surgical revision ranged from 9 to 24% and varied according to the type of initial surgery and the category of obesity. Initial gastroplasty with the smaller collar more often necessitated surgical revision, and superobese patients were more likely to require reoperation, perhaps because excessive eating was more often a problem for them than for the morbidly obese patients. Third, Mason et al. failed to report the percentage of patients who were lost to follow-up. Without such information, it is difficult to get an accurate and comprehensive picture of the actual effectiveness of bariatric surgery. Some researchers (Makarewicz, Freeman, Burchett, & Brazeau, 1985) have suggested that patients who fail to return for follow-up evaluations should be considered treatment failures, along with those who show inadequate weight losses. Using these stringent criteria, the "hard failure rate" for gastroplasty has been calculated at 42% in one sample (Kral, 1989) and 48% in another (Makarewicz et al., 1985). Kral has cautioned, however, that patients may be lost to follow-up either because they are feeling well and see no need for a visit or because they are experiencing medical complications and are afraid their physician will suggest a reversal or "takedown" of the gastric procedure.

Sugerman et al. (1987) conducted a randomized prospective trial of gastric bypass versus vertical-banded gastroplasty. They found that the gastric-bypass procedure produced significantly greater weight losses than the gastroplasty procedure at evaluations conducted 1, 2, and 3 years after surgery (see Table 3.3). Patients who were "sweets eaters" (i.e., those who, before their surgery, reported eating more than 15% of calories as sugar) had poorer outcomes (versus non–sweets eaters) with the gastroplasty procedure but not with the gastric bypass operation. This finding was understandable because in patients who have the gastric-bypass surgery, consuming sweets results in specific aversive consequences (i.e., the "dumping syndrome"). Sugerman et al. (1987) concluded that the gastric-bypass procedure was the preferred operation for sweets eaters, whereas gastroplasty was the preferred procedure for non–sweets eaters. In a second *non*randomized study, Sugerman et al. (1989) showed that the gastric bypass produced greater weight loss than the gastroplasty but was associated with more serious postoperative complications.

Weight losses resulting from surgical treatment often produce substantial improvements in obesity-related illnesses, including hypertension, arthritis, hyperlipidemia, pulmonary dysfunction, and diabetes (Brolin, 1987). Moreover, surgical treatment of obesity also results in improved quality of life. Stunkard, Stinnett, and Smoller (1986) have documented dramatic improvements in vocational and psychosocial functioning following bariatric surgery, including decreased body-image disparagement and enhanced marital and sexual satisfaction.

However, it is important to note that a substantial number of patients

TABLE 3.3   WEIGHT LOSS AFTER ROUX-EN-Y GASTRIC BYPASS (RYGBP) VERSUS VERTICAL-BANDED GASTROPLASTY (VBGP)

	RYGBP		VBGP	
	n	mean	n	mean
Percentage over ideal body weight				
Before surgery	20	113	20	125
One year	19	38*	18	76
Two years	18	39*	17	78
Three years	18	42*	16	80
Weight loss (pounds)				
One year	19	96**	18	71
Two years	18	96**	17	67
Three years	18	91*	16	60
Percentage decrease in weight				
One year	19	33**	18	22
Two years	18	33**	17	22
Three years	18	32*	16	20

Source: Sugerman, H. J., Starkey, J. V., & Birkenhauer, R. (1987). A randomized prospective trial of gastric bypass versus vertical banded gastroplasty for morbid obesity and their effects on sweets versus nonsweets eaters. *Annals of Surgery, 205,* 613–624. Adapted with permission.

*$p < .01$

**$p < .001$

who undergo surgical treatment for obesity have operations that are technically successful but fail to produce expected weight losses due to either physiological or psychological reasons. Plateaus in weight loss are often reached 6–12 months after surgery, and the majority of patients remain 40–80% over ideal weight (Hocking, Kelly, & Callaway, 1986; Sugerman et al., 1987). In some cases, the excess numbers of fats cells associated with morbid obesity may impose physiological barriers to further weight loss. In other instances, behavioral or psychological factors may lead to unsuccessful long-term outcome. Many patients who have had gastroplasties compensate for the restricted size of their stomachs by consuming large amounts of calorically dense liquids or soft, sweet, creamy foods. Poor outcome attributable to "soft calorie syndrome" may be as high as 30% (Kral, 1989). The problem of self-sabotage indicates the postoperative need for comprehensive long-term care, including psychological as well as dietary counseling.

SUMMARY AND CONCLUSIONS

Conservative treatments represent the first line of care in the management of obesity. These relatively safe methods of intervention generally are tried before implementing more aggressive interventions, which entail greater risks for negative side effects. Conservative treatments include conventional low-calorie diets, commercial weight-control programs, self-help groups, and comprehensive behavioral treatments. When utilized under the best of circumstances, these approaches generally produce moderate amounts of weight loss (i.e., 10% reduction in body weight). For the most part, the weight losses produced by conservative treatments are not well maintained over the long run.

Retrospective self-reports suggest that many mildly obese individuals diet effectively on their own and successfully maintain long-term weight losses of 20 to 30 pounds. Research including *documented* evidence of weight changes by overweight individuals has shown, however, that the actual percentage of "self-cures" of obesity is probably less than 10%. Moreover, self-reports of dieting success appear to be inflated by inaccurate recall. Obese people report losing more weight than documented records show.

Commercial weight-control programs using low-calorie diets produce average losses of 10–20 pounds, but the significance of such reductions is minimized by high rates of attrition (i.e., 80% over a 1-year period) and poor maintenance of weight loss. Similarly, self-help groups for weight loss are also limited by high dropout rates and very modest initial weight losses.

Low-calorie diets administered by health-care professionals on an outpatient basis appear to result in average weight losses of about 18 pounds, with approximately 25% of patients losing 20 pounds or more. Little information is available about the long-term efficacy of low-calorie diets, but available data suggest that weight losses are not well maintained.

Comprehensive behavioral interventions regularly produce either weight losses of 20 pounds or 10% reductions in body weight. Attrition rates are relatively low (i.e., less than 15%), and negative side effects of treatment are virtually nonexistent. During the year following behavioral treatment, participants typically regain about 40% of their initial weight losses. Follow-up evaluations conducted 4 or 5 years after behavioral treatment generally show poor maintenance of weight loss. Fewer than 20% of participants maintain half their posttreatment weight losses at 4-year follow-up.

Aggressive approaches to the treatment of obesity include pharmacotherapy, VLCDs, and bariatric surgery. The use of an anorectic drug in conjunction with dieting enhances the rate of weight loss by about 0.5 pounds per week over 12 weeks. Unfortunately, drug-induced weight losses are rapidly regained when the drug is withdrawn, and combining behavior therapy with pharmacotherapy seems to impair rather than enhance maintenance of weight loss. Thus, there appears to be little benefit in the short-term use of anorectic agents in the treatment of obesity. Some researchers have suggested that the long-term use of anorectic drugs may improve the maintenance of weight loss, but further research is needed before such an approach can be advocated.

Under proper medical supervision, VLCDs safely produce large and rapid reductions in weight. The magnitude of these losses—33 to 55 pounds—exceeds all conservative treatments for obesity. Unfortunately, VLCD-induced weight losses are very poorly maintained. During the year following treatment, patients often regain two thirds of their end-of-treatment weight losses. Combining the use of VLCD with behavior therapy increases initial weight loss and fosters better maintenance of weight loss during the year following treatment. Nonetheless, long-term results with VLCDs with or without behavior therapy are discouraging. Follow-ups of 2–5 years show that the majority of patients treated with VLCDs regain the entire amounts initially lost in treatment. A particularly troublesome issue regarding VLCDs centers on the long-term consequences of large fluctuations in weight. As noted in Chapter 1, mounting evidence suggests that losing and regaining large amounts of weight may be detrimental to physical health. In addition, there may also be negative psychological effects experienced by the individual who loses a large amount of weight, only to regain it shortly thereafter. Even though the experience of losing and regaining weight may be common in obese persons, the dramatic weight losses and weight gains induced by VLCDs may do particular damage to an individual's self-confidence and self-esteem.

Gastric bypass and vertical banded gastroplasty, the two most common current surgical treatments for obesity, produce very large weight losses but entail a much higher degree of risk than alternative treatments of obesity. Severely obese patients typically lose 20–35% of their preoperative weight within 1 year of surgery, and these weight losses appear to be maintained relatively well at 2- and 3-year follow-up evaluations. The risks of surgery, however, include postoperative complications that require surgical revisions in 9–24% of patients, and the operative mortality rate associated with bariatric surgery is approximately 0.5% (Hocking, Kelly, & Callaway, 1986; Kral, 1988; MacLean, Rhode, & Shizgal, 1983; Mason et al., 1987). A substantial minority of patients who undergo surgical treatment for obesity have operations that are technically successful but fail to produce expected weight losses, due to either physiological limitations or poor behavioral adherence. The problem of self-sabotage following bariatric surgery may be as high as 30% and suggests that after surgery, many patients need comprehensive long-term care, including psychological as well as dietary counseling.

One overarching conclusion can be drawn from this selective review. At present, there is no safe and reliable means of producing large and lasting weight loss. Surgical interventions come the closest to meeting this objective, but serious risks associated with surgery limit its use to those very severe cases representing less than 1% of all obese individuals. Many of the current treatments for obesity do produce positive short-term results. For example, comprehensive behavioral treatment is safe, has a low rate of attrition, and results in sufficient weight loss to reap benefits in both physical health and psychological functioning. Furthermore, the combination of behavior therapy plus VLCD produces even more impressive short-term weight losses. Unfortunately, long-term evaluations consistently show that weight reductions are poorly maintained, regardless of whether the weight loss was initially attained through dietary, behavioral, or pharmacological means.

Perhaps we should not be surprised by the poor long-term outcome associated with treatment-induced weight losses. Virtually all of current treatments are in effect short-term interventions that leave the obese individual inadequately prepared to meet the challenge of a relentless physiology ever-primed for weight gain (see Chapter 2). When on their own, most obese individuals cannot sustain the substantial degree of psychological control necessary to override these compensatory biological mechanisms. Thus, it is quite apparent that initial treatments for obesity need to be supplemented with programs of follow-up care, specially designed to enhance the long-term maintenance of weight loss. In the following chapter, we address this issue in greater detail, and we describe the impact of maintenance programs on the long-term management of obesity.

4

Effectiveness of Weight-Loss Maintenance Programs

After completing treatment for obesity, most patients will regain weight. Indeed, as we described in the previous chapter, long-term follow-up studies generally show that the *majority* of patients regain most of the weight that they initially lost during treatment. Such findings have led reviewers of the obesity-treatment literature, such as Jeffery (1987) to conclude that "the most pressing continuing challenge is maintaining weight loss . . . obesity should be viewed as a chronic condition requiring long-term supportive care" (p. 20). In this chapter, we examine the problem of poor maintenance of weight loss from a biobehavioral perspective, which posits that physiological and psychological factors interact to hinder the long-term maintenance of weight loss. We describe how a cognitive/social-learning framework has guided our development of interventions to improve the long-term management of obesity, and we summarize a series of studies that tested the effectiveness of specific interventions designed to enhance the maintenance of weight loss. Finally, we present the results of one of the few studies in the literature to investigate the long-term impact of a *continuous-care* approach to the management of obesity.

Poor maintenance of treatment-induced weight loss appears to stem from the interplay of biological and behavioral factors. As we described in Chapter 2, weight loss triggers physiological mechanisms, such as AT (adaptive thermogenesis) and increased production of adipose tissue LPL (lipoprotein lipase), that dispose the obese person to regain weight. Moreover, continuous exposure to an environment rich in fattening foods and a heightened sensitivity to palatable foods induced by dieting are additional ingredients in a recipe guaranteed to result in relapse. Short-term treatments of obesity often fail because they do not adequately equip the patient to deal with relentless physiological processes that serve to compensate for weight loss.

When obese patients are on their own following weight-loss treatment, many become discouraged by the significant difficulties that they encounter in trying to maintain weight loss. More often than not, they attribute their lack of success to personal failings. Such attributions frequently lead to a host of negative emotions, including feelings of frustration, guilt, anxiety, depression, and anger. In attempting to reduce these distressful feelings, many patients use ineffective means of coping. Often, they resort to rationalizations and avoidance, saying to themselves, for example, "I'm too stressed out to deal with a diet just now, but come Monday, I'll get back on the wagon." The effect of such an approach is to give themselves permission to deviate even further from behaviors needed to sustain their weight loss. An accumulation of broken resolutions to resume appropriate eating behaviors eventually precipitates abandonment of the entire weight-loss effort; as a consequence, many obese patients end up regaining much or all of the weight that they lost during treatment.

The long-term failure of short-term treatments for obesity prompted us to investigate the effects of providing patients with additional care during the period following an initial phase of obesity treatment. Aware that compensatory physiological mechanisms make long-term success difficult to achieve, we sought to develop posttreatment strategies that would enable patients to sustain the behavioral changes (i.e., decreased energy intake and increased energy expenditure) required for the maintenance of weight loss. We investigated a variety of maintenance strategies, including (a) professional guidance in the form of continued therapist contacts after initial treatment; (b) skills training to prepare patients to more effectively manage the challenges of the posttreatment period; (c) social-influence programs, to supply increased social support after treatment; (d) increased physical activity, to provide patients with positive physical and psychological benefits that may enhance long-term success; and (e) multicomponent interventions, which combine several procedures to assist patients in weight-loss maintenance.

In our research on the development of weight-loss maintenance strategies, we conducted a series of six randomized, prospective experiments. In each study, all patients were treated initially with a conservative program consisting of behavior therapy and low-calorie diet and were then assigned randomly either to an experimental maintenance program or to a control condition with no additional therapeutic contact. Subjects in the control conditions in each of the studies received no further contact following treatment except for follow-up evaluations. The patients in our studies were mildly and moderately obese volunteers who responded to announcements of a weight-loss research program. Our typical subject was a 45-year old, middle-class, married, white woman who at the start of treatment weighed approximately 200 pounds and was about 50% over ideal body weight.

STUDY 1. CONTINUED PROFESSIONAL CONTACT AND SKILLS TRAINING

Booster sessions have been the most commonly used approach to foster maintenance of weight loss. Following treatment, clinicians often suggest that their patients return for occasional treatment sessions during the follow-up period. These sessions are typically used to review and reinforce the behavioral changes accomplished in treatment, on the premise that overlearning will contribute to lasting habit changes. This approach makes intuitive sense. It seems reasonable that additional sessions following the termination of treatment would boost patients' adherence to the habit changes required for the maintenance of weight loss. However, the findings from several carefully designed studies have failed to demonstrate that booster sessions are an effective means of maintaining weight loss (e.g., Ashby & Wilson, 1977; Beneke & Paulsen, 1979; Hall, Hall, Borden, & Hanson, 1975).

Looking back, it is simple to understand why the booster session approach was unsuccessful. In most cases, only 3 to 6 booster sessions were scheduled during the posttreatment period, and the sessions were often spaced 1 to 3 months apart. Consequently, the amount of professional contact may have been too meager to supply patients with adequate advice and support at the times when they required it most. Furthermore, booster sessions often consisted solely of a review of weight-loss techniques already presented during treatment, yet difficulties unique to the posttreatment period may be the cause of maintenance problems. Thus, the strategies necessary to *maintain* behavior change may differ substantially from those required to *initiate* behavior change (see Wadden & Bell, 1990).

After treatment has ended, loss of motivation often contributes to poor maintenance of the habit changes needed to sustain weight loss. Thus, a simple review of initial treatment procedures may be inadequate to meet the special needs of patients who have already completed a preliminary course of weight-loss treatment. Professional contacts during the posttreatment period may be more effective if they offer frequent opportunities for advice and guidance, and they provide training in strategies aimed specifically at sustaining the behaviors needed to maintain weight loss. Therefore, in the first study in our series (Perri, Shapiro, Ludwig, Twentyman, & McAdoo, 1984), we investigated whether the maintenance of weight loss could be enhanced by posttreatment professional contacts, as well as by skills training targeted at relapse prevention.

As most clinicians are aware, when patients complete weight-loss treatment, they are confronted by a major challenge. In order to avoid regaining weight, they must maintain a life-style that requires lowered caloric intake and greater energy expenditure than they are used to or comfortable with. To address this challenge, patients must maintain an active awareness and enhanced vigilance regarding critical aspects of their eating and exercise patterns. Posttreatment professional contacts encourage such vigilance by helping patients to be continuously mindful of their progress. When these contacts are used to restructure the patients' experiences in a positive, constructive, and hopeful fashion, the motivation to sustain behavior change can be enhanced. Furthermore, when difficulties in maintaining weight loss arise, posttreatment contacts can also provide an opportunity for therapist-directed problem solving.

Therapist contacts by mail and telephone represent one approach that may be employed to provide professional support and advice during the period following initial weight-loss treatment. Patients' vigilance and maintenance of behavior change may increase when they mail self-monitoring data with information about their eating, exercise, and weight to their therapists (Hall, Bass, & Monroe, 1978; Hall et al., 1975). Furthermore, promising findings have suggested that frequent posttreatment telephone contacts between therapists and patients may serve as an effective maintenance strategy for a range of problems (see Spevak, 1981). Therefore, in our first study, we examined the effectiveness of posttreatment professional contacts as a maintenance strategy by having patients mail in relevant self-monitoring data, and by having the therapists contact patients via telephone to discuss progress and problems in weight control.

Although frequent therapist contacts may help patients to maintain habit changes begun during an initial treatment phase, an effective maintenance program may require additional components, such as providing patients with the skills to anticipate, avoid, and cope with those circumstances that increase the risk of a relapse (Brownell, Marlatt, Lichtenstein, & Wilson, 1986; Marlatt & Gordon, 1985). Marlatt and colleagues' relapse-prevention model provides the most comprehensive conceptual framework for understanding and dealing with the maintenance problem in the treatment of addictive behaviors. This model is quite relevant to understanding the difficulties experienced by obese individuals who have succeeded in losing weight during therapy.

Some time after treatment, these individuals will be confronted by situations that tempt them to exceed a prescribed calorie goal or otherwise to deviate from the strategies learned in treatment. Without the skills necessary to negotiate this "high-risk situation," the individual may slip or have a lapse in self-control. Furthermore, if the individual views the lapse as proof that he or she is unable to exert self-control, he or she is likely to experience a feeling of hopelessness and a reduction in self-efficacy. This initial slip then grows into a full-blown relapse, in which the individual abandons the habits developed in therapy, reverts to prior eating patterns, and regains weight. In contrast, if the person is prepared with the coping skills necessary to effectively confront the high-risk situation, he or she is likely to experience a greater sense of self-efficacy, and to continue with the positive changes developed in treatment.

In order to prevent or reduce the risk of relapse following treatment, Marlatt and Gordon (1985) have recommended several specific therapeutic procedures. First, it is important that patients be taught to recognize and identify those situations that represent a high risk for relapse. Second, problem-solving techniques can be employed to generate coping strategies for high-risk situations. Next, patients must have an opportunity to practice coping in vivo with high-risk situations. Finally, patients need to learn cognitive strategies to master the negative feelings and sense of failure that often accompany lapses in self-control. Practically every patient will experience some form of slip during the posttreatment period. Nonetheless, the therapist can teach patients to interpret slips as learning experiences, individual events to be overcome in the future through appropriate coping responses.

Thus, in our first study, we evaluated the impact of posttreatment professional contact and skills training on weight-loss maintenance. We examined the effectiveness of relapse-prevention training and of posttreatment therapist contacts by mail and telephone in the long-term management of obesity.

The participants in our first study were 129 volunteers who were mildly and moderately obese and averaged 195 pounds and averaged 57% over ideal body weight prior to treatment. Through random assignment, subjects were placed in one of six conditions in a 3 x 2 factorial design. This factorial design consisted of three therapy conditions (i.e., nonbehavioral treatment, behavior therapy, behavior therapy combined with relapse-prevention training), crossed with two maintenance-period conditions (i.e., either no additional contact or therapist–patient contacts through both telephone calls and mail).

All initial treatments involved 15 weekly 2-hour group sessions. The nonbehavioral treatment consisted of exchange plan diets, recommendations for exercise, and group sessions focusing on understanding the "underlying reasons" for overeating. The behavior therapy sessions emphasized the various self-control techniques commonly employed in behavioral programs for weight reduction (Johnson & Stalonas, 1981). The behavior-therapy-plus-relapse-prevention-training condition supplemented the behavior-therapy program with specific training experiences intended to minimize or prevent relapse, and to encourage the maintenance of habit change and weight loss. Patients were taught to identify those situations and circumstances with increased risk for slips, and they were trained in problem-solving skills (D'Zurilla & Nezu, 1982) to help them develop the coping strategies necessary to overcome high-risk situations. Two high-risk situations provided patients with in vivo practice of coping skills: dining out in an Italian restaurant with a limited number of low-calorie foods, and socializing at a potluck party, which included high-calorie snack foods. Furthermore, patients were taught cognitive strategies to cope with the guilt feelings and sense of failure that accompany slips. Therapists directed patients to interpret a slip as a *learning experience*—a single individual event to be overcome in the future through an appropriate coping response.

Following the 15-week treatment, contacts between therapists and participants were discontinued in three of the six experimental conditions, except for periodic assessments. Patients in the posttreatment contact condition were directed to monitor and record daily weight-related information on postcards specially prepared for them to mail weekly to their therapist during the first 6 months following the initial treatment. The therapists in turn contacted each patient by telephone to discuss briefly (approximately 5–10 minutes) the information received and to provide support and advice. These contacts, although tailored to the individual, remained consistent with the patient's original treatment condition. For the first 3 months following treatment, telephone contacts were made weekly, then were faded during the second 3-month period. The final patient–therapist contact by telephone and mail occurred 6 months after the end of the initial treatment.

This project's primary outcome measure was change in body weight, which was evaluated immediately after treatment, and again at 3-, 6-, and 12-month follow-up assessments. In addition, questionnaires at posttreatment and follow-up sessions were employed to examine participants' use of weight-loss techniques.

The results showed that all treatments resulted in substantial initial weight losses (mean = 18.7 pounds), and that no significant between-group differences existed at the end of the initial treatment. Over the course of the 12 months of the follow-up period, a significant three-way interaction effect for Time X Initial Treatment X Maintenance Condition emerged ($p < .05$). Figure 4.1 illustrates the pattern of net mean weight losses for each condition over the course of the study. As the figure shows, posttreatment contact had differential effects that varied according to the

Mean Weight Losses (lbs.)

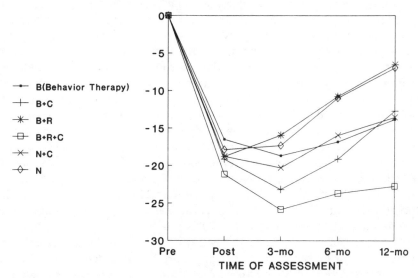

R = Relapse Prevention
C = Therapist Contact
N = Non-behavioral Therapy

FIGURE 4.1. Net mean weight losses (pounds), from pretreatment, for the following conditions: nonbehavioral treatment, nonbehavioral treatment plus posttreatment therapist contact, behavior therapy, behavior therapy plus posttreatment therapist contact, behavior therapy plus relapse-prevention training, and behavior therapy plus relapse prevention training plus posttreatment therapist contact. Based on data from Perri, Shapiro, et al., 1984.

participants' initial type of treatment. Posttreatment patient–therapist contact by telephone and mail improved the maintenance of weight loss for groups that received nonbehavioral treatment or behavior therapy plus relapse prevention. However, the posttreatment contact strategy did not enhance maintenance for the groups that received behavior therapy only.

Only one condition—behavior therapy plus relapse-prevention training, combined with posttreatment contact—both maintained its mean posttreatment weight loss and avoided significant relapse during the 12-month follow-up period. This combination of initial treatment and maintenance strategy was the only one that provided patients with both specific coping strategies to prepare for posttreatment difficulties, and supervised practice in applying those strategies during the actual follow-up period. Self-report data indicated that participants in this condition may have experienced greater success because during the follow-up period, they made greater use of key weight-management strategies, including self-monitoring, stimulus control, and exercise.

The group that received behavior therapy plus relapse-prevention training *without* posttreatment contact demonstrated a surprisingly poor performance. Perhaps, the relapse-prevention training provided during the initial treatment did not provide patients with the experiences necessary to become proficient enough in the various cognitive strategies for effective independent use during the posttreatment period. Alternatively, patients may have interpreted the relapse-prevention training experiences as permission to experiment with deviations from the recommended eating and exercise habits. For example, rather than appropriately using cognitive coping strategies, some patients may have used them to rationalize a sustained series of slips (e.g., "My therapist expected that I would slip up once in a while—this doesn't necessarily mean I'm off the program for good!"). Unfortunately, without confronting feedback from a therapist, repeated slips resulting from such rationalizations can snowball to the point that some patients never resume the eating and exercise habits needed to sustain weight loss. Thus, relapse-prevention training may only be helpful as a maintenance strategy if it is combined with a therapist's posttreatment guidance to ensure appropriate implementation.

The interaction of the posttreatment contact strategy with relapse-prevention training strongly suggests that the *content* of patient–therapist interactions is crucial to posttreatment success. For example, providing advice about specific coping techniques may have been instrumental in helping patients manage slips and avoid relapses. Thus, the *combination* of training targeted at the specific difficulties of the maintenance period together with therapist contact by mail and telephone appears promising as an effective maintenance strategy.

STUDY 2. SOCIAL SUPPORT AND A MULTICOMPONENT PROGRAM

A *multifaceted* set of posttreatment strategies may be necessary to maintain behavior changes successfully. Stuart (1980) hypothesized that, to be effective, maintenance programs should consist of a combination of strategies, such as continued self-monitoring, frequent posttreatment contacts with the therapist, and patient involvement in self-help groups. Our first study included two of the three key maintenance program elements recommended by Stuart: namely, continued self-monitoring of relevant weight-control strategies, and continued therapist–patient telephone contacts during the posttreatment period. In our second study, we supplemented the maintenance program with Stuart's third element by instructing subjects to develop their own self-help groups during the posttreatment period. We then evaluated how effective this multicomponent program was for long-term maintenance of weight loss (Perri, McAdoo, Spevak, & Newlin, 1984).

The participants in our second study were 56 mildly and moderately obese patients who were randomly assigned to one of two conditions: behavior therapy plus booster sessions or behavior therapy plus a multicomponent maintenance program. Initial treatment for both conditions consisted of 14 weekly group sessions of behavior therapy for obesity. Upon completion of the initial treatment, patients in the behavior-therapy-plus-booster-session condition participated in 6 biweekly booster sessions, which reviewed and reinforced strategies implemented during treatment. Other than 5 follow-up assessments, these were the only contacts scheduled with therapists or other group members.

After the initial treatment phase, patients in the behavior-therapy-plus-multicomponent-maintenance-program condition attended six biweekly sessions focusing on strategies to enhance weight-loss progress during the maintenance period. These patients also received instructions about developing their own peer self-help groups. Self-help group meetings followed the structure and procedures of problem-solving treatment. Patients learned to monitor each other's weight, to reinforce weight-loss progress with praise, and to problem solve as a group, to assist members experiencing difficulties in their efforts at weight loss (D'Zurilla & Nezu, 1982). Therapists encouraged these self-help groups to meet regularly throughout the year after treatment. Furthermore, therapists asked patients in the multicomponent maintenance program to mail weekly postcards providing information about their weight-loss progress; the therapists in turn telephoned these patients to provide additional support and guidance during the year after treatment (as in our first study).

Four subjects in each of the two conditions dropped out during the initial treatment. Although no additional subjects dropped out of the multicomponent-maintenance-program condition, five participants did drop out of the behavior-therapy-plus-booster-session condition during the 21-month follow-up period. This difference in posttreatment dropout rates was statistically significant ($p < .05$). During the follow-up period, patients in the multicomponent program, on average, participated in 8.5 self-help group meetings, mailed in 22.5 postcards describing weight-loss efforts, and received 26.9 telephone calls from their therapists.

The two conditions resulted in equivalent weight losses at the conclusion of the initial treatment period. Figure 4.2 presents the pattern of net mean weight losses, by condition, over the course of the study. As the figure illustrates, a significant interaction effect is evident for Time X Posttreatment Condition ($p < .05$). According to post hoc comparisons, these between-group differences were not significant at either the 3- or 6-month follow-up sessions. However, at the 9-, 15-, and 21-month follow-up sessions, patients in the multicomponent maintenance program were significantly more successful at maintaining weight loss than were subjects in the behavior-therapy-plus-booster-session condition (see Figure 4.2). Thus, our second study's most important conclusion was that during

Mean Weight Losses (lbs.)

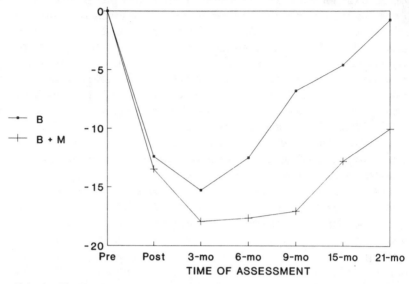

B • Behavior Therapy
M • Multicomponent Program

FIGURE 4.2. Net mean weight losses (pounds), from pretreatment, for behavior therapy only and for behavior plus a multicomponent maintenance program. Based on data from Perri, McAdoo, et al., 1984.

posttreatment, a multicomponent program consisting of social support, self-monitoring, and patient–therapist contacts significantly improved weight loss maintenance. However, it is important to note that only a modest amount of weight loss was maintained, and that a substantial amount of therapist time was required to provide telephone contacts throughout the year after treatment.

STUDY 3. AEROBIC EXERCISE AND A MULTICOMPONENT PROGRAM

The third study in our series (Perri, McAdoo, McAllister, Lauer, & Yancey, 1986) evaluated whether behavior therapy for obesity might be more effective if supplemented by an aerobic exercise regimen during treatment, and by a multicomponent maintenance program after treatment. The first goal of this study was to increase the amount of weight initially lost in behavioral treatment. The second goal was to enhance weight-loss maintenance by replicating the results in our second study's multicomponent program.

The focus of behavioral treatment has typically been to reduce food consumption through habit changes. Despite the fact that inactivity may be a major contributor to obesity, the importance of energy expenditure has been acknowledged to the extent that patients are exhorted to "exercise more." Recent research has demonstrated that, compared to normal-weight people, obese individuals may not consume more calories but are significantly less active (Brownell, Stunkard, & Albaum, 1980; Garrow, 1986; Stern & Lowney, 1986). Because of this evidence and the modest impact of dietary interventions, several reviewers have concluded that exercise holds promise for improving the management of obesity (Brownell & Stunkard, 1980; Epstein & Wing, 1980; Foreyt, 1987; Thompson, Jarvie, Lahey, & Cureton, 1982). Furthermore, post hoc data from several studies have suggested that one of the few consistent correlates of long-term success in weight management is exercise (e.g., Colvin & Olson, 1983; Gormally & Rardin, 1981; Katahn, Pleas, Thackrey, & Wallston, 1982; Kayman et al., 1990).

Exercise exerts its impact in weight loss by increasing the rate of fat loss while reducing the loss of lean body tissue. The increase in metabolic rate associated with exercise may also facilitate weight loss. This increase may serve to counteract an adaptive slowing of basal metabolism that accompanies restricted caloric intake (Donahoe, Lin, Kirschenbaum, & Keesey, 1984). In addition to possible improvements in weight loss, aerobic exercise improves coronary efficiency, blood pressure, and glucose tolerance (Bjorntorp, 1978; Martin & Dubbert, 1982). Furthermore, regular exercise can enhance psychological functioning by improving mood and self-concept and by increasing an individual's sense of well-being (Folkins & Sime, 1981).

Prior to 1985, few experiments had examined whether increased physical activity enhances the effectiveness of behavior therapy for obesity. One study suggested an additive effect for the inclusion of exercise in behavioral treatment (Dahlkoetter, Callahan, & Linton, 1979). Two experiments did not find an exercise effect during initial treatment (Harris & Hallbauer, 1973; Stalonas, Johnson, & Christ, 1978) but found that exercise appeared to improve the maintenance of weight loss during the posttreatment period.

In our third study, we tested whether initial weight loss would be enhanced by an aerobic program consisting of brisk walking and stationary cycling, with set levels of intensity, duration, and frequency. These particular aerobic activities were chosen because they involve high energy output and minimal equipment, and they have reduced risk of injury. In addition, we evaluated whether our multicomponent maintenance program, consisting of ongoing self-monitoring, frequent posttreatment therapist contacts, and patient involvement in peer self-help groups, would improve the long-term maintenance of weight loss.

At pretreatment, the 90 mildly and moderately obese subjects averaged

203 pounds and averaged 60% over ideal body weight. Through random assignment, participants were placed in one of four conditions in a 2 x 2 factorial design. This design involved crossing the two treatment conditions (i.e., behavior therapy or behavior therapy plus aerobic exercise) with the two posttreatment conditions (i.e., no posttreatment contact or a multicomponent posttreatment maintenance program). Initial treatments occurred over the course of 20 weekly group sessions. In accordance with typical behavior-therapy protocols, the participants in the behavior-therapy condition were encouraged to increase their activity levels (e.g., to use stairs rather than elevators). In this condition, patients did not receive a specific program of exercise, but they were provided with lists of the caloric expenditure of a number of physical activities. Participants received instructions to add 800 calories to their weekly energy output.

The behavior-therapy-plus-aerobic-exercise condition supplemented the standard behavioral treatment with therapist-led demonstrations and actual practice of an aerobic regimen in each therapy session. The exercise routine entailed (a) a warm-up, to stretch the muscles and gradually increase the heart rate; (b) a conditioning period, to stimulate the heart rate to the aerobic training range; and (c) a cool-down, to gradually decrease the intensity level after the conditioning phase. Initially, the minimum exercise level was set at 32 minutes per week. Each week, an additional 4 minutes were scheduled until reaching the minimum target level of 80 minutes per week (i.e., 20 minutes per day, 4 days per week).

After the 20 sessions of initial treatment, subjects in two of the conditions were seen for assessment at follow-up sessions scheduled 3-, 6-, 12-, and 18-months posttreatment. These patients had no other contacts with their therapists. Subjects in the other two groups participated in the multicomponent maintenance program described in our second study.

Figure 4.3 presents net mean weight losses by condition over the course of the study. The initial treatment period resulted in substantial weight losses (mean - 20.8 pounds) for subjects in all conditions. Those subjects who participated in the behavior-therapy-plus-aerobic-exercise program lost significantly more weight (mean - 23.3 pounds) than those in the standard behavioral treatment (mean - 18.0 pounds). Thus, the aerobic exercise program exerted a net effect of 5.3 pounds lost during the 20-week treatment period. This is a 29% improvement beyond the weight lost in the behavior-therapy-only condition.

During the 18-month posttreatment period, a significant Time X Maintenance Condition interaction effect emerged ($p < .001$). At all four follow-up evaluations, participants in the multicomponent maintenance program had significantly greater weight losses than subjects in the groups without posttreatment therapist contact (see Figure 4.3).

The aerobic-exercise regimen in this study entailed brisk walking and/or stationary cycling. The choice of these particular activities, and the specific fashion in which they were used may have had a significant

Mean Weight Losses (lbs.)

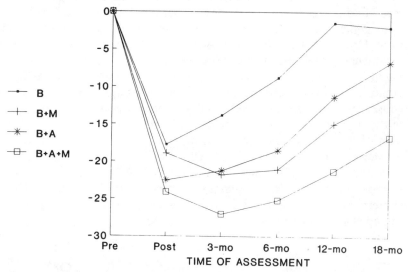

B • Behavior Therapy
A • Aerobic Exercise
M • Multicomponent Program

FIGURE 4.3.   Net mean weight losses (pounds), from pretreatment, for the following conditions: behavior therapy, behavior therapy plus aerobic exercise, behavior therapy plus a multicomponent maintenance program, and behavior therapy plus aerobic exercise plus a multicomponent maintenance program. Based on data from Perri et al., 1986.

impact on the overall effectiveness of the aerobic-exercise program. Indeed, according to self-reports, subjects adhered well to the prescribed routine; in fact, during the initial treatment period, 80% of the participants exceeded the recommended minimum routine of 20 minutes per day, 4 days per week. Several factors may have contributed to this relatively high degree of adherence. The exercises selected were simple activities of moderate intensity, which did not result in excessive physical pain or stress. In addition, increases in exercise occurred very gradually and were adapted to each patient's ability. Each session included a therapist-led exercise period, and participants could measure their progress by monitoring their heart rate during the in-session exercise.

During the 18-month posttreatment period, self-report data indicated that the mean amount of aerobic exercise dropped from more than 100 minutes per week to less than 30 minutes per week. Moreover, by the time of the 18-month follow-up, 42% of the participants reported that they had ceased all exercise. To maintain exercise changes after treatment, it may be necessary to develop procedures specifically designed to increase adherence during the posttreatment period. For example, long-term adherence to aerobic regimens may increase if coronary efficiency is routinely monitored and if group exercise opportunities continue to be offered.

In general, subjects tended to regain weight during the follow-up period. However, the multicomponent maintenance program enhanced weight-loss progress. At the 18-month follow-up, subjects who participated in the multicomponent posttreatment program maintained, on average, 84% of the mean weight they had lost at posttreatment, whereas subjects who were not offered a maintenance program sustained only 21% of the mean weight loss they had shown at posttreatment. The effectiveness of the maintenance program may be attributed to its participants' greater adherence to behavioral self-control procedures (see Stalonas & Kirschenbaum, 1985). Thus, both adherence to behavioral changes and improved maintenance of weight loss seemed to be facilitated by the combination of continued self-monitoring, frequent phone contacts with therapists, and peer-group support.

STUDY 4. THERAPIST CONTACT VERSUS PEER SUPPORT

In our second and third studies, we showed that a multicomponent posttreatment program significantly enhanced the maintenance of weight loss. The multicomponent maintenance program provided support and advice through both peer-group support meetings and patient–therapist contacts. In our fourth study (Perri, McAdoo, McAllister, Lauer, Jordan, Yancey, & Nezu, 1987), we compared the effectiveness of peer support versus therapist contact as approaches to weight-loss maintenance. The primary issue that we addressed was whether, compared to a no-post-treatment-contact condition, maintenance programs of peer support or therapist contact would result in greater success in maintaining weight loss.

Eight-five moderately obese adults volunteered to serve as subjects. All patients participated in 20 weeks of standard behavioral treatment that included the aerobic exercise regimen employed in our third study. After the initial treatment, patients were placed through random assignment in one of two maintenance programs or in a control condition, which had no further contact with therapists.

Participants in the peer-support-group program met biweekly for 15 maintenance sessions over the 7 months after initial treatment. These self-help group meetings followed the structure and procedures of problem-solving treatment. Patients learned to monitor each other's weight, to reinforce weight-loss progress with praise, and to problem solve as a group, to assist members experiencing difficulties in their efforts at weight loss.

The therapist-contact program also entailed 15 biweekly maintenance sessions, scheduled over the 7 months after initial treatment. These groups of patients were seen by the same therapists who had treated them in the initial phase of the study. The biweekly sessions consisted of weigh-ins, reviews of self-monitoring data, and therapist-led problem solving of difficulties in maintaining habit changes in eating and exercise.

Figure 4.4 presents the net mean weight losses for each condition over the course of the study. Following the 20 sessions of initial treatment, the mean weight loss across all participants was 23.5 pounds. No statistically reliable differences among the three conditions existed. During the 18-month follow-up period, an overall significant Time X Posttreatment Condition interaction effect was observed ($p < .05$). Significant between-group differences were observed at 30 weeks posttreatment (i.e., at the conclusion of the maintenance programs). Participants in the therapist-contact condition were significantly more successful in their weight-loss efforts than subjects in the peer-support and control conditions ($p < .05$; see Figure 4.4). During this period, both the peer-support group and the no-posttreatment-contact group regained weight, and the amounts regained were equivalent. In general, subjects in all the groups regained weight between the 7- and 18-month follow-ups. However, compared to the

Mean Weight Losses (lbs.)

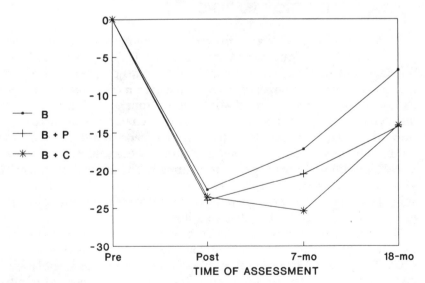

B = Behavior Therapy
P = Peer Support
C = Therapist Contact

FIGURE 4.4.   Net mean weight losses (pounds), from pretreatment, for behavior therapy, behavior therapy plus posttreatment peer support, and behavior therapy plus posttreatment therapist contact. Based on data from Perri et al., 1987.

control group, both the therapist-contact and the peer-support programs demonstrated greater maintenance of weight loss (see Figure 4.4).

According to adherence questionnaires, at the 7-month follow-up, participants in the therapist-contact program made significantly greater use of behavioral self-control strategies than patients in the peer-support and the control conditions ($p < .05$). By the 18-month follow-up, self-reported adherence to weight-control procedures had declined significantly from posttreatment levels for subjects in all conditions. Moreover, the significant between-group differences favoring the therapist-contact condition were no longer apparent.

The posttreatment progress attained by participants in the therapist-led maintenance program occurred only while they were under the supervision of their therapists. After the therapist-led maintenance program ended, its participants began to regain weight and to display the same relapse pattern that occurred for subjects in the peer-support condition. Nonetheless, the 18-month results of this study suggest that posttreatment programs consisting of either peer group or therapist contacts can foster better long-term weight-loss progress, compared with therapy that does not include a posttreatment maintenance program.

STUDY 5. THERAPIST CONTACT VERSUS RELAPSE-PREVENTION TRAINING

This study evaluated relapse-prevention training versus frequent therapist contacts as weight-loss maintenance strategies (Perri, McKelvey, Schein, Renjilian, Viegener, & Nezu, 1990). The major question we examined was whether, compared to a no-posttreatment-contact condition, increased weight-loss progress would result from *yearlong* posttreatment maintenance programs consisting of either (a) comprehensive training to prevent and overcome relapse or (b) a high frequency of therapist contacts.

The subjects were 88 mildly and moderately obese volunteers who were 25–99% over ideal body weight at pretreatment. The patients completed 20 sessions of behavioral weight-loss therapy. After this initial treatment, subjects were randomly assigned to one of the two maintenance programs or to a no-further-contact control condition.

The relapse-prevention maintenance program was conducted during the year after initial treatment and consisted of 26 biweekly group sessions. The program focused on training participants (a) to identify situations that pose a high risk for relapse, (b) to learn skills needed to effectively handle such circumstances, (c) to practice coping in actual high-risk situations, and (d) to develop cognitive strategies to overcome lapses in self-control. The therapist-contact maintenance program was also conducted during the year after initial treatment and consisted of 26 biweekly group sessions. These sessions, which entailed weigh-ins and reviews of progress, were focused on therapist-led problem solving directed at helping participants to maintain the behavioral changes that they had accomplished during the initial treatment.

Figure 4.5 illustrates the pattern of net mean weight losses for each condition over the course of the study. Following the initial 20 weeks of treatment, the mean weight loss for the entire sample was 19.1 pounds, and no significant between-group differences were apparent. However, during the year following initial treatment, a significant Time X Posttreatment Condition interaction effect was observed ($p < .0001$), and mean weight losses differed significantly among the conditions at both the 6- and 12-month follow-up evaluations. Post hoc tests revealed that participants in both maintenance-program conditions demonstrated significantly greater weight-loss progress at 6 and 12 months posttreatment than subjects in the no-posttreatment contact condition. In addition, post hoc testing showed that the relapse-prevention and therapist-contact maintenance conditions produced equivalent effects on weight loss (see Figure 4.5).

The results from this study showed that weight-loss maintenance can be enhanced through structured posttreatment programs. Moreover, the

Mean Weight Losses (lbs.)

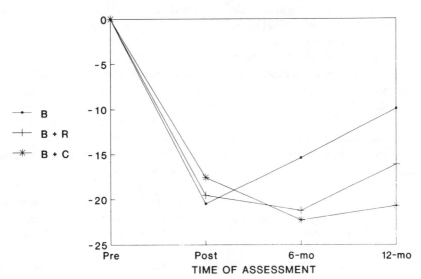

B • Behavior Therapy
C • Therapist Contact
R • Relapse Prevention

FIGURE 4.5.   Net mean weight losses (pounds), from pretreatment, for behavior therapy, behavior therapy plus posttreatment therapist contact, and behavior therapy plus relapse prevention. Based on data from Perri et al., 1990.

findings indicated that frequent posttreatment sessions consisting of therapist-led problem solving may help patients to maintain weight loss as effectively as a comprehensive program of relapse-prevention training.

STUDY 6. THERAPIST CONTACT, SOCIAL INFLUENCE, AND EXERCISE

In our sixth study, we examined the impact of four yearlong maintenance programs, which were developed from strategies that showed promise in our earlier studies (Perri, McAllister, Gange, Jordan, McAdoo, & Nezu, 1988). Thus, we evaluated the effectiveness of the following maintenance procedures: (a) a therapist-contact program consisting of 26 biweekly posttreatment sessions that focused on therapist-led problem solving; (b) an aerobic exercise maintenance program that raised recommended exercise levels from 80 to 180 minutes per week; (c) a social-influence maintenance program that provided group contingencies for attendance and weight-loss progress; and (d) a combination of the aerobic exercise and social-influence maintenance programs.

Ninety-one mildly and moderately obese volunteers served as subjects. The study employed a constructive-treatment research design, wherein maintenance components were added to the basic treatment regimen to evaluate whether the additions increased the effectiveness of the basic treatment. Thus, all subjects participated in 20 sessions of a behavioral weight-loss program ("B"), which included the aerobic exercise procedures described in our third study. After the initial treatment ended, participants were randomly assigned to one of four maintenance programs or to a no-further-contact control condition. All four maintenance programs involved 26 biweekly 2-hour sessions scheduled during the year after the initial treatment ended; that is, even when additional components were added, the time in treatment remained equal across groups. For subjects in the control condition, except for assessments, no additional therapist contacts occurred after the initial treatment period.

The behavior therapy plus posttreatment contact condition ("B+C") consisted of the initial behavioral program followed by a posttreatment maintenance program involving 26 biweekly therapist contacts. At these maintenance program sessions, the therapists weighed the participants, reviewed their self-monitoring data, and led group problem solving of obstacles to maintenance of behavioral changes and weight loss. The therapists instructed the subjects in this condition to continue their aerobic exercise at 80 minutes per week (i.e., 20 min/day, 4 days/week).

The behavior therapy plus posttreatment contact plus social-influence maintenance program ("B+C+S") consisted of the initial behavioral treatment, the posttreatment therapist contact procedures, and a multifaceted program of social-influence strategies. The social-influence procedures, which were designed to enhance motivation and to provide incentives for continued weight-loss progress, included monetary group contingencies for program adherence and continued weight loss, active participant involvement in preparing and delivering minilectures on maintaining weight loss, and instructions on how to provide peer support through ongoing telephone contacts and peer-group meetings during the posttreatment period.

The behavior therapy plus posttreatment contact plus aerobic exercise maintenance program ("B+C+A") consisted of the initial behavioral treatment, the posttreatment contact procedures, and an aerobic exercise maintenance program involving new exercise goals and therapist-led exercise bouts during the posttreatment sessions. The maintenance program gradually raised the recommended frequency and duration of aerobic exercise from 20 minutes per day, 4 days per week, to 30 minutes per day, 6 days per week (i.e., from 80 to 180 min/week).

Participants in the fourth experimental condition ("B+C+A+S") received the initial behavioral treatment, the posttreatment therapist-contact procedures, and both the aerobic-exercise and social-influence maintenance programs previously described.

Figure 4.6 shows the net mean weight losses for each condition over the course of the study. At the end of the initial 20 sessions of treatment, the mean weight loss for the entire sample was 27.4 pounds, with no significant differences among the five conditions. A significant interaction effect for Condition X Time emerged during the 18-month follow-up period ($p <$ .05). At the 6-month follow-up, participants in the four conditions with posttreatment maintenance programs maintained significantly more weight loss than subjects in the no-further-contact condition (for all conditions, $p <$ .05). Moreover, the participants in the B+C+A+S condition achieved a significant *additional* mean weight loss of 9 pounds ($p <$ .05).

At the 12-month follow-up, subjects in all four experimental conditions maintained significantly more weight loss than patients in the behavior-therapy-only condition, who experienced a significant weight *gain* (mean = 11.3 pounds) during the year after initial treatment ($p <$ .05). Moreover, compared to subjects in the no-further-contact condition, participants in the four maintenance conditions also demonstrated significantly greater maintenance of weight loss at the 18-month follow-up (see Figure 4.6). On average, participants in the posttreatment programs maintained 82.7% of their mean posttreatment losses, whereas subjects in the behavior-therapy-alone condition maintained only 33.3% of their initial weight loss. There were no significant differences among the four experimental conditions at any of the follow-up evaluations.

These findings indicate that posttreatment maintenance programs can have a significant beneficial impact in the management of obesity. Indeed, the magnitude of weight losses sustained by maintenance-program participants at the 18-month follow-up (mean = 23.4 pounds) compares favorably with results reported in the obesity literature. These findings show that intensive, therapist-led programs, targeted at the specific problems of

Mean Weight Losses (lbs.)

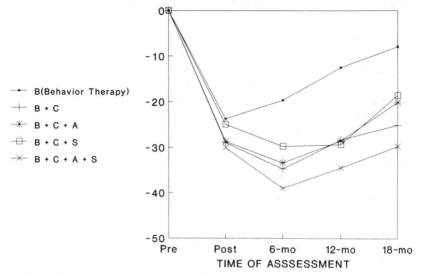

- ━•━ B(Behavior Therapy)
- ━+━ B + C
- ━✱━ B + C + A
- ━☐━ B + C + S
- ━✕━ B + C + A + S

C = Therapist Contact
A = Aerobic Exercise
S = Social Influence

FIGURE 4.6. Net mean weight losses (pounds), from pretreatment, for the following conditions: behavior therapy, behavior therapy plus posttreatment therapist contact, behavior therapy plus posttreatment therapist contact plus aerobic exercise, behavior therapy plus posttreatment therapist contact plus social-influence program, and behavior therapy plus posttreatment therapist contact plus aerobic exercise plus social-influence program. Based on data from Perri et al., 1988.

the posttreatment period, can substantially improve the long-term maintenance of weight loss.

The effectiveness of the therapist-contact maintenance programs may have resulted from participants' increased adherence to weight-loss strategies during the months immediately following the initial behavior-therapy period. The therapist-directed problem-solving strategies used in maintenance sessions may have helped participants to overcome high-risk situations, which, when experienced cumulatively, often lead patients to revert to previous eating and exercise habits (see Perri, 1989). Furthermore, the continuing therapist demand may have influenced subjects' adherence as well. Participants in the posttreatment maintenance program showed better overall adherence to self-control procedures than subjects who had no contact with their therapists during the posttreatment period. Thus, the longer that patients continue in contact with their therapists, the longer they adhere to the behaviors recommended by their therapists as being necessary for weight loss (see Bennett, 1986; Perri, Nezu, Patti, & McCann, 1989).

The social-influence program used in this study improved participant adherence during the year following treatment. However, the greater degree of adherence reported by subjects in the social-influence condition was not accompanied by significantly better weight-loss progress. Furthermore, when the various incentives and social supports for weight loss were removed, a significant decrease in adherence was observed (see Brehm & McAllister, 1980; Kramer, Jeffery, Snell, & Forster, 1986).

This study also examined whether long-term weight loss would be enhanced by supplementing the posttreatment therapist contact program with an increased amount of aerobic exercise. At the 6-month follow-up assessment, participants in the high-exercise maintenance conditions reported significantly more exercise (means = 149.5 and 142.1 min/week for the B+C+A and B+C+A+S, respectively) than patients in the low-exercise maintenance conditions (means = 83.2, 61.6, and 80.4 min/week for B+C+S, B+C and B, respectively; $p < .05$). However, the greater amounts of self-reported aerobic exercise were not accompanied by significantly greater mean weight losses, and the higher exercise levels were not maintained at the 12- and 18-month follow-ups. Many subjects reported difficulty in maintaining the weekly goal of 180 minutes of aerobic exercise on a regular basis, particularly during periods of seasonally inclement weather. In addition, failure to achieve the program's stringent exercise requirements may have prompted many patients to develop negative self-statements about their ability to maintain other self-management strategies as well (see Brownell & Foreyt, 1985). Indeed, self-report data indicated that overall adherence for participants in the B+C+A condition dropped significantly between the 12- and 18-month follow-ups, whereas adherence levels for patients in the B+C condition remained stable during the same period.

The final question addressed in the sixth study was whether the addition of *both* the aerobic exercise and the social-influence maintenance programs would increase the effectiveness of the posttreatment therapist-contact intervention. Between posttreatment and the 6-month follow-up, the B+C+A+S condition was the only condition to accomplish a significant amount of additional weight loss (mean = 9.0 pounds; net mean weight loss from pretreatment = 39.1 pounds). Furthermore, the B+C+A+S condition sustained 99% of its mean posttreatment weight loss at the 18-month follow-up. Collectively, these results indicate that combining high-frequency aerobic exercise with intensive support from peers and therapists represents a promising multifaceted approach for improving the long-term management of obesity.

EXAMPLE OF A CONTINUOUS-CARE APPROACH TO OBESITY MANAGEMENT

Research on helping patients to sustain the behavioral changes required to maintain weight loss is in the early stages of development. Our work represents an initial foray that has suggested directions for future investigations. In many cases, successful long-term management of obesity may require maintenance programs involving years rather than months of follow-up care. There is little research available on the effectiveness of maintenance programs that extend beyond 1 year. One exception is an investigation by Bjorvell and Rossner (1985, 1990), who have examined the impact of a comprehensive 4-year, continuous-care approach to the management of obesity.

Bjorvell and Rossner (1985) argued that successful management of obesity would require long-term care and a multifaceted approach to treatment. Thus, they constructed an intensive, comprehensive, and long-lasting treatment regimen, including behavior therapy, nutritional training, and supervised exercise, and they examined its effects over a period of 10 years. (Using a nonrandomized design, these researchers compared their comprehensive treatment to an alternative treatment, jaw wiring, and to a control condition consisting of a short-term weight-loss intervention; we limit our summary to the results reported for the comprehensive treatment.)

Participants in the comprehensive treatment program included 53 women who, at the start of treatment, averaged 245 pounds and averaged 69% over ideal body weight. Initial treatment was conducted during a 6-week period of inpatient hospitalization. Treatment was conducted in small groups of 5 patients. Participants had two behavioral treatment sessions per week, which included standard behavior-therapy techniques, plus training in relapse-prevention strategies, and they had three supervised exercise sessions per week, plus a program of additional activities that included walking and swimming. The subjects also received extensive training from a dietitian regarding techniques of low-calorie cooking. In addition, during the 6-week course of their hospitalization, the patients were placed on a VLCD consisting of approximately 600 calories per day (including 60 g of protein, 16 g of fat, and 54 g of carbohydrate).

Following this initial phase of treatment, participants received a 4-year maintenance program. All patients were expected to attend one of two group sessions that were offered each week. Therapists made vigorous efforts to contact any patient who missed a scheduled appointment. Post-treatment contacts by both telephone and mail were used to keep patients actively involved in participating in the maintenance sessions. Finally, whenever it appeared that a patient was in jeopardy of a relapse, the investigators had the individual return to the hospital for short-term (i.e., 2-week) "refresher" courses of treatment. Over the 4 years of the investigation, virtually all the participants returned for at least one course of rehospitalization.

Figure 4.7 presents the pattern of net mean weight loss over 10 years for the women who underwent comprehensive treatment in the Bjorvell and Rossner (1985, 1990) study. The findings in this study are impressive. That

Mean Weight Losses (lbs.)

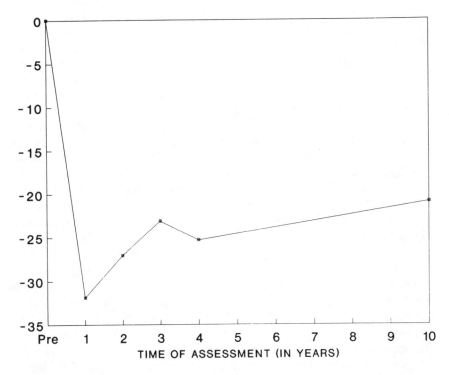

TIME OF ASSESSMENT (IN YEARS)

FIGURE 4.7. Net mean weight losses (pounds), from pretreatment, for women who participated in a 4-year, comprehensive treatment program for obesity. Based on data from Bjorvell and Rossner, 1985, 1990.

the women in the study lost a significant amount of weight after 6 weeks of inpatient treatment is not surprising. What is both surprising and heartening are the long-term results. At 1 year, the subjects had improved their initial weight losses on average by 50%, and at the 4-year assessment, the participants had maintained 77% of their peak losses. Even more impressive are the 10-year results, showing that the subjects succeeded in maintaining an average weight loss of more than 20 pounds 6 years after the end of active treatment (see Figure 4.7). These findings strongly suggest that providing obese patients with an intensive program of continuous care can result in successful long-term management of obesity.

SUMMARY AND CONCLUSIONS

In this chapter, we have argued that the ineffectiveness of obesity treatments stems from a failure, by clinicians and patients alike, to recognize that *obesity is a chronic condition requiring continuous care*. Most weight-loss treatments are in effect "short-term" interventions that leave the obese individual inadequately prepared to meet the challenge of a relentless physiology ever-primed for weight gain. When on their own, the majority of obese individuals cannot sustain the substantial degree of psychological control necessary to override these compensatory biological mechanisms. Therefore, we believe that it is essential that treatments for obesity be supplemented with programs of ongoing care, specially designed to enhance the long-term maintenance of weight loss.

In this chapter, we described the results of a series of studies in which we tested the effectiveness of various weight-loss maintenance strategies, including ongoing professional contact, skills training, social support, physical activity, and multicomponent programs. Our results included both positive and negative findings. The bad news is quite evident: Unless initial weight-loss treatments are supplemented with interventions targeted at the problem of maintenance, successful long-term management of obesity is unlikely. According to our results, if patients are not provided with a posttreatment maintenance program, they are very likely to abandon the self-control strategies learned in treatment and to regain weight.

On the other hand, the good news is also quite clear: Participants in posttreatment maintenance programs exhibit greater adherence to weight-control strategies and demonstrate better maintenance of weight loss. Our studies consistently showed that structured programs of posttreatment therapist contacts successfully helped patients to sustain weight-loss progress. Posttreatment contact seems to be helpful because the longer that patients remain in contact with health-care professionals, the longer they sustain the eating and exercise habits necessary to maintain weight loss (see Perri et al., 1989).

To be effective, maintenance programs require multifaceted sets of strategies. After initial treatment, ongoing self-monitoring of eating and exercise behaviors, along with a high frequency of patient–therapist contacts, appear to be prerequisites for continued weight-loss progress. Indeed, most patients require professional help to deal effectively with the many obstacles that impede the maintenance of weight loss. The use of a problem-solving approach can provide therapists with a conceptual framework to assist patients in coping with the challenges of the posttreatment period.

Our studies suggest that skills-training and social-support strategies by themselves may not be sufficient to help patients maintain weight losses on their own (Perri, Shapiro, et al., 1984; Perri et al., 1987). Moreover, a comprehensive yearlong program of relapse-prevention training was no more effective than the simpler program of therapist-led problem solving (Perri et al., 1990). Similarly, the program of posttreatment therapist contacts was more effective than the social-support intervention of peer-group self-help meetings (Perri et al., 1987). Nonetheless, both skills-training and social-support strategies may be useful as components of multifaceted maintenance programs (Perri, McAdoo, et al., 1984; Perri, Shapiro, et al., 1984; Perri et al., 1986; Perri et al., 1988).

For a variety of reasons, exercise can play a major role in obesity management. Initial weight loss can be enhanced by a program of regular physical activity (Perri et al., 1986). Moreover, the results from our sixth study (Perri et al., 1988) demonstrated that a posttreatment program combining therapist contact, social support, and a high frequency of aerobic exercise not only enhanced maintenance but also produced significant *additional* weight loss during the period following initial treatment.

Weight-loss progress in our studies occurred only during those time periods when participants were actively involved in either the treatment or the maintenance programs. Thus, clinicians must convey to obese patients an appropriate awareness of the long-term implications regarding the management of obesity. Obese individuals need to know that, similar to patients who are diabetic or hypertensive, they may never be "cured" of their "disease." Instead, they must focus their efforts on controlling their condition through active self-management efforts for the *rest of their lives.*

Health-care professionals should also be aware of the daunting long-term implications of obesity treatment. In addition to acknowledging that obesity is a chronic problem, clinicians must develop treatments that will provide patients with lifelong assistance in managing their obesity (see Perri, 1989). The successful management of obesity will, in most cases, require multiple stages spanning very long periods of time. Thus, the health-care professional's role is to serve as an *active problem-solver* who systematically and continuously aids the patient in identifying effective strategies to sustain the behavioral changes needed for long-term success. Long-term success is unlikely unless the obese patient develops a life-style that sustains the decreased energy intake and increased energy expenditure necessary to maintain a lower weight. Equipped with a variety of strategies designed to enhance the maintenance of behavior change, clinicians will be better able to assist patients in the long-term management of their obesity. In the next two chapters, we present a continuous care/problem-solving model for the management of obesity, and we describe how this framework can guide clinical decision making in the long-term care of the obese patient.

PART II

A CONTINUOUS-CARE/ PROBLEM-SOLVING MODEL

5

Toward a Continuous–Care/Problem–Solving Model of Long-Term Obesity Treatment

Thus far, we have essentially presented the reader with a good news/bad news scenario regarding the long-term treatment of obesity. Along the lines of good news, an ever-increasing body of scientific information is being obtained concerning the variety of causes and ramifications of obesity. In addition, research has also underscored the effectiveness of various clinical interventions in terms of short-term weight loss. Unfortunately, the bad news is easily summed up in two words—*poor maintenance*. Even programs that are geared to facilitating the maintenance of treatment gains have had to concede that long-term weight loss is not easily achieved (see Chapter 4). Moreover, studies have found that continuous fluctuations resulting from unsuccessful repeated attempts to lose weight (i.e., the so-called yo-yo effect) may have a detrimental impact on health (Hamm et al., 1989; Lissner et al., 1991).

As health-care professionals, one possible reaction to such bad news is to continue to implement treatment approaches that have the highest success rates and hoping for the best, while continuing to pose new research questions regarding areas that significantly relate to the issue of maintenance. For example, across the various addictive disorders (i.e., obesity, smoking, alcoholism, drug abuse), Brownell, Marlatt, Lichenstein, and Wilson (1986) advocate an increased empirical focus regarding the phenomena of lapse and relapse. According to these researchers, a better understanding of the process of relapse can lead to the identification of more effective strategies to facilitate maintenance.

However, even if this promise is fulfilled in the future, in the absence of such specific information at this time, the health professional treating obese clients must do so with the implications of the bad news about obesity treatment weighing heavily on their therapeutic shoulders. For example, as Foreyt and Goodrick (1991) recently noted, "After decades of research, effective and long-lasting treatments have not been found. . . . With success rates so low, it is difficult to determine whether the few successes are due to a treatment effect or whether these few came to treatment with greater motivation or a more favorable physiological disposition to lose weight" (p. 292). In other words, the *definitive* answer to the question posed by the health-care professional—"What treatment should I use to help this obese client lose *and* maintain weight loss?"—is not readily available.

Another approach to compensating for this lack of conclusive answers to obesity treatment involves matching clients to different available treatments, depending upon the particular type of obesity a client presents. For example, according to Guy-Grand (1987), "failure of one method in a given patient . . . does not necessarily indicate that another method will also fail. . . . the old question about treatment for obesity should be replaced by a new one that considers treatments for different kinds of obesity. The clinicians, faced with his patients, should find a treatment for each of them" (p. 313).

Marlatt (1988), for example, suggests that one method of matching patients to treatment should entail an assessment of problem severity. In other words, treatment should be graded in intensity and should be appropriate to the magnitude of the presenting problem. To illustrate this approach, Marlatt draws from research concerning treatment decisions for hypertension, which he suggests are geared toward the severity of one's problem. For mild hypertensives, treatment may initially consist of lifestyle changes, such as reduction of salt intake, increases in regular exercise, and/or avoidance of alcohol. Increased severity of the problem, however, may require increased intensity of treatment, where the next step upward may involve mild (e.g., diuretics) or more intensive (e.g., beta-blockers) medications.

Focusing on the dimension of the severity of obesity, Stunkard (1984) developed a classification system in order to provide initial treatment guidelines. Treatment recommendations would include behavior therapy for mild obesity (20–40% overweight), low-calorie diet plus behavior therapy for moderate obesity (41–100% overweight), and surgery for severe obesity (>100% overweight) (see Wadden & Bell, 1990).

More recently, Brownell and Wadden (1991) have expanded this classification system, which also may be used as a means of guiding treatment selection. Their system includes four levels: Level 1 (5–20% overweight); Level 2 (21–40% overweight); Level 3 (41–100% overweight); and Level 4 (100%+ overweight). Treatment decisions using this system are based on judgments concerning intervention efficacy and cost/benefit analysis of health risk (i.e., iatrogenic effects of the intervention itself). For example, they suggest that VLCDs may only be used with individuals who are in Levels 3 and 4 due to the potential health risks involved that may not be justifiable for people who are only mildly overweight (i.e., persons in Level 1 or 2).

Another perspective concerning a graded, stepped approach to treatment decisions for obesity comes from the public health arena. For instance, Black and his associates provide evidence to support a stepped approach to weight-loss interventions (Black, 1987; Black, Coe, Friesen, & Wurzmann, 1984; Black & Threlfall, 1986, 1989). Minimal interventions, such as self-help manuals, are used as an initial strategy, after which the intensity of the treatment increases in graduated steps, based on the client's individual performance or perceptions of success. In other words, rather than basing treatment decisions on the severity of the problem (i.e., level of obesity), this approach advocates that such judgments be based more on the individual's ability to implement a clinical self-help strategy. Whereas such overall approaches appear to offer promising avenues for continued research and empirical study, the clinician treating obese patients is left again with the question originally posed by Paul (1969) regarding psychotherapy in general—"What treatment, by whom, is most effective for this individual with that specific problem [i.e., obesity], under which set of circumstances?" Unfortunately, because a set of variables has not yet been identified that reliably predicts successful weight loss (Foreyt & Goodrick, 1991), attempts to match individuals to treatment are bound to rely more heavily on the clinician's judgment than on the empirical literature.

We have argued elsewhere that under such circumstances, the need especially exists for therapists to use a formal model of decision making to help guide the difficult process of making clinical judgments and treatment recommendations (Nezu & Nezu, 1989). In response to the bad news about obesity treatment noted previously, we begin in this chapter to delineate our *continuous-care/problem solving model* of clinical interventions for obesity. In describing this approach, we draw heavily from the problem-solving model that we have previously articulated concerning the process of clinical decision making in the practice of behavior therapy in general (Nezu & Nezu, 1989). The desirability to adopt such a problem-solving approach to obesity treatment planning is related to the general lack of a treatment handbook.

NONEXISTENCE OF A TREATMENT HANDBOOK

A clinical-intervention handbook does not currently exist for people in general, whereby health-care professionals can look to a comprehensive index to locate *the* treatment strategy to implement for a given patient. Even among individuals suffering from the same problem, such as obesity, heterogeneity is the rule rather than the exception. Interindividual differences exist along a wide range of parameters, including *demographic variables* (e.g., age, sex, ethnic background, socioeconomic status), *disorder-related dimensions* (e.g., presence of additional physical and/or mental health problems, severity of obesity, previous dieting history, age of onset, symptom duration), *psychosocial variables* (e.g., coping ability, social support, personality factors), *cognitive factors* (e.g., knowledge of basic nutritional information), *behavioral aspects* (e.g., eating habits, exercise habits), and *biological factors* (e.g., number and size of fat cells, metabolic rate, presence of medical complications). More important, each of these elements potentially can affect the efficacy of a given treatment strategy.

For example, inattention to social support issues for Bob, an obese patient, may not be important, due to the presence of strong support from his wife to begin a weight-loss program. However, for Jane, an obese patient whose husband has often undermined her efforts to lose weight in the past, due to feelings of jealousy, addressing such issues may be imperative for treatment ultimately to be successful.

In addition, it is important to acknowledge the multidimensional nature of obesity, underlying its potential variety of distal and proximal causes. In other words, the etiology and pathogenesis of a given person's obesity problem is likely to be pluralistic in nature. To use problem-solving terminology, the obstacles to goal attainment (i.e., weight-loss maintenance) are multiple and varied. This strongly suggests that any theory attempting to explain obesity that focuses on a unitary causal factor is likely to fall short of clinical reality. Moreover, any clinical intervention for its treatment that incorporates only a single technique is also likely to fall short of success. Thus, simple, textbook cases are rare.

Emphasis on Continuous Care

The necessity of a *continuous-care* paradigm emanates from the consistent findings from most of our structured research programs that continuous contact with a health-care professional is essential to successful weight-loss maintenance. Specifically, as discussed in Chapter 4, it is crucial that therapists orient obese patients to understand and accept the long-term implications of weight *management*. Similar to the diabetic or hypertensive patient, many obese individuals may never be cured of their health problem. Instead, it would be important for both the obesity therapist and the obese patient to adopt the perspective that this condition is kept under control through active efforts at self-management *throughout the patients' life*. As we have advocated previously, in addition to acknowledging that obesity is a chronic problem, it is incumbent upon health-care professionals to structure treatments that will provide patients with *lifelong* assistance in managing their obesity (Perri, 1989).

In addition, the variability regarding causal and maintaining factors of being overweight may not just exist *among* differing obese persons, but also can exist *across an individual's life* at different points in time.

For example, Janet may have had an easier time maintaining a weight loss as a single, young adult, as compared to when she becomes older, married, and a mother. The realistic probability is that such major life-style changes can limit her time, energy, and opportunities to engage in optimal weight-management strategies, such as daily exercise. As such, the type of clinical advice given to Janet at 21 years may be different than when she is 42 years old.

Given such intra- and interindividual differences, the therapist must seek the most effective and appropriate treatment strategy for a given patient, under a specific set of circumstances. Our continuous-care/problem-solving model of obesity treatment has been developed to help the health-care professional in accomplishing this difficult clinical task.

OBESITY TREATMENT AS PROBLEM SOLVING

In delineating a model of decision making when formulating clinical interventions for the treatment of obesity, we adopt a problem-solving framework. This paradigm incorporates those principles of problem solving that are the basis of *social problem-solving training*, as described by D'Zurilla and Goldfried (1971) and by D'Zurilla and Nezu (1982). The original model was offered as a prescriptive approach, the goal of which was to enhance the *individual's problem-solving ability* to cope more effectively with stressful life circumstances (see Nezu & D'Zurilla, 1989; Nezu, Nezu, & Perri, 1989), whereas the present model focuses on enabling the *health-care professional* to be the *problem solver* (Nezu & Nezu, 1989; Perri, 1989).

According to this perspective, when clinicians begin the process of treatment planning with a prospective patient, they are faced with a "problem." Nezu and Nezu (1989) define this problem as

> a clinical situation in which a therapist is presented with a set of complaints by an individual for which help is sought to reduce or minimize such complaints. This situation is considered to be a problem since the current state of affairs (i.e., presence of complaints) represents a *discrepancy* from the individual's *desired* state (i.e., goals). A variety of impediments (i.e., obstacles or conflicts) exist that prevent or make it difficult for the client to reach his or her goals at the present time without a therapist's aid. Such impediments may include variables relevant to both the patient (e.g., behavioral, cognitive, and/or affective excesses or deficits) and/or his or her environment (e.g., lack of physical and/or social resources; presence of aversive stimuli)
> . . . . treatment, then, represents the clinician's attempt to identify and implement a *solution* to this problem situation. (p. 36)

An *effective* solution within this framework is represented by the clinical interventions that reduce or minimize the initial complaints. Such treatment plans might include components aimed at (a) changing the nature of the impediments or obstacles, (b) reducing the negative impact that these impediments exert on the patient him or herself, or (c) both. Part of the overall task of the clinician as problem solver is to decide which of these general goals should become the focus of treatment for a given patient. Remember that the same treatment protocol may not be effective for all obese persons, due to individual differences.

In addition to representing obesity treatment globally as a problem-solving process, we further suggest that a variety of important subproblems exist, each of which requires the active decision making of the health-care professional. These include target problem selection, treatment planning, treatment implementation, and treatment evaluation. To a large degree, the success or effectiveness of the clinician's decision making during each of these clinical tasks affects the relative success of subsequent activities. In other words, there is a synergistic relationship among each of the outcomes of these clinical processes. For example, if the therapist inaccurately identifies the relevant factors underlying the etiology and/or maintenance of the patient's obesity problem, then it is likely that subsequent treatment plans would be ineffective. Therefore, in order for treatment to be successful, each of these subproblems also must be effectively solved.

To illustrate this approach, consider Paula, a 22-year-old, mildly obese woman, who is seeking treatment to lose weight at an outpatient clinic. Using problem-solving terminology, the impediments or obstacles (i.e., factors that are causally or functionally related to the presenting problem) that prevent or make it difficult for Paula to attain such a goal on her own can be quite varied: lack of knowledge concerning nutrition, poor assertiveness skills when dealing with family members who insist that she eat larger quantities or less appropriate food than she should, ineffective coping skills in dealing with stress, minimal exercise, poor self-control skills when eating in social situations, large number of fat cells, high percentage of fat intake, and so forth (or any combination of these factors).

Given these various causal and maintaining factors, an initial subproblem that the therapist needs to address is the accurate identification of such variables *with specific regard to Paula*. After identifying these impediments, the clinician can begin to develop an overall treatment plan that might address any or all of these target areas. For Paula, after a comprehensive assessment phase, it might be determined that an overall intervention plan should include (a) limiting her daily caloric intake through self-monitoring, (b) assertiveness skills training as a means of increasing her ability to say "no" at family gatherings, and (c) rearranging her diet to decrease its percentage of calories from fat.

For another client, Nathan, who also is seeking help to lose weight, a comprehensive assessment might indicate that his spouse's continuous reinforcement of his overeating serves as a major impediment to goal attainment. More specifically, Nathan's wife, who is overweight herself, is afraid that their marriage may change if he loses weight. Hence, the treatment plan for him might involve marital therapy first. Some clinicians may be qualified to provide such services themselves; others may suggest instead a referral to an appropriate professional.

For yet a third client, Joanne, evaluations of potential causal and maintaining factors of her obesity might reveal a combination of variables, such as poor social skills, ineffective coping skills, limited physical capability to engage in exercise, poor eating habits, lowered self-esteem, and inadvertent peer reinforcement for overeating. Therefore, it is likely that a treatment plan for Joanne should include intervention strategies aimed at each of these important problem areas.

After developing an overall treatment plan, based on the unique features of a particular case, the therapist then needs to carry out the various clinical intervention strategies, in addition to monitoring their effects. Continuous scrutiny of the patient's progress is necessary in order to determine whether the implemented treatment plan is, in fact, an "effective solution." If progress leads to overall goal attainment, then treatment can be terminated, with the clinician's problem having been solved. If the goals are not reached, the therapist should then recycle through the various problem-solving tasks in order to determine what changes, if any, are required at this juncture.

As noted earlier in this chapter, simple cases do not exist. Some problems may only be identified once treatment has begun. Additional complications may occur as a function of changes in a client's goals, resulting from a lack of rapid progress (e.g., strong negative emotional reaction to slow progress leads to poor adherence to treatment recommendations).

Because clinical reality suggests that such complexities are the norm, our model of clinical decision making emphasizes the need for flexibility in treatment planning. Moreover, the therapist should always be cognizant of the reciprocal influences among treatment goals, effects, choices, and decisions (Nezu & Nezu, 1989).

To summarize, we conceptualized obesity treatment within a problem-solving framework, where the discrepancy between a patient's initial state and his or her ultimate goal state was presented as the problem for the health-care professional to solve. In addition, given our bias toward a social-learning perspective regarding clinical interventions, we identified several specific subproblems that the clinician must address in order to ameliorate this discrepancy. These include target behavior/problem selection, treatment selection and design, treatment implementation, and treatment evaluation.

In essence, our model of clinical decision making suggests that the health-care professional views him- or herself as an active problem solver in attempting to address each of the aforementioned components of case formulation, treatment planning, and treatment implementation and evaluation. We advocate the use of various problem-solving principles as a means of optimizing the effectiveness of these clinical endeavors. Before we describe in detail the application of this approach in Chapter 6, the remainder of the present chapter will describes the five major components underlying our general model of the overall problem-solving process.

THE PROBLEM-SOLVING PROCESS

We conceive of the overall problem-solving process as containing five specific skills rather than a single unitary ability. These components include (1) problem orientation, (2) problem definition and formulation, (3) generation of alternatives, (4) decision making, and (5) solution implementation and verification. Each is viewed as making an important and distinctive contribution toward effective problem resolution (Nezu et al., 1989).

Before we briefly describe each of these components (see D'Zurilla & Nezu, 1982, and Nezu et al., 1989, for a more complete description of these problem-solving processes, as well as research supportive of their effectiveness in training programs), it should be noted that this model is prescriptive in nature and does not represent how expert problem solvers or clinicians address problems in real life. In addition, though we depict these five processes sequentially herein, we do not imply that problem solving always proceeds in such an orderly, unidirectional manner. Rather, effective problem solving is more likely to involve continuous and reciprocal movement among the five components before the overall problem becomes adequately resolved.

Problem Orientation

This first problem-solving component is defined as the response set that individuals use in relation to understanding and reacting to problem situations in general. These orienting responses include a general sensitivity to problems, as well as a host of relatively stable beliefs, assumptions, appraisals, values, and expectations concerning problems and one's own general problem-solving ability. Depending upon the specific nature of these cognitive variables, this orientation may have either a facilitative or a disruptive effect on later problem-solving activities. For example, if a clinician holds the belief that obese persons simply lack willpower, it is likely that this judgmental attitude will influence treatment recommendations.

More generally, problem orientation emphasizes the influence of the clinician's worldview on both assessment and treatment planning. Worldviews incorporate cohesive philosophical frameworks within which people attempt to understand the way in which the world works (Pepper, 1942). For health-care professionals, a worldview centers around the manner in which *people work*. In other words, worldviews provide a particular perspective that helps the clinician to understand, predict, and explain human behavior and psychopathology. It incorporates several underlying assumptions concerning cause–effect statements pertaining to thoughts, emotions, behavior, and the evironment, and the interrelations among these.

For example, various theoretical models of addictive disorders represent differing professional worldviews. A *moral model* of addiction would suggest that "poor moral fiber" and a "weak willpower" are veridical causal explanations for the development of an addiction such as alcoholism. Alternatively, a *self-control* model would invoke "faulty learning" as the major etiological variable. In addition, as shown in Table 5.1, such worldviews also lead to advocacy of specific treatment recommendations.

For purposes of our continuous-care/problem-solving model, we advocate adoption of a worldview that emphasizes a *multiple-causality* perspective within a biopsychosocial framework. This framework stresses the plurality of potential paths by which a particular clinical problem (such as obesity) can eventually become expressed, and it presumes that a variety of biological (e.g., genetic, neurochemical, physiological), psychological (e.g., affective, cognitive, overt behavioral), and social (e.g., social and physical environment) factors may act or *interact* as causal and/or maintaining variables (Nezu & Nezu, 1989). This perspective is consistent with recent calls for multivariate analytic frameworks within which to understand psychopathology or deviant behavior in general (see Craighead, 1980; Hersen, 1981; Nezu et al., 1989).

In addition, such a framework can be viewed as an example of *planned critical multiplism* (Cook, 1985; Shadish, 1986), which is a conceptual meth-

TABLE 5.1   WORLDVIEWS OR MODELS OF ADDICTION

Worldview model	Causal assumptions	Treatment recommendations
Moral model	Poor moral fiber, weak willpower	Abstinence; group support; acceptance of "higher power' control over self (e.g., AA)
Disease model	Underlying physiology and biochemistry; physical illness	Hospitalization; medications
Self-control model	Maladaptive habits; inappropriate learning	Self-management training (e.g., behavior therapy, relapse prevention)
Continuous care/ problem solving	Interaction of a variety of biological, psychological, and social factors	View therapist as a problem solver who must systematically and continuously aid the patient in identifying effective treatment strategies to facilitate idiographic applications

odological approach whereby attempts are made to minimize the biases inherent in any univariate search for knowledge. In this context, *multiple* can refer to both independent and dependent variables, to methods for measuring these variables, and to general constructs (e.g., multiple methods to assess a variable, multiple variables being assessed, multiple statistical procedures used to analyze these data, multiple hypotheses tested simultaneously). Therefore, this framework would encourage the problem solver to attend to the broad array of variables that are potentially causally related to a patient's obesity problem.

Within our model of clinical judgment, these variables, or *focal problem areas* embedded within the biopsychosocial conceptualization, are characterized as impediments to achieving the clinician's goal (i.e., reducing or eliminating the patient's presenting problems). The fundamental subproblems to be solved by the health-care professional involve the accurate identification of both the relevant causal variables and those strategies that would be effective in changing them.

In emphasizing the perspective of multiple causality, we are not suggesting that the clinician must conduct a haphazard and time-consuming search for *all* possible causal factors. Rather, we underscore the notion of *planned* multiplism. In identifying potential causal variables relevant to a given patient, we suggest that the experimental literature can serve as a rich source of information that provides guidelines to delimit such a search.

Related to the multiple-causality perspective is the view that clinical interventions are a set of strategies rather than a set of tactics. A *strategy* is conceptualized as an overall general approach that includes statements regarding subgoals and/or focal problem areas, such as anxiety reduction, anger management, coping skills training, contingency management, and relationship enhancement. In contrast, *tactics* are defined as specific means by which such strategies can be implemented (i.e., by which the subgoals are achieved). With regard to an anxiety-reduction strategy, tactics might include muscle-relaxation training, biofeedback, flooding, exposure, cognitive restructuring, and diaphragmatic breathing.

Practically speaking, if various strategies are considered initially, a wide range of tactics can then be identified. However, if clinical interventions are viewed only as a set of techniques unrelated to broader goals and strategies, it becomes more likely that a particular tactic can be misapplied. For example, automatically advising the obese client to begin a jogging program without consideration of a wide range of factors (e.g., individual differences in physical ability, previous history, life-style opportunities) can potentially lead to treatment failure.

Last, in regard to problem orientation, we again advocate the perspective that obesity treatment be conceptualized as an ongoing process that continues across a person's life span. If successful weight loss is achieved initially, the clinician's task is to help problem solve an effective short-term maintenance program specific to this given patient. If this maintenance goal is also achieved, a long-term maintenance protocol, again idiographically designed, would be implemented next. This might consist of annual or biennial check-ups.

If the patient is unsuccessful at any of these points, then the therapist attempts to problem solve a new or revised clinical intervention appropriate to the particular phase. At present, for obesity treatment to be successful over the long term, this perspective must permeate all aspects of the initial treatment for weight loss.

Problem Definition and Formulation

Whereas the problem orientation component can be viewed as a general attitude or approach to problems, the next four problem-solving processes should be viewed as specific skills or tasks. The purpose of this first task, problem definition and formulation, is to identify (a) the specific aspects of the situation that make it a problem for a given individual, and (b) a realistic set of goals or objectives for that individual. The importance of this process for effectively guiding later problem-solving activities cannot be overemphasized. More specifically, a well-defined problem is likely to positively affect the generation of relevant solutions, improve decision-making effectiveness, and contribute to the accuracy of solution verification (Nezu & D'Zurilla, 1981a, 1981b).

Within the overall model of clinical decision making, the health-care professional needs to accurately define and formulate each of the various subproblems compromising the treatment enterprise (e.g., problem identification, target problem selection, treatment design, and treatment evaluation; see also Chapter 6 regarding the processes related to "Stages of Change"). Thus, the overall goals for all patients already may be specified, according to the nature of the particular task within the problem-solving model; for this component of the model, the goal is to accurately identify the most important variables maintaining the current level of obesity. Nonetheless, given the individual differences among patients, each of these subproblems should be idiographically defined; that is, the specific goal of problem definition and formulation is to accurately identify the most important problems for *this* particular patient, with *this* particular set of presenting complaints, given *this* particular set of circumstances and conditions.

In order to increase the probability of accurately defining the problem, the health-care professional needs to engage in the following specific activities: (a) seek *all* available facts and information about the problem; (b) describe these facts in clear and unambiguous terms; (c) differentiate relevant from irrelevant information and objective facts from unverified inferences, assumptions, and interpretations; (d) identify those factors and circumstances that actually make the situation a problem; and (e) set a series of realistic and attainable problem-solving goals (D'Zurilla & Nezu, 1982; Nezu et al., 1989).

Generation of Alternative Solutions

The purpose of this third problem-solving task is to make available as many solution alternatives or ideas as possible and to maximize the likelihood that the best or most effective one(s) will be among them. An *effective* solution is defined as one that (a) achieves the specified goal(s), (b) maximizes possible positive consequences, and (c) minimizes potential negative consequences. The theoretical underpinnings associated with this problem-solving task are related to the brainstorming method of idea production, which is based on two general principles: (1) the quantity principle, and (2) the deferment-of-judgment principle. In addition, we also advocate the use of the strategies–tactics approach, described later in this section (see D'Zurilla & Nezu, 1982).

According to the *quantity* principle, the more alternatives that individuals produce, the more likely they are to arrive at the ideas with the best potential for solving the problem. The *deferment-of-judgment* principle states that more high-quality ideas can be generated if an individual initially defers critical evaluation of any particular alternative until after an extensive list of possible solutions and combinations of solutions has been compiled. At the point of generating ideas, consideration of the value or the effectiveness of the alternatives should be avoided completely, with the one exception of the *requirement* that the idea be relevant to a given problem.

The *strategies-tactics* approach suggests that individuals initially conceptualize *general* means or strategies for solving a problem and then subsequently produce various *tactics* or specific ways in which the strategy might be implemented. In this manner, a greater variety or range of ideas might be produced.

Decision Making

The goal of the decision-making component of problem-solving is to (1) evaluate the available solution possibilities, (2) select the most effective alternative(s) for implementation, and (3) develop an overall plan for solution.

To make the best decision possible, the problem solver should first assess the *utility* of various alternatives and then choose the one alternative or group of alternatives that is associated with the greatest utility. *Utility*, within our model, is defined as a joint function of both the *likelihood* of that alternative actually achieving a particular goal and the *value* of the outcome.

To estimate the likelihood that a particular alternative will achieve a particular goal, the clinician should ask, Will it work? Of equal importance is an assessment of the feasibility of the problem solver being able to implement the alternative in its optimal form. A given solution might be an excellent theoretical idea but might have practical limitations due to additional constraints. The individual clinician must therefore assess each patient's assets and liabilities to determine the feasibility of a given idea. In addition, the therapist must evaluate the effectiveness of a given treatment approach in terms of his or her ability optimally to implement that particular intervention strategy, based on the therapist's personal levels of competence and experience.

In making judgments about the *value* of an alternative, four categories of consequences must be considered: (1) short-term or immediate consequences, (2) long-term consequences, (3) personal consequences (effects on oneself), and (4) social consequences (effects on others). *Short- and long-term consequences* involve those obesity-related factors described in earlier chapters, as well as the personal and social consequences described herein. *Personal consequences* might involve the time and effort required to implement a particular alternative, personal and emotional costs versus gains, consistency with one's ethical and moral standards, and physical well-being. Specific *social consequences* may include effects on the patient's family, friends, or community.

Because individual patients differ in their personal values, goals, and commitments for change, it is impossible to develop a standard set of criteria against which to evaluate consequences for each type of clinical problem situation. As such, it might be important for the therapist to brainstorm all the potential consequences and effects of a given alternative, especially when the situation is particularly novel.

In evaluating the various costs and benefits associated with each alternative, the problem solver could use a rating system to indicate estimates of the utility for each idea. After rating each alternative, a comparison can then be made concerning the different *overall* cost/benefit ratios associated with each potential solution. It is important to assess the total picture, rather than the valence of any specific outcome criterion. For example, a solution might be judged as extremely favorable concerning two criteria but might be rejected because the overall expected costs outweigh the overall expected benefits. Based on this comparison, the clinician should then choose those alternatives for which the expected overall outcome most closely matches the problem-solving goals. If only a few ideas appear to be potentially satisfactory, then the problem solver may need to go back and engage again in the previous problem-solving tasks.

Relevant to a multiple-causality perspective, our bias is to promote a pluralistic approach to treatment. Specifically, we advocate that a variety of potentially effective treatment strategies be implemented that simultaneously address a variety of treatment objectives and subgoals. As shown in Table 5.2, several treatment strategies can be initiated to attain one goal simultaneous with the implementation of several additional strategies to attain another goal. This method increases the likelihood that overall treatment can be successful.

TABLE 5.2   TREATMENT GOALS AND STRATEGIES FOR HYPOTHETICAL OBESE PATIENTS AT A PARTICULAR TIME

Problem	Goal	Treatment strategy
a. No or little exercise	To increase aerobic exercise	1. Training in time management, to increase opportunities to exercise 2. Training in exercise per se 3. Developing a contingency management protocol to reward success
b. Little or no social reinforcement of progress	To increase positive social support	1. Identify various related support groups 2. Developing a "buddy system" 3. Developing a therapist–patient telephone system

This is not to advocate that all clients engage in an all-encompassing, shotgun-approach treatment protocol. Rather, the overall intervention should include only those strategies that are considered particularly relevant and effective for a given patient, as a function of a comprehensive, problem-solving assessment.

Solution Implementation and Verification

The major function of this last problem-solving task is the comparison between the anticipated and the actual consequences that occur as a function of solution implementation. Even though a problem may be hypothetically solved, the effectiveness of a solution or the accuracy of a decision has not yet been established. By carrying out the solution (or by actively making a decision or choice in some cases), it is possible to evaluate and verify the solution's effectiveness (or accuracy). Within a general problem-solving framework, this procedure encompasses (a) *performance* (implementing the solution), (b) *monitoring* (observing the actual consequences that follow implementation of the solution), and (c) *evaluation* (assessing the effectiveness of the solution) (D'Zurilla & Nezu, 1982). These key operations can serve as a basis for the problem-solving therapist to extrapolate when evaluating the effectiveness of critical clinical decisions.

Although the *performance* step of this process involves the actual implementation of the solution plan, this step does not necessarily involve an overt behavioral response, depending on the nature of the problem task. Instead, this step may involve making a decision or a choice. For example, the clinician might simply identify and select important patient target behaviors. Implementation of this solution would not require any overt therapist response beyond the verification process.

The second step in this process, *monitoring*, involves more than simply attending to the global effects of the implemented solution. It entails measurement of the solution's outcome at varying levels. At times, in order to obtain accurate information concerning the outcome, it may be necessary to include an objective recording procedure. In clinical situations, such a procedure might involve periodic measurement of a patient's behavior or symptom change in order to assess the outcome of a particular treatment procedure being implemented.

Thus, although the most likely global outcome measure would appear to be pounds or kilograms lost (or gained), we strongly advocate inclusion of additional measures during this process, in order to evaluate whether changes in the hypothesized moderating factors led to changes in obesity level. Such measures might include attendance at support groups, changes in eating and exercise habits, assertiveness in food-related situations, knowledge of nutrition, and/or caloric intake (see also Chapter 7).

During *evaluation*, the problem solver compares the observed outcome with the desired outcome, as specified initially during the problem-definition-and-formulation process (i.e., the various problem-solving goals). If this match is satisfactory (i.e., the discrepancy between the expected outcome and the actual outcome is minimal), then the problem can be considered resolved. Given our premise that weight-loss management is a continuous process, ongoing monitoring and evaluation becomes crucial. This would be similar to dental check-ups or annual physical examinations.

On the other hand, if the match is *not* satisfactory, the clinician then needs to discover the source of this discrepancy. The actual difficulties may involve suboptimal performance of the solution response, misapplication of some aspects of the problem-solving process itself, or both. In either case, one major option is to return to one or more of the previous problem-solving operations, in an attempt to identify a more effective solution plan. In other words, it is possible that the problem(s) were not adequately defined and formulated, or that various mediating factors were not previously identified that contribute negatively to treatment outcome. Additionally, it is possible that insufficient ideas were initially generated or that the consequences of the solution were not evaluated accurately. Essentially, this type of discrepancy between the expected outcome and the actual outcome highlights the need to continue to engage actively in the problem-solving process.

If the discrepancy is due to deficient performance, however, the problem solver can either recycle through the problem-solving process or attempt to improve upon the actual solution implementation. The problem-solving therapist may need to assess the performance of both him- or herself and the client. For example, if a cognitive-restructuring approach to assertiveness training, as a treatment strategy, does not appear to be effective in enhancing the patient's ability to regulate eating in social situations, one type of evaluation within the verfication process would be twofold. First, the clinician needs to assess whether the patient has learned how to implement this solution correctly; second, the therapist should also evaluate whether he or she adequately trained the patient in these skills. In either case, the therapist may want to identify either an alternative method of implementing the same strategy (e.g., behavioral rehearsal to increase assertiveness), or perhaps even another alternative strategy altogether (e.g., avoidance of social situations involving food).

SUMMARY

A general model of the problem-solving process has been briefly described, which encompasses five components: problem orientation, problem definition and formulation, generation of alternatives, decision making, and solution implementation and evaluation. Problem orientation represents an individual's general attitude or approach to problems, which includes the concept of a worldview. As a theoretical model, we advocated adopting a worldview that emphasizes (a) the concept of multiple causation (i.e., that the etiology of obesity is varied and that the particular path for a given patient needs to be idiographically assessed); (b) the view that clinical interventions should be characterized as strategic, rather than as a set of tactics or techniques; and (c) the importance of adopting a continuous-care perspective.

The remaining four major problem-solving tasks were described as providing very specific goal-directed guidelines for health-care professionals to use in attempting to solve problems encountered within the clinical arena. Each of these tasks was described as having an important and unique contribution to the overall problem-solving process. Additionally, the dynamic and synergistic nature of the problem-solving process was underscored. Effective application of these problem-solving components across a multitude of clinical tasks reflects the essence of our clinical decision-making model. The focus of the next chapter is a detailed application of this model to obesity treatment planning.

6

Applying the Problem-Solving Model to Obesity Treatment

INTRODUCTION

Any comprehensive approach to the treatment of obesity must distinguish between *weight loss* and *weight-loss maintenance* (Jeffery, 1987; Perri, 1987; Wadden & Bell, 1990). Although similar intervention strategies may be implemented across both treatment phases, substantial differences between the two warrant their special consideration as separate stages. As noted elsewhere, "Getting clients to lose weight is only the first half of the battle. . . . the second half . . . involves equipping them to maintain their weight losses over the long run. Without a structured program, clients abandon behavioral techniques, experience relapses, and regain much of the weight they lost in treatment" (Perri, 1989, p. 215). In this light, it is crucial to conceptualize weight-loss maintenance treatment as a separate problem for the clinician to solve, as compared to the clinical problem of planning for initial weight loss.

Within the problem-solving framework, both phases of obesity treatment (i.e., initial weight loss and weight-loss maintenance) involve four major process stages of therapy: (1) patient screening, (2) problem analysis, (3) intervention-plan design, and (4) intervention implementation and evaluation (see Nezu & Nezu, 1989). Within each therapeutic intervention stage, the problem-solving clinician must actively and effectively make a multitude of decisions. These clinical decisions range from whether a particular therapist should treat a given patient to which type of long-term maintenance program would be required to prevent relapse or recurrence of obesity. As noted previously, the effectiveness and validity of the decisions in one stage have direct implications for the probable success of those attempted during other stages throughout treatment.

At this point, it may be difficult to differentiate among the various processes, phases, and stages of the continuous-care/problem-solving model. To aid in differentiating among these three aspects of the model, we use distinctive terminology for each aspect, as briefly summarized here:

The two parts of the treatment process—(1) initial weight loss and (2) weight-loss maintenance—are termed *phases*.

The five problem-solving processes—(1) problem orientation, (2) problem definition and formulation, (3) generation of alternative solutions, (4) decision making, and (5) solution implementation and evaluation—are termed *steps*.

The four major processes of therapy—(1) patient screening, (2) problem analysis, (3) intervention-plan design, and (4) intervention implementation and evaluation—are termed *stages*.

Using this terminology, the present chapter focuses on applying our continuous-care/problem-solving model to obesity treatment. The chapter specifically guides clinicians in using the five problem-solving steps to handle the clinical tasks of each of the four stages of the therapy process, throughout both phases of obesity treatment.

APPLYING THE PROBLEM-SOLVING MODEL TO INITIAL WEIGHT-LOSS TREATMENT

Screening

During this first stage of the initial phase of therapy, a broad-based overview of the nature of the patient's obesity problem should be obtained. The overriding purpose at this juncture is for the health-care professional to pose and answer the general question, "Given this particular patient, as well as the specific parameters of the presenting obesity problem, will I be able to help this patient achieve his or her goals?" A definitive answer at this point is likely to be premature. However, the clinician needs to consider and respond to this general question, instead of *automatically* assuming that "every obese patient that comes to treatment can be helped by me!"

Essentially, attempting to answer this question can be considered an initial screening procedure. Based on information gathered during this therapy phase, the clinician can begin to answer this question and can make informed and deliberate decisions regarding the likelihood that continuation into the next therapy stage would prove fruitful. Blindly prescribing a treatment protocol at this point might engender iatrogenic effects.

Initiation Difficulties.   Before progressing further, the clinician must seriously consider the various obstacles or impediments that currently exist, which could affect treatment decisions. These have been labeled *initiation difficulties* because their presence may impede the initiation of further assessment and formal treatment (Nezu & Nezu, 1989).

In general, three categories of initiation difficulties can be identified: those related to (1) the patient, (2) the patient's significant others, and (3) the therapist. Individually or collectively, these obstacles can impede successful continuation into the next clinical intervention stage.

Difficulties Associated with the Client.   One important initiation difficulty relating to the patient concerns his or her level of motivation, cooperation, and commitment to therapy. If the patient comes to treatment as a function of spouse or family coercion, he or she may be generally uncooperative. Even if the patient initially presents a high degree of motivation, he or she may not be fully committed to undergo the time and effort in treatment necessary to result in meaningful behavior change.

A useful approach in conceptualizing client motivation is the *Stages of Change* model developed by Prochaska and DiClemente (1982, 1984) to describe addictive behavior change. Based on the premise that changes in addictive behaviors are not an all-or-nothing phenomenon, they suggest that people undergo several different stages during the process of change. Research with smokers helped these investigators to identify five basic stages of change: (1) precontemplation, (2) contemplation, (3) decision making, (4) active change, and (5) maintenance (Prochaska & DiClemente, 1982).

In applying these stages to weight-loss interventions, these stages of change refer to (1) being relatively unmotivated to lose weight, (2) thinking about losing weight, (3) becoming determined to lose weight, (4) actively modifying habits related to weight loss, and (5) maintaining these new habits for successful weight management.

An important aspect of this model is the notion that in order to achieve success in self-control, individuals need to negotiate effectively each stage of change. Furthermore, the clinician needs to assess where the patient is in this process, in order to determine the appropriate timing for implementing a given intervention. Similar to several approaches discussed earlier in Chapter 5, this model also advocates matching treatments to patients. However, the stages-of-change model suggests that the relevant dimension on which to base this match involves patient motivation, or readiness. It would be inappropriate, therefore, to attempt to teach behavioral self-management strategies to help modify the eating habits of an obese patient who is still in the contemplation stage. Rather, for such a person, intervention strategies should be geared to help move the patient in the right direction toward successful negotiation of the decision-making stage (i.e., to make a commitment to change); these strategies would be more appropriate and—thus—more effective.

This stage-of-change model has not been extensively applied to obesity treatment protocols (however, see Southard et al., in press, for a description of the National Cholesterol Education Program, which is a primary-care effort to treat hypercholesterolemia and is based on the stages-of-change model). Nonetheless, this model does underscore two important points relevant to the present discussion: (1) the necessity of addressing issues of motivation and commitment, and (2) the desirability of matching the patients to the clinical intervention strategies, based on this assessment. Moreover, consistent with our own problem-solving model of clinical decision making (Nezu & Nezu, 1989), Prochaska and DiClemente (1982, 1984) also highlight the reciprocal and interactive, rather than linear, nature of the model.

Related to a patient's level of motivation is her or his reasons for wanting to lose weight and his or her expectations regarding weight loss treatment. For instance, consider the following client's response when asked why she wanted to undergo a weight-loss program. In early September, she applied to one of our structured university-based research clinics: "I have my 25th high school reunion coming up. I need to lose 40 pounds by November 1, or I won't be able to fit into the dress I plan to wear" (Perri, 1989, p. 198).

This reaction typifies the quick-fix attitude of many individuals seeking treatment, who want immediate help. They are often more concerned with achieving a quick loss rather than what might be entailed in order to achieve such a goal (a belief often reinforced by unscrupulous advertisements for commercial weight-loss products).

In essence, it is important to assess the patient's overall motivation, willingness to commit to treatment, reasons for wanting to lose weight at the time of the initial request, and expectations regarding anticipated rate of weight loss. If any of these areas appear to adversely affect the potential success of the treatment, the clinician should question the desirability of immediately implementing behavior-change procedures.

A second type of patient-related initiation difficulty involves patients who have severe medical or physical problems. It is important initially for such a patient to consult a physician who can assess the health risk and then determine the advisability of engaging in any weight-loss program and/or exercise protocol.

The presence of some mental health problems also may impede successful clinical problem solving in two ways. First, if the patient is suffering from a severe mental health problem requiring psychotropic medication, special consideration is warranted, especially if his or her medication is associated with weight gain. In such cases, the stabilization of weight (i.e., preventing additional weight gain) may be a more appropriate goal than weight loss while the patient continues to take the medication.

Second, a variety of psychological problems may serve directly to interfere with weight-loss treatment. For example, if a patient tends to overeat when depressed, it may be more therapeutic to help this individual with the mood disorder before initiating weight-loss treatment. A downward spiral of despair can occur if the patient's depression negatively affects his or her ability to be committed to a demanding treatment protocol; this then may lead to treatment failure, thus leading to a further decrease in mood and self-esteem, and so forth.

Difficulties Associated with the Patient's Significant Others.   Differences in goals between the patient and her or his significant others can also serve as a pool of potential initiation difficulties. The spouse and/or family, for example, may resent the changes and disruption in life-style that can be a part of participating in a weight-loss program (e.g., fewer snacks in the house, less-frequent dining out at restaurants, more time away from the family while exercising). As such, these individuals can serve to hinder, or even undermine, a patient's attempts to lose weight. In addition, the presence of marital or family problems independent of such goal differences may also serve as potential obstacles to successful treatment.

Initiation Difficulties Associated with the Therapist.   A final set of potential impediments to goal achievement that should be addressed during this initial therapy phase relate specifically to the therapist. An initial assessment of personal competence or experience with a particular clinical problem represents an important decision issue. For example, the therapist with little or no background in marital therapy who identifies a significant relationship problem between a patient and his or her spouse should undergo such a self-evaluation. We are not advocating that all clinicians should practice only within an overly restrictive specialty. However, we suggest that the health-care professional be ethically bound to assess whether he or she can be, at a minimum, as helpful to a particular patient as another therapist with specialized training in a different field.

Another therapist-related factor concerns his or her emotional reactions to the patient. At times, patients and/or their presenting problems may serve as discriminative stimuli for a given therapist (being only human) in eliciting emotional responses. Examples may involve racial, cultural, or religious differences between the therapist and the patient that engender an affective response on the clinician's part. Such reactions can be either prejudicial or overly solicitous in nature. We are not suggesting that a therapist's strong emotional reaction should automatically preclude successful treatment. However, it can serve as an impediment and must be considered when determining the optimal treatment for a given patient.

Applying the Problem-Solving Method to Screening. As with all the clinical tasks that the health-care professional encounters during the process of obesity treatment, we advocate the use of the problem-solving model as described in Chapter 5 as a means of addressing these initiation difficulties. (See Table 6.1 for a brief review of the activities associated with each of the five problem-solving steps.)

The following clinical example illustrates how to apply the problem-solving model to the decisions involved in this initial weight-loss phase of therapy:

Kevin, a 44-year-old moderately obese male, was referred to our outpatient clinic by his physician, who was concerned about Kevin's hypertension. During the initial sessions with Kevin, the therapist noted that he seemed to be somewhat unmotivated. Specifically, several appointments were missed, initial intake questionnaires were never filled out, and a daily caloric-intake log was consistently incomplete. Only with some encouragement did Kevin reluctantly decide to continue.

Kevin's overall lack of motivation and commitment to treatment was therefore identified as an important initiation problem to solve. In the therapist's attempts to better understand the nature of this impediment, she presented this concern to Kevin for discussion. Kevin's reply was, "I guess I should be trying because my doctor told me to come here . . . but this seems like so much work! . . . I thought that you might hypnotize me or something and I'd stop craving food. . . . I don't know. . . . I should lose weight, but this is harder than I thought!" At that point, the therapist needed to ask herself the following goal-oriented question: "How can I get Kevin to become more motivated and actively involved in treatment?"

Using the various brainstorming principles, Kevin's therapist generated the following alternatives: (a) have Kevin sign a deposit-refund contract (i.e., Kevin would put a sum of money to be refunded, con-

TABLE 6.1   ACTIVITIES ASSOCIATED WITH THE FIVE MAJOR PROBLEM-SOLVING PROCESSES

Problem orientation
1. Adopt a worldview emphasizing the continuous-care/problem-solving approach
2. Adopt a perspective of planned critical multiplism
3. Adopt a framework of treatment involving strategies rather than a scattering of tactics or techniques

Problem definition and formulation
1. Gather all available facts about the problem
2. Describe these facts in clear and unambiguous terms
3. Differentiate between facts and assumptions
4. Identify those factors that make the situation a problem
5. Set a series of realistic problem-solving goals

Generation of alternatives
1. Generate as many alternative solutions as possible
2. Defer critical judgment
3. Generate alternative strategies first, then think of as many tactics for each strategy as possible

Decision making
1. Evaluate each alternative by rating (a) the likelihood that the alternative, if implemented optimally, will achieve the desired goals; and (b) the value of the alternative in terms of personal, social, short-term, and long-term consequences
2. Choose the alternative(s) that have the highest-rated utility
3. Design solution strategies that contain several tactics, in order to simultaneously address various subproblems

Solution implementation and verification
1. Carry out the chosen plan
2. Monitor the effects of the implemented solution
3. Compare the predicted and the actual effects
4. Exit the process if the match is satisfactory; recycle through the process if the match is unsatisfactory

tingent upon attendance and/or completion of homework assignments), (b) ignore the problem, (c) discontinue treatment at this point, (d) attempt to obtain minor clinical changes (i.e., improve Kevin's mood) as a means of demonstrating the potential efficacy of treatment, (e) improve the therapist–patient relationship, (f) use paradoxical-intention strategies (i.e., convey the belief that Kevin should remain uncooperative), (g) record progressive small changes, (h) encourage the use of positive self-statements focusing on making a commitment to change, (i) enlist support from Kevin's wife, (j) encourage him to visualize himself as being thinner, and (k) have Kevin make a list of pros and cons of extending his effort into the current weight-loss program.

Kevin's therapist then evaluated the utility of each of these alternative solutions, according to the criteria specified in the problem-solving model, with specific relevance to Kevin: (a) likelihood of each alternative contributing to the achievement of the problem-solving goal, (b) likelihood of each alternative being optimally implemented, (c) Kevin's personal consequences, (d) his social consequences, (e) his short-term effects, and (f) his long-term effects. Each alternative solution was then rated according to each criterion, using a simple rating system (e.g., "+" = positive; "–" = negative; "0" = neutral). Procedures chosen to implement as a means of increasing Kevin's initial motivation for treatment included those alternatives that had the highest associated overall set of ratings (i.e., the most "+" ratings and the fewest "–" ratings). Specifically, in attempting to solve this initiation problem, Kevin's therapist decided to use the following alternatives: enlist his wife's help, have him visualize being thinner, use a deposit-refund contract with him, and have Kevin develop a decision analysis (pros versus cons) of active participation in weight-loss programming.

After implementing these alternatives, Kevin's therapist then monitored their effects. This evaluation included formally noting the increases in Kevin's general attendance, increases in his overall attentiveness (as defined by increased eye contact and appropriate body posture), his completion of the intake questionnaire, his completion of homework assignments, and decreases in his frequency of "I don't know" responses. Because such changes did occur, treatment was then ready to proceed to the next therapy stage (i.e., problem analysis). However, if no changes had occurred, Kevin's therapist should have recycled through the various problem-solving steps to identify a more effective solution plan. If repeated attempts ended in failure, it would be appropriate at this point to refer Kevin to another therapist, thus terminating treatment.

It should be noted that such intervention strategies were aimed solely at increasing Kevin's motivation to participate actively in treatment and were not geared toward weight loss per se. Using the stages-of-change model, it is possible that Kevin was in the contemplation stage, thus remaining uncommitted. Had his therapist not considered Kevin's lack of motivation to be a problem, it is possible that immediately engaging Kevin in a behavioral-treatment protocol would have led to his dropping out.

It is important to highlight the changing and shifting nature of the therapeutic enterprise. Initiation difficulties are not always identifiable during the initial few sessions. In addition, at any time throughout treatment, events may occur or pieces of information may emerge that change the nature of the therapist's overall game plan. Thus, some of the difficulties that were described as "initiation problems" can and do occur throughout the various stages and phases of therapy. We suggest that a similar procedure to the aforementioned be applied under these circumstances, as well.

Problem Analysis

During this stage of obesity treatment, the health-care professional seeks to obtain a detailed understanding of the patient's obesity problem, as well as those factors or variables that are etiologically or functionally related to this patient's being overweight. Initial treatment goals are also identified. Essentially, the problem for the therapist to solve at this point can be represented by the following set of goal-related questions: "What is the specific nature of this patient's difficulties?" "What are those factors or circumstances that have resulted in these problems?" and finally, "What are the specific treatment goals for this patient?" In attempting to answer such questions, we again advocate applying the problem-solving model. In this section, we discuss specific issues related to the use of the five major problem-solving steps during the problem-analysis stage.

Problem-Orientation Issues.   To a large degree, the content areas of assessment depend on the clinician's worldview. As such, the therapist's own problem orientation can powerfully affect the manner in which the patient's obesity problem is conceptualized and defined. As was suggested in Chapter 5, we strongly advocate that health-care professionals who work with obese patients adopt a problem-orientation worldview that emphasizes the following aspects: (a) a multiple-causality framework, (b) an assessment of the patient's social environment, (c) a general-systems conceptualization, and (d) a focus on key behaviors.

Multiple Causality.   As argued earlier, a health-care professional's worldview should highlight the plurality of variables that are causally or functionally related to a presenting problem. Such a clinician recognizes that the cause of obesity is *not* unidimensional. Multiple factors serve as initial etiological and/or maintaining variables regarding maladaptive behavior. A clinician who treats a monosymptomatic patient or a unitary target behavior is misrepresenting clinical reality (Nezu & Nezu, 1989).

In this context, the actual scope or range of such variables should be expansive enough to embrace all the evidence provided by the actual individual case. Yet it should also be somewhat restricted to only those empirical findings relevant to the problem(s) experienced by the patient; many etiological factors would be inapplicable for most patients. We distinguish this orientation from one that addresses only *target behaviors*; we have adopted instead the term *focal problems* or *focal problem areas*, which reflects those variables or factors that represent the patient's idiosyncratic impediments to his or her goal attainment (Nezu & Nezu, 1989).

Focus on Social Environment.   Consistent with a multiple-causality viewpoint, we advocate that the search for meaningful focal problems be expanded to include areas beyond the individual patient alone. Specifically, we suggest that assessment be geared to include the patient's social environment. This might include spouse, parents, siblings, relatives, and friends. Such individuals may serve either as potential sources of support or as impediments to goal attainment.

General-Systems Approach.   The manner in which these variables interact with each other to produce a patient's obesity problem is a key component of effective problem analysis. As such, we adopt a general-systems framework that emphasizes the potential interplay among a variety of psychological, environmental, and biological events in a person's life. Each variable does not exist in isolation; rather the reciprocal influence among them is underscored. In this light, in addition to assessing each of these focal problem areas, it is also important to evaluate their intricate interplay (i.e., the system as a whole). As illustrated by the cases of Paula, Nathan, and Joanne in Chapter 5 (pp. 12–13), the differences in these system interactions often necessitate idiographic approaches to assessment (Nezu & Nezu, 1989).

Focus on Key Behaviors.   Adoption of a systems approach to treatment also implies that intervention should focus on those areas or processes that hold key positions within the complex system (see Kanfer, 1985). These key areas or *key behaviors* can affect other behaviors throughout the system's network of behaviors. Moreover, priority should be given to those areas that can have a clinically significant impact on the probability of attaining the client's goals. The most relevant focal problem areas are those variables that can help the client most effectively reach his or her goals. This involves more than the simple removal of only the hypothesized causative factors. For example, coping-skills training might be used as a means of increasing the client's adaptability to stressful life situations that might engender a relapse. This approach emphasizes increasing the patient's future ability to function, in addition to helping him or her to overcome some of the originally identified obstacles to goal attainment (Kanfer, 1985).

Applying the BBATS Model. Problem Definition and Formulation Issues.   At this point, the therapist is ready to identify the areas of the patient's life that should be assessed in relation to his or her obesity problem. For this, we recommend that the level of assessment after screening involve a broad-based investigation of possible focal problem areas, using our three-dimensional BBATS model, as depicted in Figure 6.1, where **B** = behavior, **B** = biological factors, **A** = affect, **T** = thoughts (and other cognitive variables), and **S** = social factors. In addition to depicting these overall problem areas as assessment categories, this model suggests that such areas also provide guidelines concerning selection of treatment strategies and the therapy evaluation targets as well.

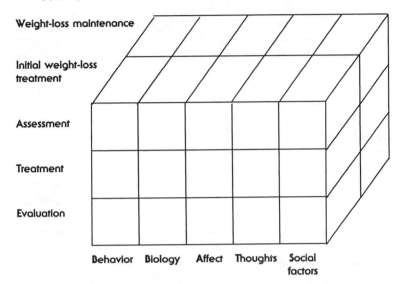

FIGURE 6.1. Three-dimensional BBATS model of assessment, treatment, and evaluation across the weight-loss and weight-loss-maintenance phases of obesity interventions.

According to this model, the clinical task (assessment, treatment, or treatment evaluation) should focus on various behavioral, biological, affective, cognitive, and social factors across both treatment phases (i.e., weight loss and weight-loss maintenance).

Behavioral factors might include a variety of molar and molecular overt behaviors under the general categories of exercise and eating habits. Exercise-behavior factors would include the type, frequency, and duration of any routine exercise program; the amount of daily/weekly walking; and any previous exercise history. Eating behavior factors would involve presence or absence of binge eating, types of foods consumed, daily caloric intake, eating patterns (e.g., eating on weekends, having snacks while driving, eating while watching TV, drinking alcohol with every meal), percentage of calories from fat (from protein, from carbohydrates, etc.), speed of eating, number of eating occasions per day, number of snacks, grocery/food shopping behavior (e.g., shopping from a list, on a full stomach, buying fast foods), storing foods, eating habits at restaurants, and previous dieting and eating behaviors.

Biological factors would involve biological and physiological variables that might be etiopathogenically related to a patient's obesity (e.g., metabolism, number of fat cells, upper- versus lower-body obesity). In addition, it is important to determine the presence of medical problems that might negatively influence or be influenced by the potential impact of any weight-reduction program (e.g., coronary heart disease, diabetes mellitus, arthritis).

Although assessment of such biological factors would be extremely difficult for the average health-care professional, it helps to obtain indirect information. For example, strict adherence to a caloric-intake goal over a period of several weeks can provide an estimate of the person's rate of metabolism depending upon how much weight is actually lost. In our research with moderately obese, middle-aged women, we have generally observed that a self-reported daily consumption of approximately 10 calories for each pound of body weight balances the average patient's energy equation. Thus, to maintain a person's weight of 200 pounds requires a daily intake of approximately 2000 calories. In order to lose 1 pound per week, this person should reduce daily intake by 500 calories because a loss of this amount generally requires a decrement of 3500 calories. After a 2- or 3-week period, assuming that the daily calorie log is accurate, the therapist can determine whether the expected loss has occurred (i.e., 2–3 pounds). If not, it is likely that the individual's biology serves as a major limitation to average weight loss. Such physiological factors can include food efficiency, fat-cell size, fat-cell number, metabolic rate, lean body mass, fat distribution, and/or adipose-tissue receptor activity (see Brownell & Jeffrey, 1987; Keesey, 1986).

Moreover, tremendous variability exists among obese persons with regard to their metabolic rate. Knowledge of such biological factors would help better understand the desirability of articulating differential treatment goals for different people. For instance, consider June and Carla, both overweight at 225 pounds:

To maintain her weight, June eats about 2200 calories per day and must reduce to about 1700 calories per day in order to lose 1 pound per week. On the other hand, Carla was found to maintain that same weight by eating only 1650 calories per day. She would have to reduce to less than 1200 calories per day in order to lose the same 1 pound per week. Obviously, Carla would have a more difficult time dieting than June, due to differences in their metabolic efficiency. Because of such differences, it would not be appropriate to designate the same calorie goals for both women. Note that patients can be referred for testing of their resting metabolic rate in those cases where no weight loss occurs despite only minimal caloric intake.

Moreover, when treating Carla, the therapist can predict that because of her potential biologically based difficulty in losing weight, relative to June, Carla's level of continued motivation might fluctuate. Therefore, Carla's therapist might design intervention strategies geared to enhance her commitment to treatment, to facilitate her ability to accept the difficulties that she will encounter, and to maximize the amount of positive social support she receives from significant others; these and other motivational tactics may be more salient and necessary for Carla than for June.

In regard to *affect*, assessment areas would include determining the particular feelings that are typically associated with eating for a given client, such as boredom, depression, frustration, anxiety, stress, loneliness, jealousy, joy, hostility, resentment, and fear. In addition, it would be important to assess the role that emotions play in general, with regard to dieting and weight management for a given client.

For *thoughts* and other cognitive variables (e.g., beliefs, attitudes, knowledge), potential focal problem areas might be knowledge about obesity, nutrition, and calories in general; fantasies regarding "thinness"; expectations of the consequences of losing weight; goal setting; self-confidence; problem-solving coping ability (e.g., ability to generate distracting activities in lieu of eating in response to stress); and negative automatic thoughts pertaining to dieting (e.g., "If I blow my diet, I might as well go ahead and *really* blow it, since I'm off it now!").

Social factors would include the client's eating behavior in social situations (e.g., parties, holiday get-togethers), possibility of positive social support, preference for "solo" or social (e.g., diet buddies) dieting, potential help or hindrance of an exercise buddy, reactions to social pressures to eat, presence of relationship problems with spouse or other family members, and presence of significant psychological problems of spouse or other family members.

The SORKC Analysis.   After assessing each of these BBATS areas, the clinician conducts a functional analysis of the patient's obesity problem. Consistent with a general-systems approach to the problem-solving model, this type of assessment involves understanding the type of relationship, or function, that each of these variables serve, with specific regard to the patient's obesity. To conduct such an analysis, the health-care professional can use the acronym *SORKC* to summarize the relationships among such factors: S = stimulus (individual or environmental antecedents), O = organismic variables that might mediate the stimulus (e.g., biological, emotional, or cognitive state of the individual, R = response, K = ratio of the consequence's frequency to that of the response, and C = consequence. This acronym was first proposed by Kanfer and Phillips (1970), to characterize the manner in which major variables can influence the probability of a response occurring. Using problem-solving terminology, this sequence, or behavioral chain, helps to identify those variables that serve as major impediments to goal attainment, as well as to highlight their interrelationships. Assessing these relationships helps to identify potential focal problems to target for change.

Hypothetically, depending on the specific nature of a case, interventions can be developed that address each of the variables within the chain. In other words, treatment can focus on changing aspects of the stimulus, the response, the consequence, the organism, and/or the operant relationship between the response and the consequence. Again, we advocate the notion that optimal treatment gains might be obtained by including several therapy strategies that simultaneously address various aspects of this chain within an overall obesity treatment protocol.

Carol, a 29-year-old, moderately obese, single woman illustrates such a behavioral chain regarding obesity. She described the following sequence of events:

A friend of mine, Laurie, was supposed to come over after lunch last Saturday and we were going to go to the movies together. After I just ate my "diet" lunch, she called to cancel because she was feeling real sick. I hate to go to the movies by myself, so I decided to stay home and watch TV [social antecedent stimulus]. Nothing was on, and I started to get bored and frustrated [affective organismic state]. I even started to get angry [affective organismic state] at Laurie because she "ruined" our plans. I thought that I deserved to go to the movies as my reward because I ate my diet lunch [cognitive organismic state]. When I start to get bored and upset, I usually eat [behavioral response] so I started reading and eating . . . reading and eating . . . eating more than reading. I started to feel bad and guilty about going off my diet [affective consequence], but I thought—Heck, I already blew it and this weekend is ruined, so I might as well eat whatever I want now [cognitive consequence *and* stimulus], which just only makes me want to eat more [response]! This pattern is pretty typical of me [ratio of consequence to response]!

As can be readily observed in Carol's description, continuation of this pattern can easily lead to a vicious cycle of overeating and inconsistent adherence to her weight-reduction program.

After a comprehensive assessment, the therapist then applies the next two problem-solving steps—generation of alternatives and decision making—as a means of selecting those focal problem areas that can be targeted for change.

Issues in Generating Alternatives and Decision Making.   In developing a list of problems to target for initial weight-loss treatment, the clinician uses the pool of potential problem areas just produced. The therapist uses the brainstorming principles to generate a list of the variables emanating from the BBATS framework that appear to be functionally related to the patient's obesity problem, based on a SORKC analysis.

Next, when *selecting* the focal problems to target for initial intervention, the clinician uses the various decision-making guidelines (i.e., the likelihood and value criteria described previously). In this way, the therapist systematically identifies the most important variables in need of change for a given patient, from among the many variables listed during the brainstorming process. Essentially, by using these criteria, the therapist assesses the overall cost/benefit ratio for each problem area listed as a potential target. Those that are rated highly (i.e., those targets that are assessed as having a high likelihood of overall positive effects and a minimal probability of negative effects) are then chosen as initial target areas. Again, we suggest that several highly rated areas be selected for targets concurrently, as a means of maximizing the potential for overall goal attainment.

Simultaneous with the process of identifying focal problem areas, the therapist and the patient also develop a list of realistic treatment goals and subgoals by following the problem-solving model. Once the therapist has listed the target problem areas, and the therapist and client have jointly listed the potential goals, the therapist then applies the last problem-solving activity: solution implementation and verification.

Issues in Solution Implementation and Verification.   At this point in the problem-analysis stage of therapy, development of the list of targeted focal problem areas and goals represents the beginning of the solution-implementation step of this problem-solving operation. Verifying the soundness of these choices initially depends on patient feedback. Regardless of the clinician's opinion, if the patient perceives this list of target problems and goals as inappropriate or irrelevant, effective treatment cannot continue. It is possible that such disagreement represents another initiation difficulty, which must be identified and addressed as such.

Once the therapist and patient agree (at least tentatively) on the appropriateness of the list of goals and target problems, the second important source of feedback only comes later in the treatment process (i.e., weight loss per se). In other words, in determining whether a particular goal is appropriate and effective for a given client (e.g., "to increase Paula's ability to say 'no' to family pressure to eat more than one helping at Sunday family dinners"), it is crucial to monitor whether reaching this goal ultimately *also* leads to the goal of weight loss. To get to a point where this can be evaluated, the clinician needs to proceed to the next therapy stage: treatment design.

Treatment Design

The major purpose of this stage of therapy is to design an overall obesity treatment plan geared to idiographically assisting the patient in achieving his or her subgoals as a means of ultimately attaining significant long-term weight loss. As with the other stages of therapy, we advocate applying the problem-solving model to help answer this stage-specific question: Given these particular focal target problems, what kind of intervention plan is necessary to best reach this particular patient's goals?

In describing treatment design, we should note that movement within the overall problem-solving process does not always flow in an uninterrupted, unidirectional manner. It is possible that even after carefully conducting a comprehensive problem analysis, new exigencies in the client's life may arise. The unexpected breakup of a relationship or the death of a family member can obviously dramatically affect a patient's outlook, as well as his or her goals. In addition to these major life events or crises, more subtle changes can occur that can also affect the therapist's game plan. For example, many patients who initially appear quite motivated for obesity treatment may become less committed as the work gets tougher. At the very least, such situations require a detour off the clinician's proposed treatment road map. Again, the clinician needs to be flexible in order to best help a patient achieve his or her goals.

Problem-Orientation Issues.   When designing the overall treatment protocol, the clinician needs to identify any differential training methods that might be necessary for optimal implementation of this plan, as well as appropriate problem-orientation perspectives. The three specific problem-orientation perspectives to underscore at this point in treatment are that (1) treatment should be based on the idiographic application of nomothetic principles; (2) multiple target problems (i.e., obesity-related contributing factors) may require multiple intervention components; and (3) effective overall treatment plans include strategies that increase a client's overall capacity to cope with future stressors in order to prevent or minimize relapse.

Idiographic Application of Nomothetic Principles.   A treatment plan should be tailor-made for a given patient in order to effectively account for the plethora of complexities associated with a particular case, as well as the variability and diversity inherent among differing groups of obese persons. Such differences include a given patient's biological vulnerability, psychological and behavioral strengths and weaknesses, age, gender, cultural background, socioeconomic status, and social network. Even in cases where an effective treatment can be identified easily, based on applying nomothetic principles in an analysis of a given patient's obesity problem, the treatment may need to be *implemented* differentially, based on these additional factors.

For example, a comprehensive assessment of Jeff's overall obesity picture may indicate that one component of treatment is to encourage and help him to exercise more. However, due to a physical disability (i.e., lower-back problems), it would be impossible for him to engage in typical aerobic exercises. Because some exercise regimen is deemed important as part of his treatment plan, the therapist needs to identify alternative ways of implementing this same strategy.

In general, the clinician should not just assess whether a given treatment strategy is effective for a given focal problem. Rather, he or she needs to assess whether that *particular intervention approach* would be effective for that *particular patient* who is experiencing that *particular difficulty*. Thus, instead of treating a disorder or problem, we advocate treating the person.

Multiple Interventions for Multiple Target Problems.   In addition to having a multivariate understanding of a patient's obesity problem, the clinician needs to incorporate several intervention components in the overall treatment plan. These components should address several different target problems, either simultaneously or sequentially. A clinician who engages in a unidimensional search for potentially effective interventions is unlikely to help the patient to attain weight-loss goals.

In developing sample behavioral chains relevant to a given patient during the problem-analysis stage, the therapist, in effect, also designated potential focal target problems. In other words, as noted previously, a comprehensive treatment plan can incorporate those clinical strategies that address each link in a patient's behavioral chain. Providing that such links are important and key problem areas, and that treatment design was based on the problem-solving model, such a comprehensive plan is likely to yield significant behavior change that is far-reaching, wide-spreading, and durable (Nezu & Nezu, 1989).

Inclusion of Future-Oriented Intervention Components.   In additional to those intervention strategies that would be geared to ameliorating specific causally related variables or to overcoming idiographic impediments to weight-loss goal achievement (e.g., training patients to modify their eating behaviors, to reduce daily caloric intake), we also advocate the inclusion of strategies that address generalized coping skills. These components would be included in order to enhance the patient's goal attainment, maintenance and generalization of treatment effects, and ability to cope more effectively with future problems or stressful circumstances as a means of minimizing the likelihood of relapse. Essentially, this reinforces the concept of a continuous-care model of obesity treatment and underscores the need to specifically program for maintenance of behavior.

For example, we often train patients to become more effective personal problem solvers, via an approach similar to the one described in Chapter 5, as one component in our overall obesity treatment package. We do this for two reasons: First, such training helps obese individuals to identify and implement alternative ways to deal with situations that might be conducive to overeating. Second, patients can apply these general skills to a wider variety of problems in living, as a means of increasing their overall coping ability. Enhanced coping skills can help to minimize the impact of future emotional distress that might otherwise impede adherence to the weight-management skills they previously acquired (see Kirschenbaum, 1987).

Based on this orientation and the idiographic patient-based information obtained during the problem-analysis stage, the clinician then continues to apply the problem-solving model and proceeds to generate alternatives.

Generation-of-Alternatives Issues. Application of this problem-solving step involves generating a list of potentially effective treatment ideas, given the problem orientation and the previously constructed list of target focal problems and treatment goals. In addition to the two general brainstorming principles (i.e., quantity and deferment of judgment), the therapist should particularly apply the strategies–tactics approach to idea production. A list of strategies or general approaches for each focal problem area should be generated first. Then, for each such strategy, a list of specific treatment tactics can be developed. Based on these sets of lists, the therapist can also combine various ideas across strategies, to enhance their overall effectiveness.

For each strategy (e.g., stress management), the clinician would generate alternative tactics (e.g., both cognitive restructuring and relaxation training), as well as different *methods* of implementing the same tactic, if relevant. For example, a given treatment tactic may need to be implemented differentially, depending upon various patient-related factors (e.g., cognitive ability). Thus, training in self-control strategies to modify eating habits is likely to be substantially different for a 13-year-old male than for a 46-year-old female college professor. In the former case, intensive therapist modeling may need to be included, whereas in the latter case, simple didactics may be sufficient.

As an illustration of this approach, Table 6.2 contains a list of potential alternatives for a particular goal (i.e., to increase exercise), along with a list of potential tactics and different methods of implementing one of the tactics. In generating potential treatment ideas, the reader can turn for aid to Part III of this book, which is replete with a variety of strategies and tactics aimed at the major focal problem areas typically associated with obesity treatment.

After such lists of potential treatment ideas have been developed, the clinician then begins the decision analysis, the next problem-solving step.

Decision-Making Issues. In order to make selections concerning the particular components to implement within an overall treatment plan, each alternative needs to be evaluated according to the various decision-making criteria, as contained in Table 6.3, concerning its utility. Based on these criteria, the therapist attempts to rate each tactic specifically in relation to the identified goal that it addresses.

Ideally, each preferred treatment alternative would have the following definitional characteristics: very effectively reaches the client's goals, espe-

TABLE 6.2   PARTIAL LIST OF STRATEGIES, TACTICS, AND METHODS GENERATED DURING THE TREATMENT DESIGN STAGE FOR A PARTICULAR GOAL

Goal: To increase calorie expenditure through increased exercise

Potential Strategies
1. Develop individualized exercise program
2. Join local sports team
3. Join armed forces unit
4. Develop "exercise buddy system"
5. Take job that requires more physical work
6. Engage in hobbies/leisure activities that require more physical work
7. Train for the Olympics

Potential tactics related to Strategy 1, individualized exercise program
1. Aerobic exercise program
2. Walking
3. Swimming
4. Jogging
5. Team sports
6. Racquet sports
7. Cycling
8. Weight lifting
9. Dancing
10. Mountain climbing
11. Rowing
12. Sailing
13. Bowling

Potential methods of implementing Tactic 1
1. At home with videotape
2. At home with spouse
3. At home with family member
4. At home with exercise buddy
5. At home with personal trainer
6. At local gym or health club (with class, friend, alone, etc.)

cially substantial weight loss; allows for easy and optimal implementation; yields results that are mostly positive in nature regarding both personal and social consequences; costs very little in terms of time, money, and effort; provides both wide- and far-reaching positive consequences; ameliorates the distress associated with the presenting problems; enhances the overall quality of the patient's life; engenders positive reinforcement from all spheres of a client's social environment; and is consistent with his or her values. However, it is rather unrealistic to believe that any treatment package can be identified for which the alternatives can fit *all* such criteria. Nonetheless, the responsibility of the therapist is to approximate this definition as closely as possible for a particular obese patient, with a particular set of associated problems, given his or her unique life circumstances.

As noted earlier in this chapter, a simple rating system can be used to help in the evaluation process, where "+" = a positive, "–" = a negative, and "0" = neutral. One or even a few negative ratings concerning any of

TABLE 6.3   DECISION-MAKING CRITERIA TO EVALUATE ALTERNATIVE TREATMENT STRATEGIES AND TACTICS

Likelihood of treatment effects

- What is the likelihood that this particular intervention will achieve the specified goal(s)?
- What is the likelihood that this particular therapist can optimally implement this particular treatment approach?
- What is the likelihood that the patient can optimally carry out a particular strategy?
- What is the likelihood of collateral participants in therapy or paraprofessional therapists being able to optimally implement a particular strategy (e.g., can the patient's spouse optimally carry out an alternative that requires his or her participation)?
- What is the likelihood that this treatment approach will contribute to the patient's ability to cope more effectively with future problems or stressful situations?

Value of treatment effects

Personal consequences

- How much of the patient's and the therapist's time and other resources would be required to implement this treatment alternative?
- How much patient and therapist effort is involved in implementing this treatment approach?
- What would be the emotional cost or gain for the patient and the therapist if this treatment were implemented?
- Is the use of this intervention consistent with the morals, values, and ethics of the patient and the therapist?
- What are the physical side effects of this treatment plan for the patient and for the therapist?
- What is the impact of this treatment approach on related patient problem areas?

Social consequences

- What are the effects of the patient's family concerning the use of a particular alternative?
- What are the effects on the patient's friends, neighbors, and/or social and work acquaintances?
- What are the effects on the patient's community?
- What are the effects on others in the client's social environment?

Short-term consequences

- What are the immediate effects of implementing this treatment approach?

Long-term consequences

- What are the long-term consequences of this treatment approach?

these criteria does not necessarily render a given treatment alternative unusable. Rather, it is the overall balance, or ratio of pluses to minuses, that best describes an alternative's utility. Thus, a high percentage of negative ratings across various criteria would probably indicate that an alternative would be given low priority on a list of choices.

Based on the results of the original decision analysis (and refinements engendered by further problem solving, if necessary), the therapist then chooses the best-rated alternatives to be the components of an overall treatment plan for a given client. Again, we suggest the inclusion of several alternatives within an overall treatment package, as a means of enhancing maintenance and generalization effects, as well as facilitating multiple goal attainment. After making such choices, the clinician then moves to the next step in the problem-solving model.

Solution Implementation and Verification Issues. Before treatment is actually implemented, the therapist should verify the choices made during the decision-making phase by eliciting the patient's feedback. As noted previously (when discussing the verification of the therapist's choice of target behaviors and treatment goals), if a patient disagrees with any of the intervention options proposed at this juncture, it is likely that treatment will fail. Such divarications between therapist and patient, however, can be solved as yet another initiation difficulty. Once the patient is in general agreement with the treatment plan, then the clinician moves on to the next major therapy stage: treatment implementation and evaluation.

Treatment Implementation and Evaluation

This last stage of the overall treatment process can be viewed as quite similar in nature to the solution-implementation-and-evaluation step of the general problem-solving model. In other words, both processes involve this procedure:

1. Actually implement a solution (i.e., treatment plan).
2. Collect information as a means of monitoring the effects of the solution (i.e., both process and outcome data).
3. Compare the predicted and the actual consequences of the implemented solution (i.e., Is the treatment working?).
4. Based on the results of Step 3, either (a) troubleshoot if the match is unsatisfactory (i.e., changing the treatment plan), or (b) exit from the problem-solving process if the match is satisfactory.

At this point, we assume that the reader has become familiar with each of the five problem-solving operations. Therefore, in this section, we simply highlight several of the important concerns involved in this therapy stage (see also Chapter 7 for a discussion of general clinical considerations).

Implementing Treatment. In implementing initial weight-loss treatment, the therapist needs to develop an initial timetable or schedule of when a specific treatment component will be conducted. Some of these intervention tactics can be implemented concurrently or sequentially, depending upon the specific client.

For example, if Kia Lee appears to be wavering in her motivation concerning therapy in general, it might be important to carry out a treatment component for a relatively easy-to-change obesity-related problem, as a means of enhancing her motivation. For Kareem, on the other hand, if his severe anxiety problem tends to inhibit his ability to benefit from training in modifying his eating habits, treatment geared to reduce this anxiety should be implemented first.

Monitoring Effects of Treatment.   In order to evaluate whether the treatment is effective (i.e., whether the solution is working), the therapist must collect information across a variety of areas as soon as possible. Beyond the sine qua non measure of actual weight loss per se, monitoring changes in those problem areas previously identified as being causally related to a patient's obesity level is imperative. For example, the therapist might assess a patient's emotional reactivity, assertiveness, interpersonal relations, actual use of self-control procedures aimed at modifying eating habits, and increases in the frequency, duration, and intensity of an exercise program.

Matching Predicted and Actual Consequences.   Based on such evaluation data, the therapist then compares how closely the *actual consequences* (i.e., effects of an intervention) match with the *predicted consequences* (i.e., those articulated during decision analysis). For example, the following questions might be asked:

"Did a daily calorie goal of 1200 lead to an average of 1–2 pounds of weight loss per week for Jim?" "Did three sessions of role-playing to increase Sally's ability to deal with family pressure to eat facilitate her refusal skills?" "Did increasing the frequency per week of Carl's walking program help him to break his weight-loss plateau?" "Has the use of a detailed shopping list helped Joan to reduce the amount of fast foods she purchases at the grocery store?"

Unsatisfactory Match: Troubleshooting.   If the match between the actual consequences and the predicted effects is unsatisfactory (i.e., a particular intervention idea does not appear to be facilitating goal attainment), then the therapist, in collaboration with the client, should attempt to identify why this discrepancy exists.

As noted in Chapter 5, unsuccessful goal attainment can occur as a function of ineffective implementation of a particular strategy, ineffective clinical problem solving, or both. If it is the former, then the clinician can attempt to problem solve alternative means by which to implement the same strategy (i.e., different tactics or different methods of conducting the same tactic). If it is the latter, then the therapist needs to recycle through the various problem-solving operations across each of the previous stages of treatment, particularly with regard to the problem-analysis and treatment-design phases.

The clinical advantages of adopting our problem-solving model is particularly salient at this juncture. This approach places on the therapist's shoulders the onus of pinpointing the reasons underlying such discrepancies between actual and predicted outcomes, rather than subtly giving the message to the client that he or she, *once again*, failed at self-control. This is especially relevant if a very different alternative cause is responsible for such a discrepancy: biological limitations.

Assuming that the patient's adherence and motivation is high (as evidence by data collected as part of the monitoring process), and the therapist is confident that the caloric intake records are valid, it is possible that the client's metabolism is overly efficient. In other words, less than 10 calories per pound of body weight are necessary in order to balance this client's energy equation. If continued efforts to reduce caloric intake and/or increase caloric expenditure does not lead to significant weight loss (again assuming the validity of self-report records and the presence of continued adherence), it may be important to recycle back to the problem-analysis stage in order to reevaluate the client's goals. For example, the amount of weight to lose may need to be readjusted in light of this new information. Moreover, it is very possible that the patient may experience treatment burnout and a decrement in motivation (e.g., "Why should I keep trying so hard if nothing happens!").

Alternatively, a different treatment goal to consider might be one that involves prevention of continued weight *gain*. Rather than becoming thinner, the objective would be to help the patient keep from becoming increasingly heavier. Again, for most patients who enter treatment with expectations of becoming slim, shifting to this type of goal requires the therapist to problem solve additional intervention strategies that are aimed at maintaining their commitment and motivation. The therapist may also need to identify ways to facilitate a client's acceptance of this state of affairs, a goal that dramatically contradicts the various commercial weight-loss programs promising that "You too can lose 10 pounds in 2 weeks if you only try the _____ way!"

Given recent research regarding the role of various biological factors that can moderate the balancing of the patient's energy equation (Brownell, 1991; Brownell & Jeffrey, 1987; Garrow, 1978), even strict adherence to the straightforward advice of "consume less and exercise more" as a means of losing weight is not that straightforward. As such, if a thorough evaluation conducted as part of this phase of treatment suggests that this perspective appears to be relevant for a given patient, the clinician then needs to reorient him or her toward a reevaluation of goals.

Satisfactory Match: Exiting from the Problem-Solving Model. On the other hand, if the comparison between the actual effects and the predicted consequences of treatment appears to be satisfactory, then therapy can proceed to the next intervention steps. During most of weight-loss treatment, this generally means moving to the next therapy or educational component. When the patient has finally reached the ultimate goal of attaining her or his ideal weight (i.e., the effects of the *overall treatment plan* has been positive), then exiting from the problem-solving process at this juncture implies completion of the initial weight-loss program and proceeding to the maintenance phase of treatment.

APPLYING THE PROBLEM-SOLVING MODEL TO WEIGHT-LOSS MAINTENANCE TREATMENT

Exiting from the initial weight-loss phase of treatment suggests that the patient has successfully achieved his or her goals (see Chapter 7 regarding goal specification). Unfortunately, however, this success implies only that half the battle has been won thus far; in addition, the patient needs to learn how to maintain both the behavioral changes and the weight loss.

Within our continuous-care/problem-solving model of obesity treatment, we suggest, similar to other behaviorally oriented approaches, that maintenance be viewed as requiring potentially different strategies than those necessitated during initial weight loss. As research has substantially documented, clinicians cannot assume that after the weight-loss phase of treatment is over, the patient will continue to faithfully and vigorously adhere to all the program regulations (see Chapter 4).

We further advocate that maintenance be viewed conceptually as the *second major phase* of the overall treatment program, and that this phase also comprises the four major therapy-process stages (refer back to Figure 6.1). If perceived in this manner, it is more likely that the clinician will seek to consider all the complexities inherent in this process, rather than to search for and attempt to conduct a standardized maintenance package. In other words, similar to the differences that exist among obese individuals concerning the optimal plan for them to lose weight, differences also exist among patients regarding maintenance issues. As such, it is important to consider such differences when idiographically designing a maintenance program for a given patient.

In attempting to do so, we again advocate applying the five-step problem-solving model to the major decisions encountered during each of the four major therapy-process stages (i.e., screening, problem analysis, treatment design, treatment implementation and evaluation). Because the process of applying the model is similar across all clinical decisions, we avoid the redundancy of delineating its application once again. Instead, we highlight areas of concern for the therapist to consider, which are specifically relevant to the maintenance phase.

Maintenance Screening

During this initial stage of the maintenance phase of obesity treatment, the therapist essentially attempts to assess the presence of any *maintenance-initiation difficulties*. Similar to those impediments the clinician may have first encountered at the beginning of treatment, several initiation problems can exist that make it difficult for the patient to begin this second major stage of treatment.

Initiation difficulties associated with the patient at the beginning point of maintenance can also revolve around issues of commitment, motivation, and cooperation. It is possible that the patient believes that continued treatment is no longer necessary once his or her goals have already been achieved. Even when it has been emphasized throughout earlier treatment, a patient may not have adopted a continuous-care framework; rather, he or she may feel, "Once I've lost 30 pounds, I can now go off the diet!"

Significant others can also represent initiation difficulties that impede effective maintenance by not wholeheartedly adopting the continuous-care model: "Why do you still have to go to that therapist now that you lost weight; is this a way for him to still get money from you?" "You've worked so hard to lose weight; you deserve to eat like a normal person now!" Such social pressures can inhibit a patient's ability to initiate maintenance treatment effectively.

Rather than beginning the maintenance phase based on the assumption that the patient will maintain a high level of commitment, and that his or her significant others will continue to provide a high level of positive social support, it is important to evaluate the presence of such initiation difficulties. Failure to do so can result in early relapse. Especially if the patient has had one or more previous unsuccessful attempts at maintaining weight loss, this recent relapse can simply reinforce the tenuous nature of his or her self-confidence. Again, in addressing such concerns, we advocate applying the problem-solving model to such clinical problems. Having done so effectively allows the therapist to move to the next therapy stage: problem analysis.

Maintenance Problem Analysis

Although attainment of the patient's initial weight-loss goals would appear, at least superficially, to be quite a positive event, we prefer to characterize this transition as a period of adjustment. In this manner, similar to recent formulations regarding the concept of stress, this major change in the client's life can be seen as potentially having both positive *and* negative effects (see Nezu, Nezu, & Perri, 1989). How the client copes with this adjustment process will, to a large degree, determine how successful he or she will be in maintaining this weight loss.

As such, the problem-solving therapist needs to answer the following types of questions during this stage of maintenance treatment: "What is the impact of losing weight on this patient?" "What are the idiosyncratic positive and negative consequences of being slimmer for this particular patient?" "What are some of the problem areas for this particular patient that can potentially have a negative impact on his or her ability to maintain this weight loss?"

In attempting to answer such questions, it is again useful to apply the BBATS model described earlier in this chapter, in order to identify potential focal target problem areas (see also Figure 6.1). In this manner, the therapist can more effectively develop a maintenance program that is specifically relevant to the given patient.

Within the *behavior* category, it would be important to assess the actual changes in the patient's behavior regarding earlier maladaptive eating and exercise patterns. For example, has the patient been consistent in applying these new adaptive patterns? What behaviors were the easiest to change? Which behaviors were the hardest to change? Are there still any maladaptive eating and/or exercise patterns? Which behaviors appear to be closely associated with weight loss?

With regard to *biological* factors, the therapist needs to assess the potential impact of the patient's metabolic rate on future maintenance. Metabolic efficiency, as noted previously, can only be indirectly evaluated by the average health-care professional. Essentially, the rate of weight loss, in relation to the changes in caloric intake, can provide a gross estimate of the efficiency of a patient's metabolic functioning.

For example, if a given patient consistently lost an average of 1–2 pounds per week, based on a decrement of approximately 500–1000 calories per day from baseline, he or she can be considered average. If, on the other hand, a different patient had several plateaus and did not lose weight consistently despite high levels of adherence to low-caloric-intake restrictions, it is likely that this other person has a greater-than-average metabolic efficiency. As such, only slight elevations in caloric intake are necessary to offset weight-loss maintenance. Such differences imply different goals and treatment strategies.

Note that the person's metabolism can also change as a function of treatment. Patients can lose or gain muscle, and the amount of muscle influences metabolic rate. As such, changes can occur over time within the same person, as well as among differing people. Therefore, goals and treatment strategies may need to be revised for the same patient over the course of his or her treatment.

By conceptualizing significant weight loss as a transition period necessitating adjustment, the therapist especially should assess the patient's emotional or *affective* reaction to this life change. One major reaction may involve anxiety and fear. Specifically, is the patient afraid that he or she might revert back again to old habits, especially if previous diets ended in failure? How emotionally vulnerable to difficult situations does the patient feel? Does the patient feel that he or she might easily lose control over food now that the weight-loss phase of treatment has ended? How discrepant is the patient's perception of control from his or her actual control over various situations?

Consider the role that fear played in Amy's reaction in her adjustment to becoming thin. Having been overweight most of her adult life, she had always been hesitant to enter into relationships for fear of being rejected. However, although having been successful in losing 41 pounds at the age of 32, she did not automatically feel comfortable with members of the opposite sex. Instead of acknowledging her discomfort due to her inexperience, she now rebuffed the attention that she was newly receiving from male coworkers, commenting, "How come they didn't like me when I was fat? I'm the same person! I can't like anyone who only thinks about how attractive a person is before they start a relationship!"

Such rationalizations led to a decreased commitment to her weight-loss maintenance program, which eventually led to significant weight increases. Amy's fear of relationships and social rejection did not automatically disappear as a function of weight loss; rather they became exacerbated. Inattention to such fears during the maintenance phase can result in other patients experiencing a similar fate to Amy's.

Another emotional reaction might involve depression. Again, even though significant weight loss would appear to be emotionally quite positive, if such goal attainment did not also engender additional positive consequences, it is possible that a patient may experience sadness.

For example, consider Caroline, a patient who successfully, through rigorous adherence to her weight-reduction protocol, lost 34 pounds in 5 months. Although this loss represented a success in her mind, she secretly harbored the fantasy that her life would drastically change in relation to being thin—"I thought that I would become beautiful and successful; that I would meet my handsome prince and be whisked away in a romantic fervor! Geez, I was sure wrong!"

Unfortunately for Caroline, such dreams did not come true. Although many of her friends responded positively to her success in losing weight, she remained depressed, which often led to bingeing episodes, which quickly led to poor maintenance. It was only after she was able to place the role of her body weight in its proper perspective that she was able to work on other goals (e.g., relationships) independent of her attempts at long-term weight loss.

Thoughts and other cognitive factors might include the patient's expectations and fantasies about being thin and its rewards, the amount of time and effort necessary to maintain weight loss, the likelihood of control in difficult or high-risk situations, and attitudes and automatic thoughts related to relapse (e.g., "If I deviate from my diet at John's party, I can go back on track tomorrow since I know what to do" versus "If I *ever* eat another piece of banana cream pie again, I just know that I'm going to lose control!").

Another major cognitive variable to consider involves the patient's self-efficacy beliefs. In essence, the degree to which the patient perceives that he or she will be able to successfully cope with this adjustment period will, to a large degree, also determine ultimate success at weight-loss maintenance. If the patient appears to have a poor sense of self-efficacy, the clinician may ask, Is this perception global and generalizable to most stressful situations? Is it specific to weight-loss maintenance issues? Is it specific to certain types of weight-related situations?

A third cognitive variable concerns the patient's perceptions of body image, particularly in relation to what the patient expected to look like after losing weight. Due to the strong impact of the various media forms on what is supposedly our cultural ideal (especially for women), patients may be quite disappointed by any perceived and/or actual discrepancies (see Brownell, 1991). Few obese (and nonobese) persons can expect to look like a movie star or a beauty-contest winner, even after goal attainment. What the therapist may need to convey is the inordinate amount of time and other resources devoted to appearance by such individuals. For the average person, it would be extremely difficult (and probably unhealthy) to match this type of commitment.

The last major category of focal problem areas within the BBATS model is *social* factors. In particular, it would be important to assess the various reactions by significant others and other members of the patient's social environment to his or her weight loss. For example, Are they supportive? Have they served as facilitators or inhibitors regarding the actual weight-loss program? Does the patient's spouse understand the need for long-term commitment to weight-loss maintenance?

A second important social area to consider involves the possibility of maintenance buddies. For some patients, going solo may be preferable; for others, adherence to a long-term weight-maintenance program is enhanced by undergoing it with another person.

Maintenance Treatment Design

In developing maintenance programs, the health-care professional who adopts our model uses the problem-solving framework in order to idiographically design an effective protocol for a given patient. Part III of this book provides a plethora of clinical strategies and tactics that should be considered as potential intervention components within a maintenance program. In selecting such approaches, with the initial weight-loss treatment, the therapist should adopt the following problem orientation: (a) Maintenance treatment should be based on the idiographic application of nomothetic principles; (b) multiple focal problems may require multiple intervention components; and (c) intervention strategies should also encompass future-oriented goals.

Maintenance-Treatment Implementation and Evaluation

As in the initial weight-loss phase of treatment, this last stage of the maintenance phase of treatment involves applying the problem-solving activities associated with the solution-implementation-and-evaluation process: (1) Implement the solution; (2) monitor the effects of the solution; (3) compare the predicted and the actual consequences of the solution; (4) based on the results of Step 3, either (a) recycle through the problem-solving process to identify the source of a discrepancy if this match is poor, or (b) exit from the process if the match is satisfactory.

The major difference between the maintenance phase of treatment and the initial weight-loss phase of treatment involves the *continuous* nature of this feedback loop. In essence, long-term weight-loss maintenance requires that the patient continuously engage in this stage throughout his or her lifetime. As noted previously, we characterize obesity as being functionally similar to other chronic health problems, such as hypertension or diabetes. In this light, the therapist needs to conceptualize treatment as being continuous over the long term.

One key concern for the therapist during this stage is to determine which aspects of the patient's BBATS profile, in addition to actual weight, should be continuously monitored. In this way, threshold levels can be developed for each of these key components, such that when the thresholds are reached or exceeded (e.g., weight gain of 2 pounds, increases in frequency of daily snacks, decreases in weekly exercise program), treatment can be reinstated, or additional intervention strategies can be implemented.

Given the failure thus far of behavioral weight-reduction programs that rely solely on the efficacy of self-control procedures (Foreyt & Goodrick, 1991), responsibility for such monitoring should be shared between the patient and the therapist. Similar to dentists who systematically send reminders to patients regarding annual dental check-ups, therapists can play a more active role in supervising the verification/evaluation stage of obesity treatment. These check-up sessions can be a review of previous treatment strategies and can be devoted to teaching the patient new techniques for maintaining weight loss.

As an illustration of this approach, consider the case of Fred, a 39-year-old male who lost 22 pounds and who is currently in the maintenance phase of treatment. During the problem-analysis stage, the therapist determined that social situations involving food, particularly holiday parties with family, continue to be high-risk vulnerabilities for Fred. In addition to weekly weigh-ins at home, Fred agreed to (a) monthly checkups with the therapist, and (b) preplanning sessions before each major holiday that Fred celebrated. By having such checkup sessions, Fred was able to feel more committed to long-term weight loss and more confident in adhering to the maintenance protocol.

SUMMARY

In describing the process of applying our continuous-care/problem-solving model of obesity treatment, we initially characterized treatment as consisting of two major phases: (a) initial weight-loss treatment, and (b) weight-loss maintenance treatment. Within each of these phases, we further identified four major intervention stages: (1) screening; (2) problem analysis; (3) treatment design; and (4) treatment implementation and evaluation.

As a means of addressing each clinical concern (i.e., "solving each clinical decision") encountered in each of these eight stages (see Figure 6.1), we strongly advocated using the entire five-step problem-solving model.

Although future advances in obesity treatment will be a better judge of the utility of this overall approach, we predict that regardless of the types of innovative intervention strategies for long-term weight loss that might be developed, a problem-solving framework will always remain critical, due to the inherent heterogeneity among obese patients. As such, rather than describing *the* single treatment program to use, we outlined a methodology by which to idiographically design and evaluate such programs for a wide variety of patients.

Part III of this book, as follows, contains a plethora of clinical strategies and tactics that should be considered as potential components of such programs for different patients. Prior to focusing on these specific areas, however, we address general clinical concerns in the next chapter.

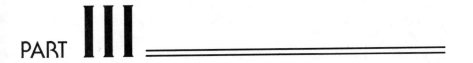

CLINICAL GUIDELINES

7

General Clinical Considerations

INTRODUCTION

Beginning with this chapter, the remainder of this book contains a pool of clinical strategies that the health-care professional can use as a resource in developing individualized programs for both initial weight loss and weight-loss maintenance. Nonetheless, this third section should not be viewed as *the* treatment manual; rather, the reader should perceive these chapters as including potential intervention components that might eventually be part of a client's overall long-term obesity treatment protocol. Depending upon the nature of a specific case, the clinician may find that other resources become necessary.

For example, in the case of Brenda, a 32-year-old, moderately obese schoolteacher, the therapist identified a severe depression problem that required treatment prior to implementation of a weight-loss program. Specifically, the therapist decided, based on careful problem analysis, that the current severity of Brenda's emotional problems would minimize the likelihood of successful weight loss. As such, the clinician needed to draw on his previous experiences with depressed patients, in addition to other relevant resources (e.g., books, peer consultation), in order to best help Brenda. Only then did he consider implementing weight-loss strategies such as those described in this section. Further, the treatment plan that was developed was in accord with the continuous-care/problem-solving model outlined in Chapter 5 and 6.

In the present chapter, we briefly address a variety of general clinical concerns, including treatment goals, the overall structure of treatment, the use of additional training strategies, the patient–therapist relationship, pretreatment assessment suggestions, and ways in which to handle common problems encountered during treatment.

TREATMENT GOALS

At first glance, it would appear that articulating a specific goal for weight-loss treatment would be relatively easy. However, as noted in Chapter 1, the use of charts such as the 1983 Metropolitan Life Insurance tables that purportedly provide verdical ideal weights is quite problematic. Moreover, the *concept* of ideal weight is also fraught with controversy. For example, individuals with hyperplastic obesity (i.e., increased number of fat cells) are unlikely to reach ideal weight even with extremely rigorous dieting (Brownell & Wadden, 1991). As such, other treatment goals should be considered.

Brownell and Rodin (1990), for example, advocate the concept of a realistic weight goal, which is the weight at which an individual "feels good about how he or she looks." Such goals are determined by considering: (a) the weight at which a person felt happy with life in general in the past, (b) the largest clothing sizes in which the person feels comfortable, and (c) the weight of family members or friends who look "normal" to the patient. Further, in selecting a realistic weight goal, Brownell and Wadden (1991) suggest that a useful rule of thumb is to choose a weight that is no lower than the patient's lowest weight that has been maintained for at least 1 year since the age of 21.

Related to the concept of realistic weight goals, another type of objective can relate to body size, as represented by clothing sizes. In other words, rather than stating the patient's goal as losing 26 pounds, the treatment objective might be to comfortably fit into a size 42 sport jacket or a size 12 dress. Again, as with weight per se, estimates of body shape and size can easily be influenced by perceptions of the ideal shape or size, rather than a realistic objective. In other words, people unrealistically might seek to look like a famous actor or actress. As noted several times throughout this volume, the patient's physiology can severely limit the realistic attainabilty of weight-related goals. This potential constraint suggests the advisability for some patients to choose non-weight-related goals.

In Chapter 1, we described several negative medical consequences of obesity. For individuals seeking weight-loss treatment due to medical complications (e.g., hypertension, cardiovascular problems, diabetes), improvements in such arenas should be monitored as part of an overall evaluation procedure. Also, substantial reduction of a significant health risk might be viewed as the *primary* treatment goal, rather than a particular goal weight.

Consideration of this alternative conceptualization of a treatment goal becomes especially salient given recent research indicating that significant health benefits can be achieved as a function of less-than-ideal weight loss. Particularly in light of the possible existence of some biological constraints on losing weight, choosing such a goal may be even more relevant for certain patients. As Brownell and Wadden (1991) note,

> A male, for example who should lose 20 kg according to the tables might have his blood pressure return to normal after only a 10 kg loss. By losing the remaining 10 kg he would be in a lower risk category, but if doing so is too difficult and places him in conflict with biological or psychological limits on weight loss, he may relapse completely and sacrifice the benefits obtained from the first 10 kg loss. (p. 159)

As noted in Chapter 6, applying the three-dimensional BBATS approach to problem analysis can be very helpful in identifying appropriate goals for a given patient (see Figure 6.1). For instance, Table 7.1 contains examples of the variety of potential therapy goals that may be appropriate for long-term obesity treatment across the five general BBATS focal areas. Such treatment goals should be considered as alternative or adjunctive to weight-related ones (i.e., number of pounds to lose).

Finally, in regard to treatment goals, it is important to articulate specific treatment objectives during both the initial-weight-loss and the weight-

TABLE 7.1   EXAMPLE GOALS FOR LONG-TERM OBESITY TREATMENT, USING THE BBATS MODEL

General area	Potential goals
Biological	• Actual weight loss in pounds • Decrease in health risk
Behavioral	• Changes in eating habits (e.g., goal of fewer calories from fat) • Increase in exercise
Affective	• Decrease in negative moods associated with obesity • Decrease in body dissatisfaction
Thoughts (Cognitive)	• Increase in self-esteem • Increase in self-acceptance • Decrease in body distortions
Social	• Decrease in responding to social pressure to eat • Increase in social contacts involving exercise

loss-maintenance phases. It is our firm belief that articulation of goal statements during the maintenance phase increases the probability of success. These goals may be attached to focal problems that might be identified specific to maintenance issues (e.g., increase perceived self-control over eating habits) or might be statements regarding the continuation of effective behaviors (e.g., continue to walk 2 miles per day, five times a week). Moreover, unsuccessful attainment of these maintenance goals can be a major source of cues that signal the decision to reenter the problem-solving process.

STRUCTURE OF TREATMENT

With regard to the structure of treatment, we address the following specific issues: individual versus group formats, length of treatment, and treatment phases. We then summarize these issues in an example protocol.

Individual Versus Group Treatment

If both options are available, the therapist needs to decide which form of treatment is best suited for a given patient. A group-therapy approach can serve as a rich source of social support and provide peer encouragement and reinforcement. A group treatment format might also serve to normalize an individual's perceptions of his or her weight problem by offering exposure to individuals struggling with similar health concerns. Other group members can also serve as positive coping models who provide for observational-learning opportunities. The group may also facilitate the process of problem solving by generating a greater range of creative coping strategies. In addition, a group treatment approach may be less costly to the individual patient. Last, evidence exists suggesting that a group approach may lead to better maintenance of habit change and weight loss achieved in treatment when compared to an individual therapy format (Kingsley & Wilson, 1977).

On the other hand, some patients may simply prefer to be seen on an individual basis rather than in a group. A group-therapy format also provides significantly fewer opportunities to tailor interventions based on an individual patient's needs. Further, some group members may serve as negative models, thus adversely affecting other members' progress. Ultimately, a careful cost–benefit analysis should be conducted to best answer this question for a given individual. At times, depending upon available resources, both approaches might be helpful.

Length of Treatment

As noted previously, in Bennett's (1986) analysis of 105 studies, which evaluated behavioral approaches to obesity treatment, the single variable that correlated most highly with success was duration of treatment. Moreover, in an experimental investigation that we conducted, it was found that the longer patients are in treatment, the longer they adhere to the behaviors necessary for weight loss (Perri, Nezu, Patti, & McCann, 1989).

These findings strongly suggest that the typical 20-week research protocol may be insufficient for many obese individuals. For example, because the average weight loss using behavioral treatment approaches usually range between 1 and 1.5 pounds per week, persons needing to lose more than 20 to 30 pounds may not even reach their goal by the end of the structured program. Therefore, the length of the initial intervention phase needs to be flexible, using the patient's degree of obesity and his or her response to treatment as guides to making this decision (Perri, 1989).

Phases of Treatment

In Chapters 5 and 6, we previously demarcated two overall major phases of long-term obesity treatment: initial weight-loss treatment and weight-loss-maintenance treatment. In addressing additional aspects of the structure of our continuous-care/problem-solving framework, based on our research programs (see Chapter 4), we find it useful to further break down the maintenance phase into three smaller subphases: initial weight-loss maintenance; faded therapist contact/maintenance; and long-term maintenance.

As noted in Table 7.2, *weight-loss treatment* (Phase I) involves approximately 20–40 sessions, conducted over a period of 5–10 months. Ideally, meetings with the therapist occur on a weekly basis. This phase ends when the initial goals are successful attained. Throughout this component, the therapist is viewed as being more responsible for making treatment decisions (e.g., identifying effective strategies, providing information about nutrition, modeling useful clinical strategies), as compared to the patient (see Figure 7.1).

Initial weight-loss maintenance treatment (Phase II, Subphase A) begins immediately after the patient's initial goals are achieved, not any sooner. During a period of 12–18 months, the patient meets with a therapist approximately once or twice a month, depending upon his or her response to this period of adjustment. As noted in Figure 7.1, the patient begins to take on equal decision-making responsibility with the therapist regarding identification of effective intervention strategies.

When the therapist and patient, via the problem-solving model, mutually agree that the patient is continuing to attain the maintenance goals, they move on to the next maintenance subphase—*faded therapist contact* (Phase II, Subphase B). This phase can be open-ended in terms of length and is geared to increasing the patient's treatment responsibility while decreasing the contact with the therapist. Nonetheless, they maintain continuing contact, the frequency of which is open-ended (e.g., once a month, bimonthly, semiannually). Therapist contact can be through the mail, by

TABLE 7.2   STRUCTURE FOR LONG-TERM OBESITY TREATMENT USING THE CONTINUOUS-CARE/PROBLEM-SOLVING MODEL

Phase I: weight-loss treatment
- 5–10 months
- 20–40 weekly sessions
- Intervention components primarily designated by therapist via problem-solving model

Phase II (Subphase A): initial weight-loss maintenance treatment
- 12–18 months
- 1 to 2 meetings with therapist per month
- intervention components chosen by both therapist and patient via problem-solving model

Phase II (Subphase B): faded therapist contact maintenance
- open-ended with regard to length of time
- continuous contact through mail or telephone; schedule also open-ended
- therapist contact can be initiated at any time
- patient assumes more decision-making responsibility

Phase II (Subphase C): long-term maintenance
- throughout life span
- annual or biennial checkup with therapist
- additional therapist contact can be initiated at any time
- patient assumes majority of decision-making responsibility

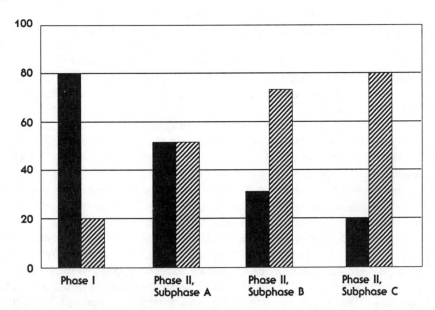

FIGURE 7.1. Responsibility for designing treatment: differences between therapist and client as a function of treatment phase.

telephone, or in person. For example, patients can be instructed to monitor and record treatment-related information (e.g., caloric intake average, fat intake, total exercise time, current weight) on specially designated postcards. These could be sent to the clinician on a continuing basis. The health-care professional can then telephone the patient to discuss such information, during which time the overall contact can be brief (5–10 minutes). Again, lack of continued success or significant relapses may spark the need for additional treatment sessions or for increased face-to-face contact with the therapist. In general, increased contact, especially when maintenance strategies are found to be ineffective, can be initiated by the patient at any time.

The last subphase, *long-term maintenance* (Phase II, Subphase C), basically continues throughout the course of the patient's life. Viewing obesity more as a chronic disease, similar to diabetes or hypertension, underscores the *continuous care* component of our overall model. It should be noted, however, that goals during this phase might change as a function of age or life-style. Contact with a therapist is in the form of annual or biennial checkups, similar to regularly scheduled dental visits or physicals. Again, additional contact with the therapist can be initiated at any time. During this phase of maintenance treatment, the patient assumes the majority of the overall decision-making responsibility, in consultation with the therapist (see Figure 7.1).

The decision regarding when to move on to the next treatment phase, or when to recycle back to a previous phase, can be made by using the problem-solving process described in Chapters 5 and 6. Similarly, the therapist-patient pair applies the problem-solving model in identifying the intervention strategies to include during each treatment phase.

Example Protocol

As an illustration, we describe here an example protocol regarding the initial maintenance phase (Phase II). This represents components of our own research efforts regarding maintenance treatment. It should be noted that this illustration is presented with the caveat that, consistent with the problem-solving model, such a plan represents only one of myriad possibilities.

Our Phase II, Subphase A, protocol comprises 52 weeks. Face-to-face meetings with the therapist are scheduled on a biweekly basis. Because our programs incorporate a group format, these 26 sessions last approximately 2 hours, in order to accommodate 6–8 patients per group. For each of these sessions, we attempt to complete the following six essential tasks: (1) obtain weight measures, and chart the results on a graph; (2) check patients' self-monitoring records (e.g., daily caloric intake, daily exercise, diet content, specific homework assignments); (3) model new exercise and/or provide an opportunity for exercise (e.g., 30-minute brisk walk);

(4) conduct problem-solving sessions focusing on patients' problems encountered that have affected progress since the last session (e.g., difficulties adhering to protocol, situational problems occuring at work that added stress); (5) review the content of a lesson provided during the last session (e.g., review of homework assignments focusing on patient's ability to integrate new information/skills); and (6) present new lessons (e.g., didatic presentation of new information, modeling of new skills).

When presenting new material, we have attempted to be concise, to offer multiple relevant clinical examples, and to provide meaningful handouts. In addition, we have found it particularly helpful to have patients bring a large three-ring binder to each session, as a means of safely storing the handouts.

With regard to content, didactic topics include realistic goal setting, relapse prevention, problem solving, dysfunctional thinking, exercise, social support, nutrition, and self-management (refer to remaining chapters). Depending on the nature of the patient's previous treatment, Phase II, Subphase A, may be a review of such topics or of their initial presentation.

One important "lesson" that is taught during this treatment phase is the need to *plan*. Planning the caloric intake for the next day, for example, helps to increase the likelihood of adherence. Planning specific activities also helps to provide structure while reducing the potential of relapse. For example, the period between coming home from work and dinner is often very difficult for an obese patient. Energy levels tend to be low, and the tendency is to use foods in order to increase energy levels. It is also a time when the person may be involved in food preparation and vulnerable to powerful stimulus cues (i.e., food smells). Careful scheduling can help patients to exert control over such situations.

> For example, Linda, a 36-year-old working mother, often had difficulty when she returned home from work. She felt tired and hungry but also felt pressure to get dinner on the table for her family as soon as possible. She would often snack on whatever foods were readily available (usually high-calorie "finger foods") just to "keep going." In an attempt to achieve more effective control over this situation, a schedule was worked out in which she planned for a small, low-calorie snack and a brisk walk before facing the demands of her family.

Last, in order to provide the consistency and therapist support crucial during this treatment stage, and to compensate for the reduction in scheduled meetings, we maintain a telephone hotline for patients to call between sessions, if necessary. Toward the end of Subphase A, sessions are devoted to help the patient to develop an individualized game plan to be implemented during the next subphase (i.e., faded contact). Patients are encouraged to use a problem-solving approach in helping to identify those strategies that will become aspects of an overall long-term maintenance program.

USE OF ADDITIONAL TRAINING STRATEGIES

Earlier, we indicated that in addition to identifying specific clinical strategies and tactics to implement as part of an overall individualized treatment protocol, the therapist, based on a given case, may also need to brainstorm various different *ways of implementing* a particular strategy (see, for example, Table 6.2). As such, we emphasize here that beyond didactic instructions (e.g., explaining the concept of "energy balance" to a patient), the therapist has access to a variety of teaching or training techniques that should be incorporated into the structure of obesity treatment. These include (a) *prompting* (e.g., providing the patient with prompts or cues during a mutual brainstorming session, in order to facilitate identification of ways to increase routine exercise times); (b) *modeling* (e.g., using films, videos, or role-plays to illustrate a given skill); (c) *behavioral rehearsal* (i.e., providing opportunities to practice a newly acquired skill); (d) *homework assignments* (i.e., facilitate in vivo applications of new skills outside the actual sessions with the therapist); (e) *reinforcement* (e.g., praising a patient's efforts at weight reduction via tangible or social reinforcement); and (f) *feedback* (i.e., providing the patient with constant and consistent information about progress).

THERAPIST–PATIENT RELATIONSHIP

As in other forms of psychosocial interventions, the therapist–patient relationship is considered important within our continuous-care/problem-solving model of long-term obesity treatment. Regardless of the proven effectiveness of any given clinical strategy, obstacles within this relationship can lead to premature attrition and poor adherence. As Goldstein (1975) suggests, without a positive therapist–patient relationship, patient change rarely occurs.

Along these lines, the clinician should display warmth, empathy, trust, and an atmosphere of genuineness. Although we are not suggesting that such therapist characteristics are the sole basis of effective obesity treatment, the caring therapist is more likely to receive more of the patient's attention and respect. Due to the emotional difficulties often experienced by obese patients (e.g., frustration, depression), the therapist who is perceived as empathetic is more likely to engender treatment compliance.

In addition, we further believe, based on our clinical experience, that it is important for the therapist to strike a balance between being an active, directive practitioner and conveying a sense of collaboration with the patient. Therefore, on one hand, the therapist needs to be able to present information in a clear, concise, and understandable manner to patients. On the other hand, the therapist has to foster a collaborative relationship with the patient that emphasizes trust, openness, and concern, especially when focusing on difficult treatment areas (e.g., unrealistic goal selection, lack of treatment progress).

PRETREATMENT ASSESSMENT SUGGESTIONS

Chapter 6 provided a detailed overview of the process and content of pretreatment assessment contained in our model of obesity treatment. As part of the overall assessment procedure, we recommended the use of the acronym *BBATS* as a means of outlining major areas of concern.

In addition, we wanted to provide the reader with specific examples of various relevant tests and measures, using this model. As such, Table 7.3 contains a brief list of potential assessment tools and/or measurement procedures that might be helpful in conducting a comprehensive pretreatment (and evaluation) assessment. In other words, such tools can provide useful information regarding potential focal problem areas to be addressed in treatment, as well as data regarding treatment progress and impact.

WAYS OF HANDLING COMMON CLINICAL PROBLEMS

Superceding any of the following specific suggestions regarding problems encountered during treatment is our general recommendation that the health-care professional apply the problem-solving model when searching for solutions. However, we offer here some ideas related to problems of poor attendance, difficulties in adhering to treatment, and responses to a progress plateau or regression.

Poor Attendance

In our experience, attendance is one of the best predictors of successful weight-loss maintenance. Therefore, the clinician needs to facilitate consistent attendance. Unfortunately, at times, a patient misses a session due to negative moods or feelings of guilt related to poor adherence to treatment suggestions. Individuals might miss a session, hoping to "get back on track" by the next meeting. However, by staying away from treatment at this critical point, the patient misses various tangible benefits (e.g., learning new treatment strategies, group support and encouragement) and runs the risk of further poor adherence.

To facilitate consistent attendance, we have found it useful to incorpo-

TABLE 7.3   PRETREATMENT ASSESSMENT MEASURES ACCORDING
TO BBATS MODEL

Behavioral
- Caloric intake: food diary (e.g., Schlundt, Johnson, & Jarrell, 1985)
- Binge eating: Restraint Scale (Herman & Mack, 1975); Binge Eating Scale ✗ (Gormally, Black, Daston, & Rardin, 1982); Three Factor Eating Questionnaire (Stunkard & Messick, 1988)
- Eating behavior: Master Questionnaire—Revised (Straw et al., 1984); Forbidden Food Survey (Ruggerio, Williamson, Davis, Schlundt, & Carey, 1988)
- Problem-solving coping ability: Social Problem-Solving Inventory (D'Zurilla & Nezu, 1990)
- Assertiveness: Rathus Assertiveness Schedule (Rathus, 1973)
- Coping skills: Coping Resources Inventory (Billings & Moos, 1981)
- Dieting history: Stanford Eating Disorders Questionnaire (Agras, 1987)

Biological
- Weight in pounds: scale; percentage over ideal body weight; body mass index (BMI)
- Body fat: skinfold calipers (e.g., Durnin & Womersley, 1974)
- Resting metabolic rate: indirect calorimetry (e.g., Feurer & Mullen, 1986)

Affective
- General distress: Symptom Checklist (SCL-90; Derogatis, Lipman, & Covi, 1975)
- Depression: Beck Depression Inventory (Beck, Ward, Mendelsohn, Mock, & Erbaugh, 1961
- Anxiety: State–Trait Anxiety Inventory (Spielberger, Gorsuch, & Luschene, 1979)

Thoughts/cognitive
- Eating attitudes: Eating Attitudes Test (Garner & Garfinkel, 1979); Eating Disorders Inventory (Garner & Olmsted, 1984)
- Body image distortion: Body Image Assessment Procedure (Williamson, Kelley, Davis, Ruggerio, & Blouin, 1985)

Social
- Stressful events: Hassles Scale (Kanner, Coyne, Schaefer, & Lazarus, 1981); ◡ Life Experiences Survey (Sarason, Johnson, & Siegel, 1978)   ◡
- Marital satisfaction: Marital Satisfaction Inventory (Snyder, 1979)

rate a contingency management component in an initial contract. Specifically, session attendance is reinforced by the return of a portion of pretreatment deposited monies. For example, a small amount of money (e.g., $1.00) is returned at each session, whereas larger amounts (e.g., $20.00) are returned for 80% attendance at points in the middle and at the end of treatment.

In addition, our philosophy has been to pursue aggressively a patient who has missed a session by calling to reschedule as soon as possible. Moreover, when patients have informed us in advance that they will miss a meeting (e.g., due to business reasons), prearrangements are made for rescheduling. In this way, structure continues to be provided to the patient; the clinician's concern and interest is also underscored.

Difficulties in Adherence

It is a gross understatement to suggest that the more a patient adheres to a treatment protocol, the higher the likelihood that he or she will be successful in reaching a goal. Therefore, incorporating strategies specifically addressing compliance behavior is also important. To facilitate adherence, we have used contingency-management principles in two ways. First, when conducting treatment in a group format, we have used the concept of "Bonus Bucks." Points are assigned for adherence to *key behaviors*, not weight loss per se. When the group achieves a certain point level, each member receives a small monetary reward. In addition to facilitating adherence, this approach also fosters group cohesiveness and a sense of "team spirit."

A second approach is the use of individual rewards for achieving specific treatment goals. Again, goals are usually defined in terms of some specific behaviors (e.g., consistently engaging in an exercise regimen for four consecutive weeks), rather than weight loss per se. Reinforcers can involve something tangible (e.g., purchasing a record album or new article of clothing) or an activity (e.g., seeing a movie, going sailing, watching television). Depending upon the reliability of the individual, such self-reinforcement may be controlled by the therapist or the patient.

Weight-Loss Plateaus and Regaining Weight

Under the best of circumstances, weight-loss maintenance requires considerable effort. One of the more difficult issues that a patient must be prepared to face is the possibility that a plateau might be reached where nothing seems to help, even those strategies that were helpful in the past. Obviously, it is very discouraging for patients to feel they are doing their best only to encounter a plateau. They may become demoralized and feel that continued progress is beyond their personal control.

When such a plateau occurs, possibly due to physiological limitations, we have often included interventions that are targeted at altering metabolic rate. These include increased exercise and alterations in the nutrient content of the patient's diet. Making adjustments in either or both of these areas has often helped our patients get past a plateau.

For example, with Carrie, a detailed analysis of her food records indicated that she obtained the recommended 25–30% of calories from dietary fats. To get beyond a plateau, we recommended that she reduce this to between 15 and 20%, while increasing the carbohydrate level of her diet. This approach, in combination with increased exercise, led to her breaking through the plateau difficulty.

In addition, the therapist should be alert to the patient's feelings of futility and questioning of the value of remaining in treatment. When such feelings are present, the health-care professional can encourage the individual to reevaluate his or her goals. Using a decisional balance sheet geared to aid the patient in determining the cost/benefit ratio of alternative treatment choices and treatment goals can be helpful in this process of reexamination (Nezu, Nezu, & Perri, 1989).

SUMMARY

In this chapter, we briefly addressed several general clinical concerns regarding the implementation of our continuous-care/problem-solving model of long-term obesity treatment, including treatment goals, the structure of treatment, the therapist–patient relationship, the use of additional training strategies, pretreatment assessment suggestions, and ways of dealing with common clinical problems. The next several chapters provide a plethora of specific clinical strategies that can be used as components of a long-term weight-loss maintenance program. We strongly recommend that the reader use the following chapters not as a treatment manual, but rather as potential aspects of a protocol that will be designed specifically for a given patient, using our problem-solving model.

8

Skills Training to Prevent Relapse

Maintenance of any form of change can often pose a different set of challenges from those faced during the beginning stages of initial treatment. Once initial goals are met, patients often express a wish to return to normal and experiment to see which behaviors are critical to continued success. They may impose less-stringent calorie goals, dispense with self-monitoring, or allow themselves to indulge in previously restricted foods. Unfortunately, reverting back to old habits quickly results in weight gain.

The realization that maintenance of weight loss requires constant vigilance may seem overwhelming at first. Although some changes made during treatment may have been easy to accomplish, it is likely that many required considerable effort. Regaining weight at this time may cause the patient to feel out of control, resulting in failure to monitor subsequent eating and further weight gain. This chapter addresses the problem of relapse by providing a range of strategies that the clinician can teach the patient for coping with the difficulties encountered during the maintenance period. We begin by briefly describing a model of relapse prevention, to provide a context for the clinician to conceptualize and apply strategies for skills training.

DETERMINANTS OF RELAPSE

The individual who attempts to change long-standing patterns of behavior must anticipate the possibility of relapse. The most comprehensive
framework for understanding relapse in individuals who have previously
made a *voluntary* choice or decision to change has been described by
psychologist Alan Marlatt and his associates (e.g., Marlatt & Gordon,
1985). Although the model was originally developed primarily for the
treatment of addictive behaviors, such as alcoholism and smoking, we
have found it to be clinically useful in the long-term treatment of obesity.

Within the relapse-prevention framework, while individuals are continuing to follow the rules of their weight-loss program (e.g., staying with
a lower-calorie limit, exercising), they are likely to experience a strong
sense of personal control or self-efficacy. The longer the period of adherence, the greater the person's sense of control. This perceived control
will continue until the individual encounters a *high-risk situation*. Such
situations are defined as events that pose a threat to the person's sense of
control while increasing the risk of possible relapse.

Research has indicated that most high-risk situations can be grouped
into three primary categories: (1) those associated with negative emotional
states (e.g., frustration, anger, depression); (2) situations involving emotional conflict (e.g., argument with one's spouse); and (3) contexts involving social pressure to engage in the "taboo" behavior (e.g., holiday parties).

An example of this third category was provided by Susan, a 31-year-
old woman enrolled in our weight-loss program: "Going to my mother-
in-law's for dinner has always been a problem. Even though I only had
to deal with it once a month, it certainly qualified as a high-risk situation. Now I can understand that there were a lot of things going on that
made it difficult for me to be there. For one thing, no one else in that
family has a problem with weight, and I've always felt they can't
understand what my husband, John, sees in me. I can never decide what
to wear when we visit there, and John gets angry with me because we're
always late. On top of that, it seems like there's never anything to eat that
isn't high in calories. Instead of watching my diet, I wind up consoling
myself with food, and acting like the pig they must think I am."

If the person is able to cope effectively with the high-risk situation (e.g.,
if Susan, in the preceding example, assertively counteracts the social
pressure to overeat), then the probability of relapse decreases significantly.
In addition, successful coping is also likely to facilitate a greater sense of
control, thus beginning a positive accumulation of future successes with
high-risk situations.

On the other hand, according to the relapse-prevention model, if the
individual is unable to cope effectively with the high-risk situation, then

the likelihood of relapse is increased, especially if the temptation exists to overeat as a means of dealing with the stress associated with the situation itself. Moreover, the person is also likely to experience a decrease in self-efficacy, feelings of personal failure, and a sense of hopelessness. This scenario also involves the tendency to react passively to future high-risk situations, thus culminating in a downward spiral of poor coping and low self-efficacy.

What contributes to ineffective coping with such high-risk situations? First, the individual may have failed to properly recognize and identify an upcoming event as posing a high degree of risk. Second, the person may lack the necessary skills required to respond effectively in a given situation. Third, although the individual may have the ability to cope with the situation, an appropriate response may be inhibited by fear or anxiety. Therefore, the therapist needs to adequately address each of these areas for a given patient, as well as to equip him or her with strategies to use if a lapse should occur.

IDENTIFYING HIGH-RISK SITUATIONS

The first step in effectively coping with high-risk situations involves prior identification. Situations that can be planned for in advance are less problematic than situations that arise unexpectedly. As such, the therapist can begin to identify those situations that are particularly relevant to a given patient in order to develop strategies appropriate to that individual. The availability of an effective response provides an alternative to old behaviors and is a prerequisite for managing the demands of these situations. Although the specific details of high-risk situations tend to be idiosyncratic, as noted previously, most fall into one of three general categories (i.e., those involving negative emotional states, those associated with interpersonal conflict, and those involving social pressure to deviate from the appropriate behavior).

For example, Grilo, Shiffman, and Wing (1989) found that although situational factors do serve to increase the risk of relapse, the variables most often associated with *overeating* involved emotionally upsetting events. In another study, Stanton, Garcia, and Green (1990) found that (a) situational cues frequently precipitated eating for individuals with a low tolerance for boredom, (b) binge eaters responded more to situational or affective cues than to hunger, and (c) dieters with depressive symptoms were most likely to eat in response to negative feelings.

High-Risk Situation Log

As such, it is important that each patient recognize situations that personally hold the highest risk for lapses in dietary control and other weight-management behaviors. One method of enhancing the patient's awareness is to have him or her create a list of all high-risk situations that occur over a specific time period (e.g., 2 weeks), as well as those situations that have caused trouble in the more-distant past. In addition to noting such events, the patients should also (a) describe their actual response to the situation, (b) rate the effectiveness of the response on a scale from 1 to 10 (1 = not effective; 10 = very effective), and (c) describe an alternative way of coping with the situation in the future. Using this format provides important information for both the therapist and the patient to use in planning more effective coping attempts.

Consider the example that one of our patients, Janet, a moderately obese, 39-year old nurse, who provided the following description of a personal high-risk situation:

Description of Event: Every Friday morning we have a coffee and bagel brunch at the medical staff meeting. Whatever is left over is brought back to the nursing station and sits on the counter near my desk until its [*sic*] gone.
Description of Response: I "pick" all day long and wind up eating several bagels and plenty of spreads by the end of the day—in addition to breakfast and lunch!
Response Rating: 1
Alternative Response: I'll decide in advance how many bagels I'll eat for the day and put that amount aside on a separate plate. In addition, I can plan to have a bagel-and-cream-cheese lunch each Friday rather than having another meal.

The situation described by Janet is one that holds a high degree of risk to proper dietary control because it is not an isolated event. Rather, it represents a regular occurrence that has a significant impact on her eating. This situation has the potential not only to affect her on that particular day, but also to leave her facing the weekend feeling out of control. She rated this situation as a "1," indicating that she recognized her usual response to be ineffective. The alternative that she proposes attempts to control the food cues in a situation in which the stimulus to eat is extremely high. Although the stimulus itself remains unchanged, the decision to set appropriate limits may provide sufficient structure to override some of these environmental cues.

Relapse Fantasy

A second assessment procedure involves descriptions of a patient's relapse fantasy. Here, the individual is asked to "imagine what it would take for you to return to the old habit pattern" (Marlatt, 1985, p. 56). In response, individuals often report that they ruminate obsessively about loss of control. Rather than being frightened by these fantasies, and allowing them to undermine their confidence, this exercise can provide an opportunity to identify the events associated with relapse. Fantasizing about a relapse can pinpoint the antecedents and consequences of problem situations, and can allow the patient to design more effective strategies for coping.

Consider the relapse fantasy of Cathy, a 43-year old secretary who lost 31 pounds during the initial phase of treatment and was now mildly obese.

I was sitting in traffic for an hour on the way home. When I finally get there, I am exhausted, and the apartment is roasting hot. I should start dinner, but I'm dying of the heat and can't bear the thought of standing over a hot stove. I remember there's a pint of chocolate chocolate-chip ice cream in the refrigerator. I'm hungry and tired and close to feeling out of control. I go to the refrigerator with a spoon and enjoy the cool mist on my face and the taste of hard chocolate and smooth cream in my mouth. I stand there eating spoonful after spoonful until it's gone. I feel exhilarated and upset, hungry and utterly full, all at the same time. There's a container of strawberry ice cream that's already opened. I dig out a spoonful with a chunk of icy fruit in it. It tastes so fresh compared to the richness of the chocolate. I love how cool it feels sliding down my throat. I stand there eating as though I'm in a trance, feeling more and more out of control.

Note that for Cathy, physical discomfort (i.e., feeling hot and tired) appeared to play a role as the initial trigger for her slip. Awareness of the antecedents that precipitate a lapse is crucial to learning how to successfully negotiate high-risk situations.

A third assessment procedure that Marlatt (1985) offers as a means of better understanding the idiographic relevance of a given high-risk situation for a particular patient involves writing a "personal relapse autobiography."

Relapse Autobiography

To provide optimally useful information, a relapse autobiography should contain: (a) circumstances that led to past relapses and weight gain; (b) thoughts and feelings that accompanied past efforts; (c) current motivation to prevent future relapses; (d) thoughts and feelings about present efforts; and (e) goals and expectations for the future.

The following excerpt is from the relapse autobiography of Laura, a 48-year old woman who has struggled with weight problems for most of her life.

I've lost weight plenty of times and started feeling pretty good about the way I looked. I even felt much better physically. I would never go swimming or play tennis when my weight was up, but after I started to lose I would be able to go out in public in a bathing suit or shorts without feeling that I looked like a freak.

It always seemed like I would get to within about 25 pounds of my goal and then things would start to go wrong. I'd be losing a pound or two a week and be feeling pretty comfortable and then, suddenly, I'd do exactly the same things and nothing would happen—absolutely nothing! At first I'd get discouraged, but I'd tell myself to just stay with it, and I'd start to lose again. People would comment on how good I looked, but instead of feeling supported, I'd hear their remarks as back-handed compliments. Every time someone would say, "You must have lost a *lot* of weight, you look really great!" I'd hear it as, "You used to look like a fat pig!" If others were so aware of the weight I lost, they'd also notice when I gained it all back again. I'd start to panic every time I stepped on the scale and still hadn't lost anything. Sometimes I'd weigh myself seven or eight times a day hoping to see some change. Then before you know it, I'd gain a pound and that would make me feel completely out of control, as if I couldn't control the things that went on with my own body. That's when everything would start to fall apart. Looking back on it I can see that I stopped doing a lot of the important things I had done while I was losing, but at the time I felt as though I *couldn't* control what was happening to me.

Once patients are able to recognize and identify idiosyncratic high-risk situations, they can then be taught to cope effectively with them. Whereas some situations can be avoided without severe negative consequences (e.g., only going to one party at work during the holidays rather than all of those scheduled), most need to be managed adequately without experiencing a significant lapse. In general, it is important for the patient to plan ahead when anticipating the occurrence of such high-risk situations. As such, patients can be taught to "set up early warning systems."

SKILLS FOR COPING WITH HIGH-RISK SITUATIONS

Setting Up an Early Warning System

Many discrete behaviors are critical to successful maintenance. The establishment of criteria regarding relapse provides an early warning system that takes into account individual goals and vulnerabilities. Developing a behavioral contract allows the patient to recognize when a lapse has occurred. For example, a weight gain of 3 pounds may be set as a limit at which to implement more stringent exercise and calorie goals. Establishing these parameters helps the individual to recognize significant violations when they occur.

It may be useful for the patient to have a backup plan to address varying contingencies. When the individual is doing well, a minimal maintenance strategy may be all that is required. However, when he or she is experiencing difficulty (weight gain can be an objective measure of this), having an alternate plan already established will help him or her to shift gears quickly with fewer self-recriminations. A contingency plan normalizes the experience of a slip and reduces the tendency for the patient to experience it as a personal failure. Having a strong sense of self-efficacy is also crucial in effectively coping with vulnerable situations.

Building Confidence in High-Risk Situations

Lack of confidence can undermine the individual's sense of self-efficacy and can spiral into a cycle of negative expectations and additional failures. Patients need to develop confidence about their ability to negotiate situations that have led to slips in the past. Identifying these problems and planning more effective strategies can break this downward spiral and increase the likelihood of a more adaptive response. The experience of success enhances self-efficacy and leads to mastery of future outcomes.

The high-risk situation described previously by our patient, Susan, had an extremely negative impact on her sense of self-efficacy and self-control. Once she was able to understand why the situation was so difficult, she was able to address both the emotional and behavioral aspects of the problem. This involved talking with her husband concerning how she thought his family perceived her and how that made her feel. In addition, she began to plan ahead about what clothes she might wear to reduce her last-minute anxiety. She then devised an eating plan for these high-risk occasions that included bringing along fresh-fruit salad as an alternative to the high-calorie desserts that her mother-in-law always served. Having this situation under control had a positive impact on her self-esteem and gave her the confidence to manage other situations throughout the week.

Despite attempts at being consistently vigilant in maintaining weight loss, slips are possible. An individual might overeat at a holiday party or skip a week of exercise due to illness. If this leads to an increase in weight beyond the predefined permissible limit (developed in the warning-system plan), what should the patient do next? According to the relapse-prevention model, how the patient perceives this slip is extremely influential in directing immediate future behavior.

Reframing: Lapse Versus Relapse

Recognizing the difference between a *lapse* and a *relapse* is essential to helping the patient negotiate the maintenance phase of treatment. A *lapse* or *slip* can be defined as a temporary disruption in self-regulation and a return to previously maladaptive patterns of behavior. When a slip occurs, the patient is taught to reframe or relabel the event as a learning experience, as an independent event that does not necessarily predict future problems in coping with high-risk situations. Any violation of the individuals's self-imposed goal should be viewed as an isolated incident, with situational and environmental determinants, rather than as a sign of personal failure. Many patients tend to catastrophize the violation, to overgeneralize its importance, and to think in increasingly negative and global terms. Reframing allows the patient to interpret the maladaptive behavior as an opportunity for learning (i.e., why the event occurred, how to prevent it in the future, what new coping strategies need to be learned in order to more effectively deal with this situation in the future, etc.). Understanding the antecedents and consequences of the event provides crucial information that enhances the client's ability to prevent future relapses.

Consider the example of Linda, a 34-year old mildly obese patient with a history of binge eating.

Linda: I almost didn't come tonight—I really blew it over the weekend! I had to go to two events, a graduation and a neighborhood barbecue—it was a double whammy!

Therapist: What went wrong?

Linda: The graduation lasted almost 3 hours, and by the time it was over, I was ravenous. Right afterwards, they had a reception in the student lounge, and I ate more than I should. I felt like I'd blown it before we even got to the party! I must have gone over my limit by at least 1000 calories by 3 o'clock in the afternoon. I just couldn't control myself! Worse yet, I still felt out of control the next day. I didn't watch myself at the barbecue at all. In fact, I even had three desserts—like the good old days!

Therapist: You felt as though you had blown your diet and reverted to some old behaviors. Let's look back and see if we can understand what happened.

Linda recognized that the problem started when she found herself in an unexpected situation—that is, being extremely hungry at a time when she had not planned to eat. She might have decided that what she ate at the reception was her lunch and compensated by not eating again until later in the day. However, the change in plans threw her off, and rather than compensating, she accused herself of having no control. She was able to recognize that if she had not become so upset, she could have adjusted her plan and still been fine. As she later realized, "I didn't really blow it until after I told myself that's what I'd done."

The greatest risk to maintenance in this situation was not the immediate behavior, but the way Linda perceived and labeled the event. If she was then able to view it as a slip, and to "chalk it up to experience," the event still would have no long-term negative effects. In fact, if she learned from the experience, it could even have positive consequences. However, if she were to catastrophize the situation and see it as being predictive of future behavior, the same event could easily lead to relapse. As such, patients often need to be taught how to counteract negative thoughts.

Countering Negative Thoughts

Countering negative thoughts with positive ones is an important step in coping with a slip. Thoughts such as "I really blew it this time, I'll never be able to keep this weight off, I'm just no good," are overgeneralizations that can be self-defeating. One approach involves teaching the patient to recall past examples of successful coping. Keeping a list of past successes enables the patient to develop a more balanced picture and to short-circuit negative thinking.

The following exercise is useful in addressing the problem. Have patients keep records of their negative thoughts related to weight management. Then model for them positive responses to counter each negative thought. Patients can also be encouraged to brainstorm their own list of possible devil's advocate statements (see Nezu, Nezu, & Perri, 1989).

For example, the following statement expresses a sense of hopelessness and negates any degree of individual control.

> *Negative statement:* "Every time I've lost weight in the past, I've just put it back on. I know I'm probably going to gain it all back this time too."

Examples of possible positive statements that can counteract this negative thought might include

> "This time I've learned to change the way I eat—that's going to make the difference this time!"

> "Thinking this way in the past only led to a big relapse! I need to think more positively!"

> "Even if I slip, it's not a relapse! I won't let myself get totally off track. I can really change this time and stay on course."

When developing such a list of positive statements, it is important to remind the patients to acknowledge that the difference between success and failure is actually under their own control.

STRATEGIES FOR ACQUIRING RELAPSE-PREVENTION SKILLS

When anticipating high-risk situations, in addition to adopting a positive mental framework, it can be extremely helpful to practice actual coping strategies prior to experiencing the event. This can involve (a) in vivo practice, (b) relapse rehearsal, and/or (c) programmed lapse.

In Vivo Practice

Placing the patient directly in the problem setting is a useful technique for effectively coping with high-risk situations. This can be done in the therapist's presence or by having the patient monitor his or her own behavior. For example, when working with obese patients in a group format, we regularly schedule potluck meals or go out to dinner at a restaurant, as an opportunity to practice coping in real situations. When the therapist is present, it is possible to observe directly the patients' susceptibility to social influences on their eating, and to provide an objective evaluation of the event. The therapist can then be better prepared to offer advice as to how best to cope with specific difficulties.

Relapse Rehearsal

In those cases where it is not practical to practice coping in real-life settings, the therapist can use imagery to help the patient rehearse coping with a high-risk situation. For example, patients can be asked to imagine themselves in a situation that would typically cause some difficulty in managing eating, such as attending a party where there are many high-calorie foods, or having the host offer a second helping of a favorite food. The patient's response to the visualized scene can provide data about the risks that individuals may face in similar real-life situations.

Consider the situation in which Susan described visiting with in-laws. The therapist helps guide her imagery in describing the scene, as well as taking the role of her mother-in-law.

Therapist: Imagine the following scene. You've gone to your in-laws for a pool party, and you're the only one who isn't wearing shorts or a bathing suit.

Susan: I stick out like a sore thumb.

Therapist: Your mother-in-law approaches you as you're sitting with several other guests and says, "You look so hot dear, why don't you jump in for a swim?"

Susan: Oh, I wish I could but I forgot my bathing suit.

Therapist: That's too bad—I'd loan you one of mine but I guess it wouldn't fit.

Susan:	I feel everyone is looking at me as if I were the original Amazon woman.
Therapist:	As soon as you can, you excuse yourself and move to a table near the pool. There is a platter of cream puffs and other pastries, as well as a plate of sliced watermelon.
Susan:	I take a piece of watermelon but the pastry looks very enticing. I'm thinking I should move before I succumb to their appeal.
Therapist:	Just as you're about to get up your husband comes over and asks you why you're sitting alone.
Susan:	I felt so embarrassed when your mother pointed out—in front of everyone—that I'm much too fat to fit into any of her bathing suits!
Therapist:	Your husband says his mother was just being truthful and tells you you're acting like a big baby. Then he gets up to go for a swim.
Susan:	Now I'm furious! I decide to dive in—to the platter of pastries! After I've eaten a few I feel angry with myself and out of control.

It is clear that emotional factors play an important role in Susan's behavior in this situation. Although the first event was upsetting, she was able to recover by leaving the situation. However, the combination of hurt and angry feelings she experienced from the interaction with her husband served to undermine her restraint.

To intervene effectively in this situation, the therapist needs to help Susan deal with her negative emotions in a way that is less self-destructive. Susan needs to be more comfortable with the way she looks so that she is less sensitive to the remarks of others. She also needs to work on the appropriate expression of anger so that she does not respond aggressively in ways that are self-defeating. Susan can actually rehearse this using imagery. Consider the following:

Therapist:	Okay. Let's try that last part once again. This time remember two important points. First, remember to be assertive and not passive and not aggressive. Second, react in a way that's good for you.
Susan:	Okay. I'll give it a try, but sometimes it's easier said than done.
Therapist:	I know—but by rehearsing here with me, you can get practice and become better. Just like practicing a musical instrument before trying out for a part in an orchestra. Okay let's try again. Remember that your husband just said that his mother was being truthful and that you are acting like a baby. How do you respond? Just like we rehearsed many times already.

Susan: Okay, okay. I guess I should tell him how I feel.
Therapist: No. Say it aloud here, as if he were here.
Susan: Okay. "John, when you say things like that, I feel hurt. I
            am trying to lose weight, and when your mother makes
            comments about my not fitting into her size, even if she is
            technically correct, that also hurts my feelings. It certainly
            doesn't help me any. In fact, it makes me want to eat more!
            I would like you to understand that, and I would like you
            to be of help to me. So please don't say things that aren't
            helpful."
Therapist: Good! Good!

Programmed Lapse

Programmed lapse is an intervention that should be used cautiously and may be most useful for the subgroup of overweight individuals who are binge eaters. These patients often ruminate obsessively about relapse and fear that an episode of uncontrolled eating will disrupt their treatment. Providing a programmed experience that allows the patient to break dietary restraint (i.e., deliberately overeat) within a structured setting has a number of advantages. In real-life situations, the circumstances in which a lapse occurs may create a halo effect that may enhance the evaluation of the event (i.e., it's expected that one will overeat at a party) and may lead to further episodes of lack of control. In a programmed lapse, the therapist maintains control over the setting and events associated with the lapse. The circumstances can be kept neutral, allowing the patient to experience the behavior apart from any positive social context and reducing exaggerated expectations that the patient may have about engaging in this behavior in the future. Feelings of guilt will be mitigated because the behavior was planned, and the patient will be less likely to make negative internal attributions, such as personal weakness or worthlessness. The therapist can encourage moderation, can help the patient to regain control more quickly, and can identify elements of personal control within the lapse situation. Moreover, the therapist is available to help the patient deal with an emotionally upsetting situation, to evaluate the benefits of the behavior objectively, to interpret reactions to having overindulged, and to do so without catastrophizing the event.

So far, we have assumed that the patient has within his or her repertoire many or all of the coping behaviors that might be necessary to manage effectively each high-risk situation encountered. In most cases, it is more likely that a personal assessment of the relapse process for a given individual will reveal a lack or deficiency of various coping strategies, and/or the presence of a strong emotional response (e.g., anxiety, depression) that serves to inhibit a coping response that the patient is capable of performing.

In the former case, the therapist may need to teach the patient the specific coping skills needed. Assessment should address the wide range of potential skill deficits that represent competencies necessary to effectively handle high-risk situations across the three general categories previously noted (i.e., negative emotional states, interpersonal conflict, and social pressure). For example, effective communication skills are necessary to successfully deal with interpersonal conflict, whereas competent assertiveness skills are prerequisites for effectively managing undue social pressure to engage in overeating. The patient's skill level in maintaining emotional equilibrium can influence the potential success of handling high-risk situations dealing with negative emotional states, especially if such negative affect inhibits the patient's performance of previously acquired coping responses.

The potential range of pertinent coping skills training protocols for a given individual might be quite vast. For example, if a comprehensive assessment reveals that a given patient's difficulty during relapse-prevention training involves the experience of depression, the underlying mechanisms may be quite varied. Etiological considerations might involve self-control deficits, an inability to engage in pleasant events unrelated to eating, ineffective problem-solving skills, negative attributions, cognitive distortions, ineffective stress-management skills, poor social skills, and dysfunctional family or marital relationships (see Nezu & Nezu, 1989). As such, a comprehensive discussion of all possible coping-skills training approaches is far beyond the scope of the present chapter. Several comprehensive texts can serve as rich sources of information in this regard (e.g., Bellack, Hersen, & Kazdin, 1990; Garfield & Bergin, 1986; Kanfer & Goldstein, 1991; Nezu & Nezu, 1989). What we would like to underscore at this point is the utility of using the problem-solving model, as described in Chapters 5 and 6, as a means of assessing which coping skills should be taught to a given patient. Moreover, the applicability of providing the patient with training in problem-solving skills as a general coping strategy should be readily apparent (see Nezu et al., 1989). Additional general coping strategies might also include relaxation training.

SUMMARY

Following the initial phase of obesity treatment, most patients will encounter difficulties in maintaining the array of behaviors needed to sustain weight-loss progress. Sometimes, the individual's best efforts meet with failure; progress in further weight loss can be exceedingly slow; and even minor behavioral digressions seem to result in a noticeable regaining of weight. In such instances, even the most motivated patients may experience frustration and may question the value of continuing in long-term obesity treatment. Clinicians can help patients to anticipate fluctuations in motivation and progress, to prepare patients to manage their feelings of discouragement and to maintain their adherence to key weight-control behaviors.

The relapse-prevention model provides the clinician with a useful context in which to conceptualize and apply strategies to help patients negotiate obstacles to long-term success. The relapse-prevention strategies involve three critical sets of skills. The first entails the identification of situational factors that pose a high risk for an initial slip or lapse in control. Negative emotional states, interpersonal conflict, and social pressure are common precipitants of initial lapses in dietary control. To identify high-risk situations that are most relevant to the particular individual, the clinician may use several sources of data, including a relapse autobiography and relapse fantasies, as well as prospective self-monitoring. The second category of relapse-prevention skills involves teaching patients to set up an early warning system to signal potential backsliding and training them to gain coping skills for handling high-risk situations, thereby enhancing both their effectiveness and their confidence. The final category of skills needed for relapse prevention entails providing patients with an adaptive cognitive framework. The use of reframing and relabeling can help the patient to develop a positive mental set so that the experience of a lapse can be viewed not as a harbinger of impending personal failure, but rather as a learning experience signaling the need for adaptive coping. Successful treatment of obesity requires that patients become experts in managing high-risk situations. To help them accomplish this objective, the clinician can draw on our continuous-care/problem-solving model as a guide to implementing skills training in the long-term management of obesity.

9

Increasing Exercise and Physical Activity

Exercise is one of the best predictors of success in the control of obesity. Indeed, numerous studies have found that the amount of exercise that an individual performs following treatment for obesity is significantly associated with maintenance of weight loss (e.g., Kayman et al., 1990; Perri et al., 1988; Stalonas et al., 1984). In this chapter, we provide an overview of the physiological, psychological, and weight-related benefits of exercise. We describe how increased physical activity can be integrated into a plan for the long-term management of obesity, and we review essential considerations in exercise planning, including the choice of activity, the benefits of routine versus programmed exercise, key principles of an exercise workout, and guidelines for determining appropriate levels of physical activity for the particular patient. We conclude the chapter by discussing problems in the maintenance of exercise, and we describe strategies to enhance long-term motivation and adherence.

EFFECTS OF EXERCISE AND PHYSICAL ACTIVITY

A compelling body of evidence indicates that regular exercise is associated with increased longevity and a reduced risk for cardiovascular disease and some types of cancer. Nonetheless, 1990 data from the Centers for Disease Control show that low levels of physical activity characterize the life-styles of the majority of Americans. Obese individuals, in particular, are often observed to be less physically active than their average-weight peers, and low energy expenditure may contribute to both the development and the maintenance of obesity.

Thus, researchers (Epstein & Wing, 1980) have long argued that exercise and increased physical activity have the potential to play a significant role in the long-term management of obesity. In addition to its effect on energy expenditure, regular exercise has a positive impact on the individual's physical health and psychological well-being. However, many obese individuals view exercise in terms of its short-term negative consequences (e.g., tiring and time consuming). Thus, providing an overview of long-term benefits of exercise can sometimes serve as a helpful first step in getting obese persons to consider exercise as a potential component of their weight-management effort. Table 9.1 provides a summary of the physical, psychological, and weight-related benefits of exercise.

Weight-Related Benefits

Numerous studies have shown that the combination of dieting plus exercise is superior to dieting alone in the treatment of obesity (e.g., Perri et al., 1986; Wing et al., 1988; for a review see Bray, 1990). The weight-related benefits of exercise are more often observed as improved *maintenance* of weight reduction rather than as additional pounds lost during

TABLE 9.1   BENEFITS OF EXERCISE FOR OBESE INDIVIDUALS

Weight-related benefits

1. Increases energy expenditure, due to activity
2. Increases thermic effect of food (TEF)
3. Decreases dieting-induced decline in resting metabolic rate (RMR)
4. Preserves lean (i.e., muscle) tissue
5. Does *not* increase appetite

Psychological benefits

1. Improves sense of well-being and enhances self-image
2. Decreases anxiety and tension
3. Reduces depression
4. Increases self-efficacy and self-confidence
5. Enhances adherence to other weight-control behaviors

Health benefits

1. Decreases heart rate
2. Decreases blood pressure
3. Improves plasma lipid profile
4. Improves insulin sensitivity

initial treatment (Dahlkoetter et al., 1979; Harris & Hallbauer, 1973; Stalonas et al., 1978, 1984). Because the contributions of exercise to increased caloric expenditure are relatively small on a daily basis (e.g., 200 calories per day), therapists must orient their patients to understand that the weight-related benefits of exercise will not be evident immediately but will accrue instead on a long-term, cumulative basis.

Clinicians often find it heartening to learn that increased physical activity is one of the few factors consistently associated with successful weight management. In a recent study, Kayman and her colleagues (1990) examined the differences between women who had lost 20% of their body weight and had kept it off for two years, versus those who had lost an equivalent amount but had regained their lost weight. The researchers found that 90% of the maintainers reported exercising regularly compared to only 34% of the relapsers. Similar findings supportive of the impact of exercise on maintenance of weight loss have been reported in other retrospective studies (e.g., Colvin & Ohlson, 1983; Hoiberg, Berard, Watten, & Laine, 1984; Marston & Criss, 1984; Stalonas et al., 1984) and in prospective investigations as well (e.g., Pavlou et al., 1989; Perri et al., 1986, 1988).

What mechanisms account for the beneficial impact of increased physical activity on weight loss? Exercise appears to improve weight loss through several mechanisms, including increased thermogenesis, the preservation of lean body mass, appetite regulation, and possibly its effect on other weight-control behaviors. We now briefly examine each of these effects.

Caloric Expenditure. Energy expenditure is determined for the most part by the weight of the individual and by the type, intensity, and duration of a particular physical activity. For example, a 250-pound person who walks for 30 minutes at 3 miles per hour will expend 234 calories, whereas a 150-pound individual walking an identical distance at the same speed will expend 141 calories. The additional calories burned up by the heavier individual are accounted for by the simple fact that more energy is required to move a larger mass than a smaller one over an equivalent distance. Table 9.2 presents the energy expenditure (by body weight) associated with various physical activities. The clinician can use this table in helping the obese patient to determine the approximate number of calories expended in different activities.

Does exercise produce energy expenditure beyond the calories burned in the activity itself? More specifically, does exercise either raise RMR (resting metabolic rate) or increase the TEF (thermic effect of food)? These questions, which have been the center of scientific debate since the early 1970s, are highly relevant to the treatment of obesity because dieting alone produces significant reductions in energy expenditure from RMR and TEF (Barrows & Snook, 1987).

TABLE 9.2   ENERGY EXPENDITURE BY BODY WEIGHT IN SELECTED PHYSICAL ACTIVITIES

Activity	Calories per min per lb body weight	Body weight (lb)			
		150	200	250	300
Archery	.030	4.5	6.0	7.5	9.0
Basketball	.063	9.5	12.6	15.8	18.9
Bicycling					
(5.5 mph)	.029	4.4	5.8	7.3	8.7
(9.4 mph)	.045	6.8	9.0	11.3	13.5
Canoeing (leisure)	.020	3.0	4.0	5.0	6.0
Chopping wood	.039	5.9	7.8	9.8	11.7
Cleaning house	.027	4.1	5.4	6.8	8.1
Climbing hills	.055	8.3	11.0	13.8	16.5
Cooking	.021	3.2	4.2	5.3	6.3
Dancing (slow)	.023	3.5	4.6	5.8	6.9
Dancing (fast)	.046	6.9	9.2	11.5	13.8
Digging (trenches)	.066	9.9	13.2	16.5	19.8
Field hockey	.061	9.2	12.2	15.3	18.3
Fishing	.028	4.2	5.6	7.0	8.4
Food shopping	.027	4.1	5.4	6.8	8.1
Football	.060	9.0	12.0	15.0	18.0
Golf	.039	5.9	7.8	9.8	11.7
Horse riding (trot)	.050	7.5	10.0	12.5	15.0
Ironing	.022	3.3	4.4	5.5	6.6
Lying at ease	.010	1.5	2.0	2.5	3.0
Mopping floor	.027	4.1	5.4	6.8	8.1
Mowing	.051	7.7	10.2	12.8	15.3
Painting (house)	.035	5.3	7.0	8.8	10.5
Racquetball	.096	14.4	19.2	24.0	28.8
Raking	.025	3.8	5.0	6.3	7.5
Running					
9 min/mile	.088	13.2	17.6	22.0	26.4
12 min/mile	.061	9.2	12.2	15.3	18.3
Sawing by hand	.034	5.1	6.8	8.5	10.2
Scrubbing floors	.050	7.5	10.0	12.5	15.0
Sewing	.011	1.7	2.2	2.8	3.3
Sitting	.010	1.5	2.0	2.5	3.0
Skiing (downhill)	.050	7.5	10.0	12.5	15.0
Standing quietly	.012	1.8	2.4	3.0	3.6
Swimming					
Backstroke	.077	11.5	15.4	19.3	23.1
Breast stroke	.074	11.1	14.8	18.5	22.2
Crawl (fast)	.071	10.7	14.2	17.8	21.3
Crawl (slow)	.058	8.7	11.6	14.5	17.4
Table tennis	.031	4.7	6.2	7.8	9.3
Tennis	.050	7.5	10.0	12.5	15.0
Typing	.012	1.8	2.4	3.0	3.6
Volleyball	.023	3.5	4.6	5.8	6.9
Walking					
3 mph	.031	4.7	6.2	7.8	9.3
4 mph	.041	6.2	8.2	10.3	12.3

TABLE 9.2   *(continued)*

Activity	Calories per min per lb body weight	Body weight (lb)			
		150	200	250	300
Wallpapering	.022	3.3	4.4	5.5	6.6
Weeding	.033	5.0	6.6	8.3	9.9
Window cleaning	.027	4.1	5.4	6.8	8.1

Note. Energy expenditure has been evaluated in terms of calories per minute. Energy values have been calculated from data presented by Bannister and Brown, 1969; Howley and Glover, 1974; McArdle, Katch, and Katch, 1986; and Passmore and Durnin, 1955.

The impact of exercise on resting energy expenditure is particularly important to obesity treatment for two key reasons: first, RMR accounts for the largest portion of daily energy expenditure (i.e., approximately 70%), and second, dieting commonly decreases RMR by 15–30% (Bray, 1969; Foster et al., 1988, 1990). Research on the effect of exercise on RMR has yielded a mixed set of findings. Some studies show an increase in RMR due to exercise (e.g., Lennon, Nagle, Stratman, Shrago, & Dennis, 1984), whereas others fail to find such an effect (e.g., Poehlman, Melby, & Badylak, 1988). Some researchers (Lennon et al., 1984) have suggested that the discrepancy in results may be attributable to the differences in the intensity of physical activities used in various studies. Moreover, the intensity of exercise required to increase RMR may be beyond what can reasonably be accomplished by most obese patients. Pi-Sunyer (1988) has concluded that levels of exercise completed by obese people in weight-reduction programs result in increases in RMR that last only 40–60 minutes beyond the completion of the exercise bout.

One potent effect of exercise may be its ability to *limit the decrease in RMR* that accompanies prolonged caloric restriction (Donahoe et al., 1984; Frey-Hewitt, Vranizan, Dreon, & Wood, 1990). For example, in a 1989 study, the addition of exercise completely reversed the decrease in RMR associated with the use of a VLCD (very-low calorie diet) (Mole, Stern, Schultz, Bernauer, & Holcomb).

In obese individuals, the increase in energy expenditure associated with nutrient consumption (i.e., TEF) is often blunted, compared to normal-weight individuals (see Chapter 2). An additional but minor benefit of exercise is its impact on this component of energy expenditure. Increased physical activity seems to enhance TEF (Segal & Pi-Sunyer, 1989).

Body Composition.   Exercise can preserve the loss of lean tissue during dieting. Obese people who reduce weight by caloric restriction alone tend to lose significant amounts of muscle tissue, in addition to fat (Hill,

Sparling, Shields, & Heller, 1987). The combination of exercise plus dieting, however, preserves lean body mass and leads to a higher proportion of weight loss from adipose tissue. In a comparison of the effects of diet versus diet plus exercise in obese men, Pavlou et al. (1989) found an equivalent weight loss for the two treatments, but the loss for the diet-only group was 36% from lean tissue, whereas the loss in the exercise-treatment group was virtually all from fat mass. For many obese patients, who often are quite concerned about appearance, findings such as these can serve as a motivational incentive to exercise. Patients are glad to learn that exercise will maximize fat loss while minimizing the loss of muscle tissue.

In addition to its positive aesthetic consequences, the effect of exercise on the preservation of muscle tissue can result in increased energy expenditure as well. Because lean body mass is the major determinant of RMR, an individual who minimizes the loss of lean tissue while dieting will experience less of a decrease in RMR. Accordingly, some researchers (e.g., Ballor, Katch, Becque, & Marks, 1988) have suggested that the combination of resistant weight training (i.e., weightlifting exercises) plus dieting may be a particularly effective means of increasing muscle mass and producing a beneficial long-term impact on RMR and energy expenditure.

Appetite.   Exercise cynics contend that increased exercise produces greater appetite and that the energy consumed following exercise often exceeds the energy expended during exercise. The impact of exercise on appetite has long been a matter of scientific debate, and conflicting results have been reported. The difficulty of accurately measuring food consumption and exercise in people who are living in their natural environment may be partly responsible for contradictory findings. However, carefully designed metabolic ward studies have now provided a clearer picture of the relationship between physical activity and appetite. Specifically, Pi-Sunyer and his colleagues (Pi-Sunyer, 1988; Woo, Garrow, & Pi-Sunyer, 1982; Woo & Pi-Sunyer, 1985) found that obese women and lean women responded differently to increases in their physical activity. For average-weight women, an increase in exercise produced a corresponding increase in caloric consumption and no change in weight. For obese women, on the other hand, an increase in exercise did *not* result in increased food consumption. Furthermore, because their calorie intake remained stable while their energy expenditure was increased, the obese women experienced significant weight losses directly due to exercise. These well-designed studies have important practical implications. Clinicians can assure their obese patients that increasing their exercise will not increase their appetite or food intake. When they exercise, obese patients can expect to lose weight in direct proportion to the amount of energy expended during exercise.

Psychological Benefits

In addition to its impact on weight, regular exercise also produces a number of significant psychological benefits. People who exercise regularly often report an improved sense of well-being associated with fitness, and research studies have shown that regular exercise improves self-concept and self-image and results in a sense of enhanced quality of life (Folkins & Sime, 1981; Hughes, 1984). For example, King, Frey-Hewitt, Dreon, and Wood (1989) documented that sedentary adults who began a program of regular exercise experienced significant improvements in perceived fitness and satisfaction with body image. In addition, exercise reduces subjective distress. Numerous studies have shown that increased physical activity has a positive impact on negative affective states, such as anxiety, tension, and depression. Exercise can reduce muscle tension and state anxiety and can alleviate many of the symptoms associated with clinical depression (deVries & Adams, 1972; Doyne, Chambless, & Beutler, 1983; Doyne et al., 1987; Klein et al., 1985; Morgan & Horstman, 1976). Regular exercise also has a positive impact on the individual's sense of self-confidence and self-efficacy (Clark, Abrams, Niaura, Eaton, & Rossi, 1991).

For patients in treatment for obesity, exercise may have an impact on adherence to other weight-control behaviors. For example, the time that patients spend exercising reduces their opportunities for eating and, immediately after exercising, people generally are not interested in eating. Moreover, many patients indicate that they feel better as a result of exercise. Anecdotally, they report that their positive affect has a beneficial impact on their motivation to limit food intake and to make healthful food choices. Thus, in addition to serving as an inhibitor of food intake, exercise may also serve as a cue to maintain moderate caloric intake and positive weight-loss behaviors. Finally, for many patients, exercise represents a symbol of positive change. Weight loss often requires that they *cut* out favorite foods and *eliminate* comfortable habits. Exercise, on the other hand, allows them to *add* something positive to their lives.

Health-Related Benefits

In addition to psychological and weight-related benefits, exercise produces important improvements in health. Exercise reduces a variety of risk factors that contribute to increased morbidity and mortality in obese people. The positive impact of exercise is most clearly demonstrated in its effects on risk factors for coronary heart disease and diabetes mellitus.

In terms of coronary risk factors, exercise decreases heart rate (Pavlou et al., 1989), reduces blood pressure (Hagberg, 1990), and leads to beneficial changes in blood lipids (Wood, Stefanick, & Haskell, 1985). For obese patients, the specific contribution of exercise has sometimes been difficult to quantify, independent of changes in body weight and food intake. However, results from nonobese subjects suggest that improvements in coronary risk factors can be substantial, provided that a threshold of exercise intensity, duration, and frequency, and length of training is exceeded (King & Tribble, 1991).

Exercise also produces significant benefits in the prevention and control of Type II diabetes in obese patients. Obese patients tend to utilize carbohydrates less efficiently due to a decreased sensitivity to insulin. Exercise enhances insulin sensitivity and leads to lower blood glucose levels. These improvements have been observed independent of changes in weight or body composition (Bjorntorp et al., 1977).

DESIGNING AN EXERCISE PROGRAM

Safety of Exercise

Before initiating an exercise program with an obese patient, the clinician needs to consider the risks of exercise in terms of the safety of the patient. Exercise itself will not produce serious medical complications in a person unless the individual has a significant underlying disease. For those persons with a known disease, such as cardiovascular disease, the absolute risks of serious medical complications during exercise are low. However, the risks associated with exercise are relatively higher than the risks associated with sedentary activities. Thus, in order to develop an individually tailored, safe and effective exercise plan, the clinician must determine whether a patient requires a comprehensive medical evaluation prior to the initiation of increased physical activity. Toward this end, the American College of Sports Medicine (1991) has recommended that potential exercise participants be classified according to the following risk categories:

1. *Apparently healthy.* This group consists of individuals who are asymptomatic and report no more than one of the following major coronary risk factors: (a) hypertension (i.e., systolic blood pressure $\geq$ 160 or diastolic blood pressure $\geq$ 90), (b) a serum cholesterol level $\geq$ 240 mg/dL, (c) cigarette smoking, (d) diabetes mellitus, or (e) a family history of coronary disease in parents or siblings prior to age 55.

2. *Individuals at higher risk.* A person is considered to be at higher risk if he or she either has two or more major risk factors for coronary disease or has symptoms suggestive of possible cardiopulmonary or metabolic disease (i.e., chest pain, shortness of breath, dizziness, difficulty breathing when lying flat, heart palpitations, heart murmur, ankle edema, or poor circulation to the legs).

3. *Individuals with disease.* This group comprises persons with known cardiac, pulmonary, or metabolic disease (e.g., angina pectoris, emphysema, or diabetes mellitus, respectively).

Once an individual's risk status has been appraised, the American College of Sports Medicine (1991) recommends that the clinician use the following guidelines to determine whether a medical evaluation and exercise testing are needed before beginning an exercise program.

For apparently healthy individuals, a program of what they call "moderate" intensity exercise (e.g., walking) may be initiated without exercise testing or medical examination, provided that the person is made aware of signs and symptoms that require medical attention. *Moderate exercise* is defined as an activity within the individual's capacity to sustain comfortably for a relatively long period of time (e.g., 60 minutes). For apparently healthy individuals, "vigorous" exercise (e.g., jogging) can be initiated without testing or medical evaluation in men under age 40 and women under age 50. *Vigorous exercise* is defined as a challenging activity, which produces a significant increase in heart rate and cannot be sustained by an untrained person for more than 15–20 minutes. It is advisable for men over 40 and women over 50 to have a medical examination and exercise testing before beginning a program of vigorous exercise.

For higher-risk individuals, a medical examination and a physician-supervised maximal exercise test is generally recommended before starting a program of increased physical activity. An exception may be made for asymptomatic individuals to begin a program of moderate exercise with appropriate guidance. For individuals with known disease, a thorough medical evaluation is needed prior to initiating any program of exercise.

Objectives of Exercise

How does the clinician design a program of physical activity appropriate to the needs of a particular obese patient? An essential starting point is to define the role and purpose of exercise in the patient's treatment. The patient and therapist should collaboratively identify the specific objectives that they seek to accomplish in developing a program of increased physical activity. These goals may differ from individual to individual. For example, the clinician may have a severely obese patient with an extremely sedentary life-style. For such an individual, the primary goal of exercise may be to increase caloric expenditure by gradually increasing daily activities that entail standing or walking rather than sitting. On the other hand, appropriate exercise goals for a mildly obese individual might include not only additional caloric expenditure but also improved cardiorespiratory fitness through a program of stationary cycling in the aerobic training range (i.e., at a level of intensity sufficient to increase cardiorespiratory endurance). A clear delineation of specific objectives, formulated jointly by clinician and patient, will enhance the patient's motivation and commitment to the exercise regimen.

Five Key Factors of an Exercise Regimen

Five factors must be considered in designing a systematic and individually tailored regimen of physical activity: (1) the mode or type of activity, (2) the intensity of exercise, (3) the duration of an exercise bout, (4) the frequency of exercise, and (5) the progression of the exercise regimen.

Type of Exercise. The type or mode of physical activity used in an exercise program will depend in large part on whether the clinician and the patient have determined that the primary goal of exercise will be caloric expenditure alone versus caloric expenditure plus increased cardiorespiratory fitness. When the major objective is caloric expenditure, the exercise program can be based primarily on increases in the amounts of routine daily activities. If, on the other hand, the objectives are broader and include improvements in cardiorespiratory fitness, then the physical activity regimen will ordinarily be based on particular periods of time specifically devoted to a program of aerobic exercise activities. In many cases, it is appropriate to fashion an exercise regimen consisting of both routine and programmed activities.

During the course of a typical day, most of the energy that an average person expends (beyond basal metabolism) is the result of routine activities of living, including sitting, standing, walking, and specific work-related tasks. Activities that involve greater movement entail a greater expenditure of energy. Thus, the various choices that patients make during the course of a day can produce meaningful increases in their caloric expenditure. For example, if a 200-pound person decided to climb stairs rather than riding an elevator for 10 minutes of each day, the individual would increase the daily caloric expenditure by more than 200 calories. During the course of a single workweek, this change would result in an increase in energy expenditure exceeding 1000 calories. If maintained over the long run, this seemingly small change in routine activity could contribute significantly to the weight-loss effort. In addition, successful changes in routine activities may help the patients to view themselves as less sedentary, as more physically active, and as more capable of initiating a program of aerobic exercise.

Aerobic exercise entails continuous rhythmic movement of large muscle groups that keeps pace with the body's demand for oxygen and can be maintained for a prolonged period. Since the early 1970s, the health benefits of programmed aerobic exercise have been widely recognized. In addition to increasing energy expenditure, individual bouts of aerobic activities increase heart rate, deepen breathing, and expand the blood vessels, enabling the circulatory system to carry greater amounts of oxygen to the muscles. Over the long run, aerobic exercise can enhance fitness by increasing cardiorespiratory endurance and by improving the proportion of lean to fat tissue (Phinney, LaGrange, O'Connell, & Danforth, 1988). Examples of aerobic activities include walking, hiking, jogging, running, swimming, skating, bicycling, rowing, and cross-country skiing. In helping obese patients to choose an appropriate type of physical activity, the clinician should keep in mind the following considerations that may increase the chances of long-term adherence (Falls, Baylor, & Dishman, 1980).

1. *Enjoyability.* Does the exercise involve an activity that the patient enjoys? Activities that individuals experience as being aversive are not likely to become lasting parts of their life-styles. Thus, it is important to have patients choose activities that they like to do. Sometimes, either varying the type of activity or the setting in which it occurs can make exercise more interesting. In addition, physical activity can be made more personally enjoyable by determining whether the patient prefers exercising alone, with a partner, or in a group.

2. *Convenience.* Does the patient have a convenient time and place to exercise? If the patient has to drive 45 minutes in rush-hour traffic to get to a health club in order to use a stationary cycle, the probability of maintenance will be low. Similarly, if access to a place for exercise is overly restrictive, or if the time for exercise regularly conflicts with other obligations, it is unlikely that the physical activity will become a part of the individual's routine. Helping patients to find a convenient time and place to exercise is essential to long-term success.

3. *Expectations.* Unrealistic expectations, whether positive or negative, can scuttle the development of an effective long-term regimen. Patients who expect too much too soon from exercise are likely to experience disappointments and dissatisfaction. Similarly, individuals who adhere to a workout philosophy of "no pain, no gain" often create for themselves an exercise program that is too aversive to be maintained over the long run. Thus, clinicians should help orient patients to reasonable expectations about the benefits of different types and amounts of exercise. Furthermore, it is essential that patients recognize that the benefits from exercise will accrue over the course of months rather than days.

The brief review that follows describes the recognized benefits and liabilities of some commonly used physical activities. The clinician may use these considerations to help the patient plan a comprehensive exercise program.

Walking. A 1991 report from the American College of Sports Medicine concluded that "many sedentary individuals would be healthier if they simply took a brisk walk for 30 to 60 minutes every other day" (p. 1). In many ways, walking is the ideal exercise for obese individuals. It provides good aerobic benefit, has a very low injury rate, is not seasonal, is inexpensive, requires no special equipment or settings, and can be done alone or with a group. Because no new skills are required, a walking program can be a positive experience from the outset. Even the first 15 minutes of a new walking program can provide as much pleasure as the hour walks the individual may eventually build up to. All too often, the reason that many people drop out of exercise programs is that they attempt activities that are beyond their physical capacity, and they wind up feeling overwhelmed and discouraged. Walking is an excellent activity with which to begin a physical-fitness program because it is noncompetitive, and individuals can proceed at their own pace. Moreover, a walking program can improve cardiovascular conditioning, enhance general fitness, and provide a sense of personal accomplishment (McArdle & Toner, 1988). In addition, walking is an effective means of energy expenditure. Walking a mile burns as many calories as jogging a mile because distance, not speed, is what counts.

Walking has become an increasingly popular activity. Almost every state has walking clubs that plan weekly or monthly outings and publish newsletters that provide information about places and times for walking with a group. In addition, throughout the country, shopping malls provide opportunities for year-round exercise. Many malls open their doors early and serve as a haven for individuals who wish to walk with a group in a temperature-controlled environment. Details about walking groups and their meeting times can usually be obtained from the general information desk in each mall.

Walking does require a couple of important accessories—a good pair of shoes. Poorly fitting shoes can cause a variety of immediate and long-term problems that can seriously limit the individual's ability to exercise and can thereby become an obstacle to long-term adherence. When shopping for a pair of walking shoes, patients should wear the type of socks that will be used during exercise, and measurements for size should be taken while the purchasers are standing. They should be aware that there are a number of key differences between shoes for walking and those for running. The foot flexes more in walking, and a good walking shoe should allow for this. To test for flexibility, the toe of the shoe should be able to be bent back toward the heel, short of the laces. Walking shoes must also provide adequate cushioning and support. The inner side of the shoe should be made of firmer material than the other parts of the sole. However, less cushioning is needed than in running shoes because the impact to the foot is not as great. In walking, the foot comes into greater contact with the ground; a thinner sole allows a better feel for the ground and reduces the possibility of tripping.

Jogging. Although jogging and running are excellent means of achieving aerobic conditioning, they are generally *not* appropriate exercises for obese patients. The risk of orthopedic injuries from jogging and running is quite high because the impact force on the knees and ankles is two to three times greater than that from walking. Thus, the potential for injuries to the joints is particularly high in obese individuals. However, if a *mildly* obese patient expresses serious interest in jogging, the clinician may consider setting a target body weight that must be achieved before a jogging program can begin. This approach may serve as an additional incentive for weight loss and may help to prevent injury as well.

Stationary Cycling. Stationary cycling can serve as an important exercise option for many obese individuals, particularly those with joint problems that may make walking painful. Stationary cycling provides many of the benefits of brisk walking and also has as low a risk of injury. In addition, it is an even more accessible an activity because it can be performed at home, in hot or cold weather, at any time of the day or night. Although stationary cycling can be somewhat boring, the variety of other activities that the individual can accomplish while cycling often compensate for this limitation. For example, the exerciser can listen to music, watch television, or read a book while cycling. Individuals who are easily deterred by even a small amount of exercise preparation frequently find stationary cycling an easy activity to initiate, and obese patients who are embarrassed about exercising in public often appreciate the opportunity to engage in a viable aerobic exercise in the privacy of their homes.

In considering the purchase of an exercise bike, the patient will need to evaluate durability and comfort, as well as expense. Stationary cycles come in a wide range of prices, with a variety of sophisticated options. Some have instruments that monitor pulse rate, as well as speed and mileage. However, it is critical to find a durable cycle that will be comfortable to use for an extended period of time (i.e., 30 minutes). Most bikes allow for adjustments in the height of the seat and the position of the handlebars, but different brands vary considerably in the sturdiness of their frame and comfort of their seat. These are particularly important considerations for obese patients. Patients should be encouraged to do comparison shopping to find a sturdy cycle with a comfortable seat. Taking a "test drive" often can help individuals to make informal decisions about the purchase of cycles that meet their needs.

Swimming. Swimming can be an excellent aerobic activity that can effectively contribute to conditioning of the entire body. Unlike walking or stationary cycling, which rely primarily on lower body movement, swimming also provides for conditioning of the upper body. Swimming is a particularly good exercise for obese individuals because the buoyancy of the water reduces any stress to the joints. Swimming does have some practical drawbacks. Frequent and regular access to a pool on a year-round basis is required, and many obese individuals are uncomfortable about being seen in a bathing suit.

Recreational Sports. Sports such as tennis, racquetball, volleyball, or handball can be beneficial when played vigorously for a sustained period of time. However, these activities often involve relatively long periods of light exercise, punctuated by moments of intense action. To produce aerobic benefit, they must be played *continuously* without significant breaks. The running that is involved, as well as the abrupt stopping and starting movements demanded by these sports, can be stressful to the joints. Thus, these activities are generally *not* appropriate for obese patients to use as the *foundation* of an aerobic training regimen. However, they certainly can be used on an occasional basis, for both fun and caloric expenditure.

Intensity of Exercise. The intensity of an activity is measured by the demand that it places on the cardiorespiratory system. Intensity is typically expressed as a percentage of maximum heart rate (HR max) or maximum aerobic capacity (VO_2 max). From a practical standpoint, heart rate or pulse can be used to gauge exercise intensity. The HR max can be estimated by subtracting an individual's age from 220. Patients can determine the relative intensity of an exercise by taking their pulse during exercise and dividing it by their HR max. For example, a 40-year-old woman would have an estimated HR max of 180 beats per minute (i.e., HR max = 220 – age). After 10 minutes of brisk walking, her pulse is 120 beats per minute. Thus, she is exercising at an intensity level equivalent to 67% of HR max (i.e., 120 divided by HR max of 180).

Exercise intensity determines its value in improving cardiorespiratory fitness. Generally, an exercise intensity equivalent of greater than 70% of HR max is viewed as the threshold necessary to produce improvements in cardiorespiratory fitness. However, for sedentary individuals who do not have a high degree of fitness, an intensity threshold of 60% of HR max can produce an aerobic training effect (McArdle & Toner, 1988). Table 9.3 presents estimated maximum heart rates and an aerobic training range (i.e., 60–70% of HR max) suitable for sedentary individuals of different ages. Most people do not find an intensity level of 60% HR max to be exceedingly strenuous. This moderate level can be comfortably maintained by most sedentary individuals for an extended period of time (i.e., 20 minutes or more).

To monitor exercise intensity, pulse rate should be taken immediately

TABLE 9.3   AEROBIC TRAINING RANGE FOR SEDENTARY ADULTS

Age (years)	Target zone 60% to 70% (beats per min)	Estimated maximum heart rate
25	117–137	195
30	114–133	190
35	111–130	185
40	108–126	180
45	105–123	175
50	102–119	170
55	99–116	165
60	96–112	160
65	93–109	155

after exercise. Except in rare cases, the number of heartbeats per minute is equivalent to the number of pulse beats per minute. Heart rate can be checked at any convenient pulse point. Generally, the carotid artery in the neck or the radial artery in the wrist are the best places for taking a pulse. The patient should be instructed to place the tips of two fingers, usually the index and middle fingers, over the carotid artery at the side of the neck. This tends to be a strong pulse point and is found under the jaw line near the ear. The thumb should not be used because it also has a light pulse that will interfere with the accuracy of this reading. To take a pulse reading at the wrist, the patient should place the tips of two fingers (e.g., index and middle fingers) on the inside of the wrist, immediately below the thumb.

Once the pulse point is found, the beats are counted for 15 seconds. The 15-second rate is multiplied by 4 to determine the rate per minute. This provides a more accurate reading than would be obtained by taking the pulse for a full 60 seconds because heart rate drops off quickly following cessation of exercise. It may take some practice before a reliable reading can be obtained consistently. Individuals who have difficulty locating their resting pulse should find that it is much stronger following a bout of exercise.

As individuals advance in their exercise programs, whether they have chosen brisk walking or any of the other aerobic activities that have been described, they are likely to experience positive changes, both in their endurance for exercise and in their sense of well-being.

Duration of Exercise.   For cardiorespiratory improvement, it is generally recommended that an exercise bout entail a minimum of 15–20 minutes of continuous aerobic activity. However, duration needs to be considered in relation to the intensity of exercise. In general, lower-intensity activities need to span longer periods of time in order to achieve an aerobic training effect. Exercise bouts of 30 minutes of moderately intense activity, such as walking, can generally produce significant aerobic benefits.

In terms of weight loss, there is a direct correspondence between exercise duration and its impact on weight change. The longer an activity is carried out, the greater the amount of energy expended, regardless of the intensity of the activity. Some researchers (Leon & Blackburn, 1983) have suggested that in order to have a measurable impact on weight loss, an effective exercise bout must last long enough to produce an energy expenditure of 300 calories.

An important caveat should be noted by the clinician. Talking to obese patients about thresholds for physical activity, such as the necessary duration of an exercise bout, can sometimes have an unintended inhibiting effect on their exercise behavior. For example, some patients may mistakenly interpret recommendations for a 30-minute, 300-calorie exercise session as meaning that any lesser amount of exercise is ineffective and therefore not worth doing. Thus, clinicians must strongly convey the message that *any* exercise activity—no matter how brief—is better than no exercise. Indeed, it is often a good idea to encourage obese patients to use "minibouts" of exercise throughout the course of each day. We regularly urge our patients to substitute 5-minute "walk breaks" in place of their morning and afternoon coffee breaks. In addition to the extra calories that they expend, patients benefit by seeing themselves as more active and energetic individuals.

Frequency of Exercise. The minimum frequency of exercise needed to achieve either aerobic fitness or weight loss appears to be *three* days per week. Additional benefits appear to be achieved with exercise frequencies of four or five times per week. For cardiorespiratory fitness, the incremental benefits of exercising more than five times per week appear to be marginal. For weight loss, however, caloric expenditure is directly related to the total amount of exercise completed. Thus, exercising six or seven times per week provides more opportunities to burn off additional calories. With high-intensity exercises such as jogging, the risk of injury increases significantly when the frequency of exercise exceeds five days per week. This issue is less of a problem for moderate exercise such as walking. Indeed, many individuals report that they find it helpful to make walking a daily habit.

Progression of the Exercise Regimen

Gradual Change. In initiating an exercise program with sedentary individuals, the clinician should be mindful that "less is better." Beginning with an amount of exercise or intensity level that is too great for the individual to comfortably complete will result in an unpleasant or even punishing experience. Moreover, recommending too much too soon can damage the individual's motivation for exercise and can lead to poor adherence. Starting with a small amount of moderate-intensity exercise and then gradually increasing the frequency and duration can provide the patient with a successful introduction to exercise. As a consequence, patients often experience an increase in self-confidence regarding their ability to accomplish exercise goals, and they come to view exercise in a more positive light as well.

In our weight-loss programs, we typically initiate exercise by asking patients to start at low levels of walking or stationary cycling. We purposely make the initial demand on the individual as light as feasible. For example, we often ask patients to begin with a 10-minute walk to be completed at a leisurely pace (i.e., ≤ 60% HR max) three times during the first week. If the walk becomes uncomfortable, they are encouraged to stop and rest. When using stationary cycling, during the first week, we ask patients to complete three 8-minute bouts, with minimal resistance set on their exercise cycles. Furthermore, in each bout, we suggest that they stop after 4 minutes. This allows time for them to take their pulse to be sure that they are not exceeding 70% of maximum heart, and it also provides them with a brief rest break. In our experience, the vast majority of patients complete the entire amount of the first week of exercise and thus get off to successful start in their program of physical activity.

Supervised Exercise.   In addition to designing a schedule that very gradually initiates patients to increased physical activity, supervision of exercise can also enhance adherence and provide an opportunity for observation of potential problems. For example, conducting the first bout of exercise in the course of an obesity treatment session will allow the clinician to model and monitor key elements of an exercise routine. The clinician can spot patients who may have a tendency to overdo exercise or to do it incorrectly, and the clinician can provide immediate corrective feedback. Similarly, the clinician can provide praise and reinforcing feedback to participants who carry out the exercise recommendations in an appropriate manner. Making exercise a regular component of each therapy session highlights for the patient its significance in the management of obesity. In addition, if some patients have not exercised since the previous treatment meeting, in-session exercise allows an opportunity to get "back on track," and patients can leave the session with a sense of having regained control of a key element in their weight-management program.

The usual progression of an exercise program involves gradual increases to higher levels of frequency, duration, and intensity. During the first phase of obesity treatment, a common prescription for sedentary adults begins initially with 10 minutes of exercise, completed 2 or 3 days per week. Then, over a 5- to 6-month period, this level is gradually increased to 30 minutes of exercise, completed 5 days per week. Table 9.4 provides a sample of how the frequency and duration of walking might be gradually increased during a 24-week program.

**TABLE 9.4   SAMPLE PROGRESSION OF FREQUENCY AND DURATION IN A
WALKING PROGRAM FOR SEDENTARY OBESE ADULTS**

Week of treatment	Duration	Frequency	Weekly total
Week 1	10 minutes	3 times per week	30 minutes
Week 2	10 minutes	4 times per week	40 minutes
Week 3	12 minutes	4 times per week	48 minutes
Week 4	14 minutes	4 times per week	56 minutes
Week 5	14 minutes	5 times per week	70 minutes
Week 6	15 minutes	5 times per week	75 minutes
Week 7	16 minutes	5 times per week	80 minutes
Week 8	17 minutes	5 times per week	85 minutes
Week 9	18 minutes	5 times per week	90 minutes
Week 10	19 minutes	5 times per week	95 minutes
Week 11	20 minutes	5 times per week	100 minutes
Week 12	21 minutes	5 times per week	105 minutes
Week 13	22 minutes	5 times per week	110 minutes
Week 14	23 minutes	5 times per week	115 minutes
Week 15	24 minutes	5 times per week	120 minutes
Week 16	25 minutes	5 times per week	125 minutes
Week 17	26 minutes	5 times per week	130 minutes
Week 18	27 minutes	5 times per week	135 minutes
Week 19	28 minutes	5 times per week	140 minutes
Week 20	29 minutes	5 times per week	145 minutes
Week 21	30 minutes	5 times per week	150 minutes
Week 22	30 minutes	5 times per week	150 minutes
Week 23	30 minutes	5 times per week	150 minutes
Week 24	30 minutes	5 times per week	150 minutes

Note. This table illustrates a gradual progression of exercise under ideal circumstances. Actual exercise goals should be tailored to the progress of the particular patient.

As patients increase the frequency, duration, and intensity of their exercise, their aerobic capacity improves, and they are able to increase the total work done per session. Specific adjustments in the progression of exercise should be tailored to the accomplishments made by the particular individual. Weekly reviews of exercise allow an opportunity to provide patients with feedback about their performance. The clinician can reinforce progress and use problem solving to deal with difficulties in exercise performance. It is generally helpful for the clinician and patient to collaboratively set *weekly goals* for exercise. These can be based on the individual's (a) exercise accomplishments during the previous week and (b) perceived ability to achieve additional increases in exercise.

Monitoring Progress. Keeping an exercise diary is a useful way in which patients can monitor their exercise progress. In addition to serving as the basis for weekly goal setting, an exercise log can serve as a powerful source of reinforcement. Charting increases in the frequency and duration of exercise often provides patients with a sense of accomplishment that can help sustain adherence to their regimen of increased physical activity.

Exercise diaries can vary in complexity and the amount of information recorded. We generally encourage participants to begin with a daily log that includes the following four pieces of information about each bout of exercise: (1) date, (2) type of activity (i.e., walking, stationary cycling, etc.), (3) duration (i.e., number of minutes of exercise), and (4) intensity (i.e., heart rate at end of exercise bout). On a weekly basis, patients tally up the number of days on which they exercised and the total number of minutes of exercise. These data are then compared to the goals previously set. If the patients have met their goals, the review of their progress provides an opportunity for the clinician to reinforce the accomplishments with ample praise. On the other hand, if the exercise log shows that patients have fallen short of their weekly goals, the clinician and patients can work together to identify obstacles to progress, and the problem-solving model can be implemented to determine a strategy to help the patients achieve a realistic amount of exercise for the following week.

In addition to duration and intensity, patients who are using walking, cycling, or swimming for exercise often find it particularly rewarding to monitor distance as well. Mileage can be established for an outdoor walking regimen by marking off the route by car. Indoor walkers who use malls for exercise will find that many malls have maps that describe the distance for a "lap" within their confines. In some instances, walkers may also find it helpful to purchase a pedometer to measure distance. A pedometer can be purchased at moderate cost (i.e., less than $20) in most sporting-goods stores. One advantage of using a pedometer is that the device can be worn throughout the day and thus can be used to monitor levels of routine activity, as well as programmed exercise. Patients who use stationary cycling as the basis of their exercise regimen can easily keep track of distance because most exercise cycles have an odometer. Swimmers can monitor distance by determining the length of the pool and keeping track of laps.

One reason why patients find it helpful to keep track of distance is that as they improve their endurance, they are able to accomplish greater distances in briefer periods of time. For example, at the start of a walking program, many moderately obese patient with sedentary life-styles require 20 to 22 minutes to walk 1 mile. After several months of a regular walking program (and weight loss), these very same individuals are often able to walk 2 miles in 30 minutes. Thus, by keeping track of distance as well as duration, many patients are truly impressed by their progress, and their exercise accomplishments often serve as a special source of pride.

Once the exercise pattern is established and a desired level of intensity achieved, the exercise log can be simplified for the sake of convenience. The easiest ways to accomplish this is to have the patient record on a daily basis either the duration or the distance of exercise. For example, the individual can simply jot down minutes (or miles) of daily exercise in an appointment book. This provides a simple and efficient record for the patient and obviates the necessity of keeping an additional book or set of papers. Weekly, monthly, or yearly totals can be readily obtained from these figures and can be used on a longer-term basis for setting goals and gauging progress.

Detraining Effects

Aerobic capacity and the other physical benefits of exercise quickly decline with lack of practice. If exercise is curtailed for just 1 week, the ability of the muscles to produce energy declines by as much as 50%. In fact, the enzymes in the muscle cells, which are essential to the production of energy, begin to decline within 3 days of the last exercise period. Regular exercise increases the number of capillaries surrounding each muscle fiber, but after 2 weeks without exercise, the number of capillaries decreases by approximately 20%. Thus, the delivery of oxygen to the muscle cells declines, contributing to a reduction in the capacity of the muscle to produce energy. Furthermore, as circulatory capacity diminishes, less oxygen is transported to the muscle cells. As a consequence, the resumption of exercise results in a quick buildup of lactic acid, thereby producing increased muscle fatigue.

The negative effects of a lapse in exercise highlight the importance of consistency in physical activity and provide justification for a continuous-care model of treatment. Lapses in exercise can be particularly problematic because as physical conditioning declines, the body is more vulnerable to the stresses of physical activity, and the resumption of exercise is often experienced as painful and tiring. These aversive consequences, in turn, decrease the chances that the individual will return to a regular routine of exercise. Many patients attribute their difficulties in resuming exercise to a loss of motivation or a lack of self-discipline. Such interpretations can have a deleterious impact not only on their exercise behavior but also on other aspects of their weight-management endeavor.

IMPROVING EXERCISE MAINTENANCE

Fewer than half of all people who begin an exercise regimen maintain it over the course of a year (Dishman, 1988). Moreover, overweight individuals as a group may be less likely to maintain fitness programs than people of average weight (Dishman, Sallis, & Orenstein, 1985). Thus, it is crucial that clinicians take active steps to help obese patients sustain their exercise regimens over the long run. The clinician can draw on many of the same strategies used to enhance maintenance of other weight-control behaviors to increase exercise maintenance as well. The most prominent of these include continuing therapist contact (including supervised exercise); the use of skills-training techniques, such as problem-solving and relapse-prevention procedures to overcome setbacks in exercise progress; and the development of social-support and social-influence strategies to prompt, model, and reinforce the maintenance of exercise (see Perri et al., 1986, 1988; also see Chapter 11).

In a recent investigation, Sallis et al. (1990) found that physical injury, loss of interest, work demands, and lack of time accounted for approximately 70% of relapses in exercise behavior. Of particular relevance to the treatment of obesity were the two factors (i.e., physical injury and loss of interest) that discriminated between those who maintained regular exercise versus those who relapsed and returned to a sedentary life-style.

Preventing Physical Injury

The greater weight of obese individuals may make them particularly vulnerable to physical injury. Thus, as we noted earlier, in order to improve the chances of long-term maintenance, it is essential that the clinician help the patient to develop a program of exercise that will minimize the risk of injury. In most cases, this means avoiding high-impact activities (e.g., jogging, running), keeping the intensity of exercise in the moderate range, and planning a gradual progression of exercise so that the demands on the body are not excessive. In addition, it is important that if an injury occurs, patients should get prompt attention from a health-care professional, preferably one who has experience in working with exercise-related injuries. In most communities, patients can locate physicians specializing in sports medicine to meet such needs. Thus, through careful planning, the clinician can help the patient to avoid or deal with physical injuries and thereby overcome one of the most significant risks of relapse from exercise maintenance.

Treating Motivation for Exercise

The second major discriminator between exercise maintainers and relapsers in the Sallis et al. (1990) study was loss of interest or motivation for exercise. As we noted earlier, to some extent, this factor may represent a post hoc explanation that patients provide for their relapse rather than a true precipitant of a lapse from physical activity. Nonetheless, it is essential that clinicians be prepared to deal with the issue of motivation in the maintenance of exercise. We have found two approaches to be helpful in this regard. The first is to build into the maintenance phase of treatment a regular series of lessons specifically designed to help patients stay motivated for exercise. The second is the use of a decision balance sheet, to help patients overcome a loss of interest or motivation for exercise.

Increasing Motivation for Exercise.   During the maintenance phase of obesity treatment, we routinely make discussion of exercise a regular part of every treatment session, both as review of the patient's progress and as a means of presenting new information or procedures that may enhance maintenance of the exercise regimen. To accomplish this objective, we recommend that clinicians consider the following motivational strategies suggested by Gibson, Gerberich, and Leon (1983):

1. Increase the patient's perceived susceptibility to obesity-related illnesses.
2. Increase the patient's knowledge about the benefits of exercise.
3. Decrease the patient's barriers to exercise.
4. Increase the patient's cues to exercise.

Increase Perceived Susceptibility to Illness.   A key question for many patients is simply why should they exercise. To deal with the impact of this question on an individual's motivation for exercise, Gibson et al. (1983) recommend having patients examine their personal susceptibility to major illnesses. Obese patients are at greater risk for coronary heart disease and diabetes mellitus by virtue of their degree of overweight. Most moderately obese individuals also have other risk factors for disease, such as hypertension, high levels of cholesterol, poor glucose tolerance, or a family history of heart disease or diabetes. Furthermore, many may already have known cardiac, pulmonary, or metabolic disease. By having participants review their personal susceptibility to these illnesses, the answer to the question "why exercise" becomes readily apparent: Exercise can help prevent the development or progression of many illnesses. An important caveat is worth noting, however. In addressing the issue of risk for disease, the clinician must refrain from the use of scare tactics as a means of motivation. Such an approach can backfire by producing high levels of anxiety and resulting in avoidance of the problem rather than active coping. Instead, the clinician should offer exercise to patients as a tangible option to reduce their personal risk of illness.

Increase Knowledge of Exercise Benefits.   Most health professionals are well aware that knowledge alone often does not result in behavior change. However, the combination of changes in behavior, coupled with information about the benefits of those changes can help reinforce the development of new habits. In the development of an exercise regimen, it is important that patients understand not only the procedural aspects (i.e., intensity, duration, and frequency) of how to set up an appropriate routine, but that they also understand both the physical and psychological effects that are likely to result from increased activity levels.

During the maintenance phase of our weight-loss programs, we carefully review the impact of exercise on health, weight, and well-being. We take the time to detail for the patient the specific processes involved. For example, we explain how regular exercise enhances insulin sensitivity and thereby leads to lower blood glucose levels and enhanced prevention or control of diabetes mellitus. We also explain how the development of exercise as a life-style habit can become a "positive addiction" with many psychological rewards. Patients appreciate the opportunity to learn about the physical and psychological mechanisms responsible for the beneficial effects of exercise. They also appreciate the metacommunication inherent in such sessions. Many patients have a history of contacts with health professionals in which they were told to change their habits "because the doctor said so." By taking the time to explain in detail *how* changes in their activity levels can have a positive impact on their health, clinicians not only provide patients with new information but also convey a sense of respect for patients as intelligent adults who are capable of integrating complex information. As a result, the esteem-building aspects of the communication between patient and clinician may facilitate the influence of knowledge on actual behavior change.

Decrease Barriers to Exercise. The fewer the obstacles to exercise, the greater are the chances of it being accomplished. It takes more motivation at the end of the workday for a person to drive across town, hunt down a parking space, change into an exercise outfit, and then begin an exercise regimen than it does to simply use 30 minutes during the lunch hour for a brisk walk. Thus, it is often helpful for clinician and patients to brainstorm about a variety of ways in which the obstacles to or costs of exercise can be minimized. By increasing the range of low-cost exercise options available to patients, the chances of continued motivation and adherence are increased. We recommend that patients develop a *menu of options* regarding the type of activity, times and places for exercise, and persons with whom to exercise. For example, patients who regularly walk for exercise might be encouraged to experiment with stationary cycling or swimming as well. Having more than one type of activity may make exercise more interesting, and the alternative activity may be available as a back-up in those instances when the individual cannot complete the usual type of exercise. Similarly, it is often very helpful for patients to have alternative times and places to exercise. Access to indoor and outdoor facilities for exercise can help individuals sustain their activity regimens throughout the year, and the flexibility of having an alternative time for exercise during the course of the day can help in coping with unanticipated scheduling conflicts. In addition, having the options to exercise with a group or with another person, such as a spouse or buddy, can have a positive impact on motivation to exercise. Indeed, our own research (Perri et al., 1988) showed that combining social-influence strategies with exercise produced significant increases in weight loss during the maintenance phase of obesity treatment (see Chapter 4).

Increase Cues to Exercise. Finally, clinicians can help patients to sustain their motivation for exercise by extensive use of stimulus-control strategies that encourage patients to continue exercise as a regular part of a daily life-style. Patients can plan ahead for physical activity by noting the times for exercise in their appointment books. They can also use environmental cues by posting graphs of data from their exercise logs in prominent places in their home or office, or they can put up signs or posters that remind them to exercise or highlight the importance of exercise. Laying out clothes or shoes for exercise in advance can also serve as a prompt for exercise, as can having a routine where exercise always occurs at the same time each day (i.e., before breakfast, during lunchtime, after clocking out at work, etc.). In addition, exercise awareness can be increased by having the individual become a positive role model or "exercise activist." Some patients find that by joining a walking club or arranging for a group of friends to exercise together that they not only increase the frequency of their exercise but also enhance the pleasure that they derive from their active life-styles.

Dealing with Loss of Motivation for Exercise: The Decision Balance Sheet. As noted earlier, it is quite common for patients who have relapsed from exercise to attribute their difficulty to a loss of motivation. Indeed, self-reported loss of motivation or interest in exercise is a distinguishing characteristic of individuals who abandon exercise and return to sedentary life-styles (Sallis et al., 1990). One approach that has shown promise in helping patients to avoid relapse from exercise is the use of the decision balance-sheet procedure. In accounting, the balance sheet lists the credits and debits of a company and provides a picture of its overall financial status. In 1975, Hoyt and Janis first described how a balance-sheet procedure could be used to increase motivation to adhere to changes in health behaviors.

This procedure entails a careful evaluation of the expected (or experienced) costs and benefits of various courses of action. Together, the clinician and patient weigh the advantages and disadvantages of various behavioral alternatives and come to agreement on a commitment to a particular course of action. The procedure is based on the premise that people are most likely to maintain a behavioral change when they perceive that they themselves have personally chosen to do so after fully considering the likely consequences of their actions.

In our work, we have adapted the decision balance sheet for use within the problem-solving framework. When patients report a lapse in exercise or a loss of motivation to continue their regimen of physical activity, the balance-sheet procedure can often help the patient and clinician to clarify the obstacles to progress. The following example illustrates this procedure.

Lynn, a 29-year old sales representative and mother of two children, ages 8 and 6 years old, entered our weight-loss program at 201 pounds.

Lynn told us that her goal was to get down to 160 pounds, and during the initial phase of obesity treatment, she made good progress, losing 27 pounds over 6 months. However, exercise was not a strong component of her weight-management effort. Indeed, Lynn had hoped to develop a *daily* walking program, but her activity diary showed that she rarely exercised more than two or three times per week. Moreover, when the second phase of treatment began, with sessions scheduled every other week rather than weekly, her walking dropped to an average of only one time per week. Lynn reported that she was frustrated by her lack of exercise progress, and she told the therapist that she was at the point where she believed it might be more beneficial for her to stop exercising altogether. She explained that the guilt feelings over not doing what she was supposed to be doing (i.e., exercising) were leading her to unplanned episodes of eating.

The therapist working with Lynn decided to use the balance-sheet procedure to help her with this problem. The therapist began by asking Lynn to draw up a list of personal advantages and disadvantages of exercise. Lynn quickly pointed out, however, that a big part of her concern about exercise had to do with its impact on her family. So the therapist adapted the procedure by asking Lynn to divide the lists of advantages and disadvantages into two groupings: first, the advantages and disadvantages to Lynn herself; and second, the advantages and disadvantages to other family members. Here are the lists constructed by Lynn:

Advantages to myself
1. Helps me control snacking
2. Helps me feel more energetic
3. Reduces my appetite
4. Helps me lose weight
5. Makes me feel more confident in myself

Disadvantages to myself
1. One more thing for me to do
2. Limits time I have for other activities
3. Disrupts the routine at work when I walk at lunchtime
4. Feel sweaty at work after walking at lunchtime
5. Feel sick when I walk in the hot sun

Advantages to my family
1. Puts me in a better mood
2. Makes me less crabby
3. Gives me more energy for the kids

4. Helps me feel more enthusiastic
5. Sets a good example for the kids

Disadvantages to my family
1. Takes time away from the kids
2. Delays making dinner when I exercise after work
3. Husband has to watch the kids when I walk at home

The next step in the balance-sheet process involved the therapist helping Lynn to categorize the various advantages and disadvantages into *types* of benefits and problems associated with exercise. The therapist suggested that Lynn first examine the lists of disadvantages for herself and family to see if any consistent types of problems were apparent. Lynn immediately noticed that the majority of disadvantages were *time-management* considerations (i.e., "one more thing for me to do," "limits time for other activities," "disrupts the routine at work," "takes time away from the kids," and "delays dinner"). Lynn further observed that a second problem with exercise seemed to be directly related to negative consequences of *walking at lunchtime* (i.e., "disrupts work when I walk at lunchtime," "feel sweaty walking at lunchtime," and "feel sick when I walk in the hot sun"). Finally, she noted a third type of problem that could be categorized as *imposition on her spouse* (i.e., "husband has to watch the kids when I walk at home").

In a similar manner, the therapist guided Lynn in categorizing the advantages associated with exercise. Lynn quickly pointed out that the major type of advantages that she experienced from exercise were psychological benefits (i.e., "more energetic," "more confident in myself," "better mood," "less crabby," and "more enthusiastic"). Another salient set of benefits from exercise for Lynn was the *positive impact on her eating* (i.e., "reduces appetite," "controls snacking," and "helps with weight loss").

Next, the therapist asked Lynn to consider the impact of two alternative courses of action. The first option would be give up exercise altogether and abandon any attempts to integrate physical activity into her weight-management program. The second course of action would be to try to come up with some new ways of integrating exercise into her life-style by dealing with the problems posed by exercise in the past. In order to make the choice between the two courses of action, the therapist and Lynn closely examined the types of advantages and disadvantages associated with exercise for Lynn. In considering the benefits and liabilities of exercise, Lynn concluded that the advantages associated with exercise clearly outweighed its disadvantages. Lynn decided to renew her commitment to giving exercise another chance.

The therapist, in turn, not only reinforced Lynn's decision but also suggested that the disadvantages identified by Lynn (i.e., time management, problems exercising at lunch time, and imposition on spouse) were crucial pieces of information that could be used to improve the likelihood of developing a lasting exercise regimen. Accordingly, the therapist suggested that problem-solving procedures be utilized to prevent these past obstacles from interfering with her future success with exercise.

SUMMARY

Exercise and increased physical activity can play a key role in the long-term management of obesity. The benefits of exercise include increased energy expenditure, the preservation of lean tissue, and improved long-term maintenance of weight-loss. Regular exercise has also been shown to reduce risk factors for coronary disease and to produce psychological benefits, such as improvements in mood and self-concept.

In designing an exercise program for obese patients, clinicians need to begin by determining whether a medical evaluation is needed. Obese patients with major risk factors or symptoms of cardiac, pulmonary, or metabolic disease require a comprehensive medical evaluation prior to initiating a program of increased physical activity. If the primary goal of exercise is simply to increase caloric expenditure, the clinician can help the patient to fashion a program based on gradual increases in routine activities of daily living (e.g., regular use of stairs versus elevators). If, on the other hand, the objective includes improved cardiorespiratory fitness, as well as increased energy expenditure, then a program of aerobic exercise will be required.

The type, intensity, duration, frequency, and progression of exercise must be considered in designing an individually tailored aerobic exercise regimen. Walking, stationary cycling, and swimming are excellent aerobic activities for obese individuals. Significant benefits can be obtained by performing these activities at moderate intensity (i.e., 60–70% of estimated HR max) for a duration of 15–30 minutes. The minimum frequency needed to achieve aerobic fitness appears to be three days per week. For weight reduction, however, caloric expenditure is directly related to the total amount of exercise completed, and a frequency of five or six times per week can improve weight loss. For obese adults with sedentary life-styles, an appropriate progression of exercise requires starting with a small amount of moderate-intensity exercise and very gradually increasing the frequency and duration of exercise.

Adherence to exercise can be increased by helping patients to find convenient times and places to perform activities that they personally find enjoyable. In addition, the clinician can enhance adherence by providing an opportunity for supervised exercise and by setting appropriate expectations for progress. Having participants keep a written exercise diary can facilitate the development of individualized weekly goal setting and can provide a basis for reinforcement of progress or troubleshooting, should problems arise.

Fewer than half of all people who begin an exercise regimen sustain it over the course of a year. Thus, in order to help patients continue exercise progress during the second phase of obesity treatment, the clinician must be prepared to take active steps to enhance exercise maintenance. Among the procedures that can be utilized are continuing therapist contacts (including supervised exercise); the use of skill-training techniques, such as problem-solving and relapse-prevention procedures to overcome setbacks in progress; and the development of social-support strategies to prompt, model, and reinforce the maintenance of exercise. In addition, during the maintenance phase of obesity treatment, adherence to exercise can be increased by using motivational strategies that (a) increase perceived susceptibility to obesity-related illness, (b) increase knowledge of exercise benefits, (c) decrease barriers to exercise, and (d) increase cues to exercise. Finally, for patients who have relapsed from exercise and have experienced a loss of interest in exercise, the decision balance-sheet procedure can be used to examine the costs and benefits of reverting to sedentary habits versus renewing the commitment to a life-style that includes regular exercise and increased physical activity. Helping patients to overcome obstacles to exercise can improve the prospects for long-term success in the management of obesity.

10

Dietary Considerations

Hardly a week goes by without a report in the national media about a "breakthrough" or a "controversy" regarding the foods that Americans should or should not eat in order to improve their health. Lively topics of debate typically center on the appropriate consumption of fats, fiber, sodium, sugar, vitamins, cholesterol, protein, and complex carbohydrates. Consumers are often faced with an array of contradictory advice about nutrition. For every proponent of a particular dietary practice, it often appears that an equally qualified expert can be found to take an opposing perspective. As a consequence, many consumers develop a skepticism about dietary guidelines, and some ignore appropriate advice because they cannot discriminate between sound and unsound nutritional recommendations. Thus, as a headline from *Newsweek* magazine recently exclaimed, "Overwhelmed by conflicting advice, most Americans have thrown in the napkin on healthy eating" (Shapiro et al., 1991, p. 46.).

For obese individuals, dietary dilemmas present an additional burden because their excess weight places them at higher risk for disease. Moreover, because obese people must consume less energy over an extended period of time in order to lose weight, the nutritional adequacy of their diet takes on added significance. In this chapter, we consider nutritional principles and dietary intake in relation to the long-term management of obesity. We begin first with the general issue of assessment and individualized dietary planning, and we address questions related to determining an appropriate level of caloric intake for long-term weight control. Next, we present dietary guidelines recommended by the American Heart Association, and we examine key concepts in nutrition and their application to weight control. Finally, we focus on strategies that we believe are essential to sound nutritional planning for the long-term management of obesity.

ASSESSMENT AND INDIVIDUALIZED PLANNING

Consider three different patients, each of whom has just completed 6 months of conservative treatment of obesity:

The first patient, Ellen, a 40-year old woman, has made good progress in treatment. Prior to the start of her weight-loss effort, she weighed 174 pounds, and at 5 feet, 5 inches tall, she had a BMI of 29.1, indicating mild obesity. Over the course of 6 months, she reduced her weight by 29 pounds, to 145 pounds. Ellen is now at a weight that both she and her therapist consider to be appropriate for maintenance. During the initial course of treatment, Ellen consumed an average of 1200 calories per day on a regular basis. During the first 3 months of treatment, this intake level produced a weight loss of approximately 1.5 pounds per week. During the second 3 months of treatment, her rate of weight loss decreased to slightly less than 1 pound per week. Ellen is now at a point where she feels that she would like to stop losing weight. She is afraid, however, that if she increases her caloric intake, she will regain weight.

Our second patient, Sylvia, a 57-year old woman, who is 5 feet, 3 inches tall, started her weight-loss effort at 212 pounds, with a BMI of 37.6, indicating moderate obesity. Over 6 months of treatment, she too averaged approximately 1200 calories per day, but she lost only 18 pounds. Her weekly rate of weight loss has been modest, about 3/4 of a pound per week. According to Sylvia's report, in previous dieting efforts, she typically has lost 20 pounds and then gained it all back when the diet ended. Both Sylvia and her therapist agree that further weight loss is a reasonable goal for the second phase of treatment, yet Sylvia feels frustrated by her slow progress. She asks the therapist whether it would be advisable for her to try to cut her caloric intake to 700 calories per day. She explains that she would like to get down to her "goal" weight of 180 pounds. She also notes that she is anxious to get to her goal weight so that she can stop "dieting" and "calorie counting."

Our third patient, Ron, is a 30-year old truck driver. When he entered treatment at 271 pounds and 5 foot, 9 inches tall, Ron (who had never tried to lose weight previously) had a BMI of 40.1, indicating severe obesity. Over the course of 6 months, Ron lost 48 pounds. His average intake was about 1800 calories per day, and he lost approximately 2 pounds per week. At 223 pounds, Ron would like to reduce his weight to under 200 pounds by continuing his intake of 1800 calories per day. His therapist agrees that further weight loss is a reasonable goal. The therapist is concerned, however, about the nutritional composition of Ron's diet. Ron, who is single, lives alone and eats most of his meals at fast-food restaurants. In reviewing Ron's eating diary, his therapist discovered that, although Ron cut his caloric intake from more than 3000 calories per day down to a daily average of 1800 calories, the "quality" of his intake left considerable room for improvement. Specifically, the therapist noted that the diet appeared to be particularly high in fats and sodium. The therapist was concerned about the potential negative impact that these factors might have on Ron's health in the long run.

Each of these three cases presents the clinician with a problem related to dietary considerations and the long-term management of obesity. For Ellen, the challenge for the clinician and patient is to determine to what degree the patient's caloric intake can be *increased*, to produce long-term maintenance of her current weight. For Sylvia, the problem is deciding whether her caloric intake should be *decreased*, to increase her rate of weight loss. For Ron, the decision facing the clinician is not whether to increase or decrease caloric intake but rather to modify the nutritional composition of the patient's current diet. Consistent with our problem-solving model, we believe that an individualized assessment (i.e., problem definition and formulation) represents an essential element in dealing with the unique challenge represented by each patient.

In formulating the diet-related problems facing the patient, the clinician will want to consider the following questions: (1) What level of caloric intake has the patient followed during the initial phase of treatment? (2) How much variability has there been in the patient's caloric intake during treatment? (3) What amount of weight loss has the patient achieved? (4) What rate of weight loss has the patient achieved? (5) Has the patient followed a nutritionally sound diet while trying to lose weight? (6) Has the distribution of *macronutrients* (i.e., proteins, carbohydrates, and fats) in the patient's diet been appropriate? (7) Has the patient's intake of *micronutrients* (i.e., vitamins and minerals) in the patient's diet been appropriate? (8) Should the diet used to achieve initial weight loss be modified for continued use during the maintenance phase?

To answer these questions, the clinician needs to know what the patient's food intake has been like, in terms of both quantity and quality. Our experience suggests that food diaries provide a rich source of information about the quantity and quality of the patient's energy intake. In some instances, however, the clinician may need to "interpret" the data presented by the patient in light of considerations about its reliability and accuracy. More faith can generally be placed in the accuracy of records that are presented on a regular basis in a detailed fashion, whereas food diaries that are sporadically kept or that show a scarcity of detail may represent only a very rough estimate of what was actually consumed.

In order to judge what changes in caloric level need to be made, the clinician also needs to know the impact of the diet on the patient's weight, physical health, and emotional state. This information can be obtained from an interview targeted specifically at a comprehensive review of the patient's progress in initial treatment. An interview of this type provides both the patient and the clinician an opportunity to look back over the progress achieved and to determine a new set of objectives for the next phase of long-term treatment.

In order to evaluate properly the adequacy of the patient's diet, in terms of quality as well as quantity, the clinician needs to be aware of relevant nutritional guidelines. This issue is of particular importance when helping patients to shape a diet pattern that they will be expected to adhere to over a long period of time. Moreover, it is also helpful to use nutritional guidelines to educate the patient about the dietary principles that guide decision making about appropriate food intake. In this way, patients will be better able to assume a greater degree of self-management in their dietary choices.

Unfortunately, when it comes to understanding information about appropriate nutrition, patients often find themselves confused by the continuous barrage of conflicting dietary advice in the popular media. As a consequence, many patients come to believe that the content of their diet is unimportant because the experts themselves disagree about which foods are healthy and which are not. This degree of diet confusion among consumers highlights the importance of making nutritional education and dietary planning a key component in the management of obesity.

Determining an Appropriate Caloric Intake

For many years, "energy balance theory" (Garrow, 1978) has guided clinicians' recommendations about levels of caloric intake needed to lose, gain, or maintain weight. The theory is based on two premises: (1) A stable weight will be maintained when energy intake is equal to energy expenditure (i.e., a balanced energy equation); and (2) a decrease (or increase) in intake of 3500 calories will produce a corresponding decrease (or increase) of 1 pound in weight because 1 pound is equivalent to 3500 calories.

In order to determine how many calories per day are need to balance an individual's particular energy equation (i.e., maintain a stable weight), the following guidelines are typically provided: Multiply the individual's weight in pounds by a factor based on their sex and activity level. For men, weight in pounds is usually multiplied by 13, 14, 15, or 16 depending on whether the individual has an activity level characterized respectively as "sedentary," "very light," "moderate," or "heavy." For women, weight in pounds is multiplied by 12, 13, 14, or 15, depending on whether the individual has an activity level characterized respectively as "sedentary," "very light," "moderate," or "heavy."

In order to lose weight, a negative energy balance must be created. Theoretically, a deficit of 3500 calories should produce a negative energy balance sufficient to result in a weight loss of 1 pound. To lose 1 pound per week through dieting would require a daily intake of 500 calories below the number of calories needed to balance the individual's energy equation. A 2-pound-per-week weight loss would require a daily deficit of 1000 calories, and so forth.

The clinician must exercise a degree of caution in using energy-balance equations to help patients decide on appropriate caloric levels for weight loss or maintenance. The limitations of this familiar, though overly simplistic, approach to predicting intake required for weight loss should be kept in mind. Obese individuals generally require fewer calories to maintain weight than the calorie totals predicted from energy balance equations, and after losing weight, their energy needs may be 15 to 20% less than such equations would predict (Geissler et al., 1987; Liebel & Hirsch, 1984). In working with moderately obese, middle-aged women who have sedentary life-styles, we have observed that approximately 10 calories per pound of body weight seems to balance their energy equation, whereas standard energy equations indicate that such individuals should require 12 calories per pound.

Moreover, as we described in Chapter 2, there is wide variability in individual responses to changes in energy intake. Physiological processes, such as AT (adaptive thermogenesis) and nutrient partitioning, often result in less weight change than would be predicted by energy-balance theory. In addition, prolonged periods of caloric restriction lead to significant increases in metabolic efficiency (Bray, 1969). This reduction in energy requirements can be explained by a number of factors, including (a) a decrease in RMR, due to a loss of lean body tissue and to AT; (b) a decrease in diet-induced thermogenesis (in proportion to the degree of caloric restriction); and (c) a decreased energy cost of movement because of lower body weight.

Thus, after a prolonged period of dieting, it is common for an obese individual not to lose weight despite rigidly adhering to a caloric intake at which energy equations would predict weight reduction. Faced with this problem, clinicians are often tempted to challenge the patient about the accuracy of self-reported adherence. In some cases, patients may indeed underreport their caloric consumption. However, it is important for the clinician to be aware that the enhanced metabolic efficiency resulting from a lengthy period of dieting may be responsible for the patient's losing weight at a rate far less than predicted by energy-balance theory. With this information in mind, we now return to the cases of the two patients who have each completed 6 months of obesity treatment but who have different goals for the second phase of treatment. Recall that each followed a 1200-calorie per day regimen over a 6-month period of time.

Ellen achieved a 29-pound weight loss and is now interested in maintaining her weight rather than reducing further. Sylvia, on the other hand, lost only 18 pounds, is far from her goal weight, and would like to reduce her intake further in order to increase her rate of weight loss. She is motivated in part by an expectation that if she achieves a 30-pound weight loss, she will be able to return to her former patterns of eating.

In the cases illustrated by our patients, Ellen and Sylvia, a key question facing the clinician concerns the level of caloric intake to recommend for the second phase of long-term treatment. In each case, the clinician can base his or her evaluation on several key pieces of information, including the food diaries completed during the initial phase of treatment, documented changes in body weight, and the patients' reports about the impact of their dieting and weight loss on their current goals for further weight change or maintenance.

For Ellen, a review of her eating diary and record of weight loss showed that she adhered well to the 1200-calorie limit that was suggested as a reasonable goal for intake during initial treatment. This level of intake provided her with a rate of weight loss of 1.5 pounds per week during the first 3 months of treatment and just about 1.0 pounds per week during the second 3 months. Based on this information, the clinician can estimate that her present intake of 1200 calories per day is approximately 500 calories per day below the amount needed to balance Ellen's energy equation. Ellen reports that she would like to stabilize her weight at its current level but is afraid about the possibility of weight gain associated with increasing her caloric intake. Ellen's goal of maintenance seems reasonable, as does her concern about weight gain. The energy-balance model would suggest that Ellen should simply add 500 calories per day to her intake in order to stabilize her weight at her current level. However, increasing her intake by 500 calories per day would represent a 42% increase in consumption. As noted in Chapter 2, significant increases in intake following prolonged dieting often result in a rapid regaining of weight (Katzeff, 1988). Thus, an appropriate strategy to employ with Ellen might entail gradual refeeding (Blackburn, Lynch, & Wong, 1986). The clinician might recommend that Ellen increase her intake up to 1300 calories per day for a 2-week period and monitor its effect on her weight. If she continues to lose weight on

1300 calories per day, then an additional 100 calories per day might be attempted until a calorie level is reached where maintenance of weight loss is achieved.

Our clinical experience is consistent with the reported findings that following weight loss, obese people typically require substantially fewer calories to maintain their body weight than individuals who have never been overweight. This sobering fact means that in order not to regain weight, most patients will have to follow a lifelong dietary regimen involving the consumption of fewer calories per day than nonobese individuals of comparable weight (see Leibel & Hirsch, 1984). It is crucial that clinicians discuss this problem with patients as they plan for caloric levels in each stage of obesity treatment. The significance of this issue is underscored by the fact that many patients retain unrealistic expectations about resuming what they consider to be normal eating once they have reached their goal weight or treatment has ended.

This problem was illustrated by the comments of our second patient, Sylvia, who indicated that she was looking forward to "ending" her diet once she reached her goal weight.

Sylvia's situation confronts the clinician with a problem that differs considerably from the concerns presented by Ellen. A review of Sylvia's food diary indicated far more variability in adherence to the 1200-calorie-per-day level of intake than was seen in Ellen's records. Indeed, Sylvia's diary showed entire weekends in which she neglected to keep eating records. In such circumstances, she typically reported that her eating was too "bad" to record and that she would be embarrassed to have the therapist see how much she had eaten. Thus, 1200 calories per day represented Sylvia's average intake during those times when she was adhering to her dietary goals. It did not include those days when her eating was "too bad" to be recorded. Further inquiry into Sylvia's eating on the unrecorded days suggested that her intake on those days may have been as high as 2500 calories per day.

This information, considered along with her age (59 years), degree of obesity (i.e., moderate), and previous history of limited dieting success, was consistent with the modest degree of weight loss (i.e., 18 pounds) that Sylvia achieved during 6 months of conservative treatment. In light of these factors, the clinician viewed Sylvia's suggestion that she reduce her intake to 700 calories per day as an unwise option for several reasons. First of all, when daily caloric intake falls below 1000 calories, it becomes increasingly difficult to ensure that the patient is consuming an adequate amount of nutrients. Second, decreases in caloric intake below 1000 calories per day are associated with significant decreases in metabolic rate. Third, such a reduction would not address two key aspects of the patient's problem: (1) the difficulty that she experienced in keeping herself from consuming large amounts of food on weekends, and (2) her expectation that when she reached her goal weight of 180 pounds that she could simply stop dieting. Thus, an appropriate approach for working with Sylvia during the second phase of treatment would involve continuing her current intake of 1200 calories per day while simultaneously using a problem-solving approach to help her (a) gain better control over her weekend eating and (b) come to terms with her unrealistic expectations about ending her diet once she reaches her goal weight.

Nutritional Considerations in the Long-Term Management of Obesity

Our third patient, the 30-year old truck driver named Ron, illustrates an important but sometimes overlooked consideration in the long-term management of obesity—namely, the nutritional quality of the diet consumed by the patient. Ron was initially referred to our program because his physician was concerned about the potential negative impact of Ron's severe degree of obesity (271 pounds, BMI = 40.1) on his health. Ron's father had recently died of a heart attack at age 57. His father had been obese, hypertensive, and diabetic, and Ron's physician was concerned that Ron might develop some of the same diseases that led to his father's death at an early age. Indeed, dietary composition alone represents a significant risk factor for many diseases, independent of the patient's degree of obesity.

As noted earlier, Ron made excellent progress over the first 6 months of treatment. He successfully reduced his daily caloric intake from approximately 3000 calories per day down to 1800 calories per day. He had a 2-pound-per-week average weight loss, and he had a net weight loss of 48 pounds. As he prepared to enter the second phase of treatment, both Ron and his therapist agreed that continued weight loss represented a reasonable goal and that maintenance of his food intake at 1800 calories per day seemed reasonable. However, in reviewing Ron's food diary, the therapist noted that Ron ate most of his meals at fast-food restaurants. The therapist became concerned about the quality of Ron's intake and decided to analyze the food records in greater detail.

Two problem areas became apparent. First, in calculating the distribution of macronutrients in Ron's typical daily intake, the therapist determined that Ron was consuming 50% of his caloric intake in the form of dietary fats. Second, in examining Ron's food records for potential problems related to intake of micronutrients, the therapist noted that Ron was consuming more than 6000 milligrams of sodium per day. The high levels of fats and sodium in Ron's diet concerned the therapist for obvious reasons. The consumption of fats, particularly saturated fats, has been linked to the development of coronary heart disease, and a high sodium intake may be problematic for a person such as Ron, with a family history of hypertension.

The clinician working with Ron expressed concern about the quality of his diet, but Ron was puzzled. He felt that he was doing a good job in managing his weight and believed he had a good grasp on the essentials of weight control. By simply cutting calories, he lost almost 50 pounds. He often joked that rather than ordering two Big Macs for dinner, he now had just one. Ron was confused about what additional changes in his diet were needed, and he asked a question often posed by obese patients—specifically, "When it comes to weight control, isn't cutting calories enough?" Ron conceded that he had largely ignored the "nutrition stuff" that was covered during the initial phase of treatment because he felt that he was making good weight-loss progress without worrying about "boring details" such as grams of fat or milligrams of sodium.

Ron's situation illustrates that two major objectives must be accomplished in helping patients to design a successful diet for the long-term management of obesity. The first objective is the development of a reasonable caloric level that promotes gradual weight loss or maintenance of weight and that prevents loss of muscle tissue or depression of metabolic rate. The second goal is to design a nutritionally sound diet that includes an adequate supply and distribution of nutrients needed to promote good health.

TEACHING PATIENTS ABOUT THE BASICS OF NUTRITION

Like Ron, many patients may "hear" what is said about the importance of nutrition, but they may not translate that information into changes in their dietary practices. Thus, the clinician's task is twofold: (1) to educate patients about proper nutrition, and (2) to help them put dietary principles into practice.

The American Heart Association (AHA, 1988) has reviewed scientific opinion about nutrition and health and has developed the following dietary guidelines for healthy adults.

1. Total fat intake (including saturated, polyunsaturated, and monounsaturated fats) should be less than 30% of total calorie intake.
2. Saturated fat intake should be less than 10% of calorie intake.
3. Polyunsaturated fat intake should not exceed 10% of calorie intake.
4. Cholesterol intake should not exceed 300 milligrams per day.
5. Carbohydrate intake should constitute 50% or more of calories, with emphasis on complex carbohydrates.

6. Protein intake should provide the remainder of calories.
7. Sodium intake should not exceed 3 grams per day.
8. Alcohol consumption should not exceed 1–2 ounces of ethanol per day. Two ounces of 100-proof whiskey, 8 ounces of wine, or 24 ounces of beer each contain 1 ounce of ethanol.
9. Total calories should be sufficient to maintain the individual's recommended weight (using the 1959 version of the Metropolitan Tables of Height and Weight).
10. A wide variety of foods should be consumed.

The AHA recommendations for prudent dietary practices provide a framework for a nutritionally sound diet that can be used in the long-term management of obesity. However, in order for patients to fully appreciate these dietary recommendations, they need to have a good grasp of basic information about nutrition. Before working to implement these recommendations with patients, it is generally helpful for clinicians to spend several sessions providing patients with an overview of the key functions of nutrients in the diet. Such a review might include information about the dietary functions and requirements for proteins, carbohydrates, fats, vitamins, minerals, and water. In reviewing such information with obese patients, we have often been surprised to find that many have a very limited knowledge base regarding nutrition. Providing them with an elementary understanding serves as an essential first step toward their recognition of the need for changes in their dietary behavior.

Protein

Dietary protein serves several key functions. First and foremost, it provides for growth and maintenance of body tissue by furnishing the amino acids needed for the synthesis of cellular tissue. Dietary protein also furnishes the amino acids needed for the production of enzymes and hormones that regulate important physiological processes, such as the regulation of blood glucose levels and metabolic rate. In order for efficient synthesis of cellular tissue, hormones, and enzymes to occur, an appropriate pattern of amino acids must be consumed. Nine of the essential amino acids for humans cannot be synthesized in the body and must be provided in the diet. The degree to which a particular food meets the body's requirements for amino acids is referred to as its "biological value." Net protein utilization (NPU) is a measure of the biological value of proteins. Eggs provide the closest mix of amino acids required in the diet (i.e., the highest NPU); hence, they are used as the standard by which other protein foods are measured. In descending order, eggs, fish, cheese, brown rice, red meat, and poultry are foods with the highest NPU ratings.

In addition to its role in the growth and maintenance of body tissue, protein provides 4 calories of energy per gram. Diets with an inadequate amount of carbohydrates or fats may cause dietary protein to be used to supply the body's energy needs and may lead to an excessive loss of lean tissue. In addition, if the supply of protein in the diet is inadequate, the body will break down tissue protein (i.e., muscle tissue) to meet its energy requirements. Thus, the individual who is attempting to lose weight should consume a balanced intake that provides an adequate quantity of carbohydrates along with an appropriate supply of high-quality protein.

How much protein is needed in the diet? The U.S. recommended dietary allowance (RDA) for healthy adults is 0.36 grams of protein per pound of body weight (National Research Council, 1989). For a healthy adult who weights 154 pounds, this amounts to 56 grams per day. Most obese patients are shocked to learn the small amount of protein that is needed per day. Indeed, as a group, Americans generally consume more than twice as much protein than is required, even though there is no benefit from consuming higher levels. In fact, an intake of large quantities of protein may be harmful. Metabolizing excessive amounts of protein can create a strain on the liver and kidneys, raise blood lipid levels, and contribute to obesity.

Carbohydrates

The major function of carbohydrates in the diet is to provide a source of energy for all bodily functions. As a fuel, carbohydrates supply 4 calories of energy per gram, either directly as glucose or indirectly by conversion to fat. The amount of carbohydrate that can be stored in the body is relatively limited. In adults, liver and muscle tissues can store roughly 250–350 grams of carbohydrate, and the circulating blood supply typically contains an additional 10 grams of carbohydrate. This modest amount of energy is generally sufficient to meet the body's needs for only a half day of moderate activity. In order to furnish the continuous energy needs of the body, a constant supply of fuel is needed. Thus, the largest portion of dietary intake should consist of carbohydrates, consumed at regular and frequent intervals. The availability of carbohydrates for energy prevents an excess degradation of fats and proteins, which in some instances can lead to a harmful state, known as "ketoacidosis." In addition to providing energy, carbohydrates also contribute to the structure of genetic material, facilitate the functioning of enzyme systems, and maintain appropriate tissue function in the liver, heart, brain, and nervous system.

Carbohydrates are classified according to their molecular structure and are divided into three groups: simple carbohydrates (i.e., monosaccharides and disaccharides), complex carbohydrates (i.e., polysaccharides), and fiber. Simple carbohydrates or sugars, such as cane sugar, fruit sugars, honey, and molasses, are easily digested and provide quick sources of energy. "Refined" sugars are those derived from cane and beet sources; "processed" sugars come from corn syrup, molasses, and honey. Much of the nutritive value of simple carbohydrates is often lost in the commercial production of refined and processed sugars. Thus, while all sugars provide glucose for the body's energy needs, naturally occurring sugars (e.g., fructose, lactose) represent a better nutritional choice because they provide many essential vitamins and minerals that are not available in processed sugars. The average American diet contains three times more refined and processed sugars than naturally occurring ones (Dunne, 1990).

Complex carbohydrates, which are found in fruits, vegetables, grains, and legumes, are *less* easily digested than simple carbohydrates. Complex carbohydrates provide energy at a slower rate than sugars and thereby help to prevent major fluctuations in the levels of glucose in the circulatory system. Current dietary recommendations suggest that more than 50% of total calories should come from carbohydrates, primarily from complex carbohydrates, with no more than 10% of total calories derived from refined or processed sugars. Currently, Americans consume only 40–45% of total calories in the form of carbohydrates, and only a quarter to a third of this amount in the form of complex carbohydrates.

Fiber consists mostly of complex carbohydrates that form the non-digestible parts of plants and is found in the skins of fruits (e.g., pectin) and vegetables (e.g., cellulose) and in the cell walls of plants. Fiber absorbs water and aids in the processes of digestion and elimination by adding bulk without adding calories. Raw fruits and vegetables provide a good source of fiber, though fiber supplements (e.g., psyllium) are commonly added to many commercially prepared foods. Bran is another acceptable way of increasing the fiber content of the diet. Many foods, especially cereals and breads, have recently added bran to attract health-conscious consumers (Kirby, Anderson, & Sieling, 1981; Mayer & Goldberg, 1990). Americans currently consume about 10–15 grams of dietary fiber per day, but many nutritional experts suggest that 20–30 grams per day represents a more appropriate level.

Fiber has particular relevance to weight-loss diets because, in addition to its potential health benefits, it has the ability to absorb fluid in the body and to produce a feeling of fullness and satiation. For example, in a recent study, participants who ate a very-high-fiber cereal for breakfast consumed fewer calories at their next meal (Levine et al., 1989). Thus, in addition to creating an immediate feeling of satiety, high-fiber foods may also have an appetite-suppressing effect that lasts several hours.

Fats

Fats, or lipids, provide the body with highly concentrated sources of energy, yielding 9 calories per gram. Small amounts of fat must be supplied in the diet in order to maintain good health. Dietary fats facilitate the absorption of the fat-soluble vitamins and play a key role in maintaining the structure of cellular membranes. In addition, food sources of fat help to maintain the adipose tissue needed for the insulation and protection of organs and bones.

Fats are commonly classified as saturated, monounsaturated, or poly-unsaturated, based on their arrangement of carbon atoms and the degree to which each is bound with hydrogen atoms. Animal sources of fat (e.g., meats, poultry, eggs, milk, etc.) generally contain more saturated fatty acids than unsaturated ones, whereas plant sources of fat typically consist largely of polyunsaturated fatty acids (e.g., vegetable oil, peanut oil). Monounsaturated fats are found in olive oil, avocados, and cashew nuts.

From a health perspective, a key relationship exists between saturated fats and cholesterol. Cholesterol is a fatlike substance that exists in animal but not plant sources of food and is essential for the production of hormones. However, the liver is fully capable of manufacturing cholesterol on its own, and there is no need for the consumption of cholesterol in the diet. Diets high in saturated fats can contribute to abnormally high levels of cholesterol in the blood and thus are often associated with high rates of atherosclerosis and cardiovascular disease. High-fat diets have also been implicated as contributors to some types of cancer.

Current estimates suggest that Americans consume excessive amounts of fats, saturated fats, and dietary cholesterol. Dietary fats currently comprise 35–40% of total calories in the average American diet, with saturated fats representing about 12% of total energy consumed (Stephen & Wald, 1990). Average consumption of dietary cholesterol is approximately 400 milligrams per day (U.S. Department of Agriculture—USDA, 1984). The National Institutes of Health (1985), the National Research Council (1989), and the AHA (1988) all agree that total fat intake should be less than 30% of calories consumed, that saturated fats should be reduced to less than 10% of total intake, and that dietary cholesterol should be limited to no more than 300 milligrams per day.

In addition to contributing to heart disease and cancer, high-fat diets have also been implicated as contributing to obesity. Moreover, decreasing the proportion of energy derived from fats appears important to weight loss. As described in Chapter 2, the composition of nutrients in the diet, as well as the total energy consumed, is crucial to the long-term control of weight (see Dreon et al., 1988; Miller et al., 1990). Fats not only contain more than twice as many calories per gram as carbohydrates or protein, but fats also appear to be metabolized differently than the other macro-nutrients. For example, although carbohydrates can be stored as fat, it takes an exceptionally high intake for this to occur. On the other hand, the majority of calories consumed as fat are immediately stored as fat and are only used for fuel when there is an inadequate supply of carbohydrate. Consequently, substantial imbalances between energy intake and expenditure are more likely to occur following the consumption of fats than the consumption of carbohydrates (Schutz, Flatt, & Jequier, 1989), and diets high in fat are likely to result in increased weight and adiposity (Lissner, Levitsky, Strupp, Kalkwarf, & Roe, 1987; Tremblay, Plourde, Despres, & Bouchard, 1989).

As a first step in reducing dietary fats, an individual must be able to identify the many forms this nutrient takes. Most people are familiar with the visible sources of dietary fat, such as butter, margarine, oil, salad dressing, bacon, and cream. Less obvious, however, are the hidden sources of fat in a wide variety of foods, including meats, fish, poultry, eggs, cheese, nuts, seeds, olives, and avocados. Hidden fats account for more than half the fats in the diet, much of which comes from the high consumption of meats in the American diet. Prime and choice cuts of meats are tender and tasty because of the marbleized streaks of fat that run through them. Some luncheon meats (such as salami) contain visible chunks of fat, but others (such as bologna and liverwurst) contain large quantities of fat that are processed into the meat and are less visible. An additional group of foods that contain hidden fats are starches and vegetables prepared or cooked with fats, including biscuits, croissants, chow mein noodles, corn bread, many types of crackers, muffins, pancakes, stuffing, french fries, and fried vegetables. Table 10.1 presents the amounts of total fat, saturated fat, and cholesterol found in some commonly used foods.

Learning to distinguish between saturated and unsaturated fats represents an additional element that is crucial to improving dietary practices. The degree to which foods contain saturated or unsaturated fats is often evident in the degree to which they range from solid to liquid states. Unsaturated fats, such as vegetable oils, tend to be soft or oily at room temperature, whereas saturated fats, such as butter or lard, tend to be solid. In some instances, the commercial processing of foods can change fats from unsaturated to saturated states. For example, hydrogenation is often used to prolong shelf life and to enhance the visual appeal of foods such as margarine. In this process, the addition of hydrogen transforms a polyunsaturated oil into a saturated fat.

Although animal fats are much higher in saturated fats than plant sources, many foods contain a mixture of both (see Table 10.1). Poultry and fish have higher proportions of unsaturated fats than red meats. Thus, poultry and fish generally represent nutritionally preferable alternatives to red meats. However, not all poultry is alike. For example, the fat content of a 3.5 ounce serving of poultry ranges from 4.5 grams for light-meat chicken to as high as 8.2 grams for domestic duck.

In recent years, there has been considerable debate over the comparative value of polyunsaturated versus monounsaturated fats. The use of polyunsaturated fats lowers total serum cholesterol more effectively but also lowers HDL (i.e., high-density lipoprotein) cholesterol. This is an undesirable effect because higher levels of HDL cholesterol appear to

TABLE 10.1   TOTAL FAT, SATURATED FAT, AND CHOLESTEROL IN SELECTED FOODS

Selected foods	Total fat (grams)	Saturated fat (grams)	Cholesterol (milligrams)
Dairy products			
Milk, whole (8 oz)	8.1	5.1	33
Milk, 2% (8 oz)	4.7	4.7	18
Milk, skim (8 oz)	0.6	0.4	5
Lowfat yogurt (8 oz)	3.5	2.3	14
Cottage cheese			
Creamed (1 cup)	10.4	6.6	34
Dry (1 cup)	0.6	0.4	10
Cheddar cheese (1 oz)	9.4	6.0	30
Mozzarella cheese, part-skim (1 oz)	4.5	2.9	16
Ice cream (1 cup)	14.4	8.8	60
Frozen yogurt (1 cup)	3.0	2.0	12
Sherbet (1 cup)	3.8	2.4	14
Meats, fish, poultry, beans, and eggs			
Beef rib roast (1 oz)	1.8	0.1	23
Ground beef (1 oz)	2.3	0.2	26
Beef liver (1 oz)	0.8	0.5	137
Pork loin (1 oz)	4.0	0.5	26
Chicken (skinless)			
Light meat (1 oz)	0.4	0.3	24
Dark meat (1 oz)	0.8	0.7	27
Turkey (skinless)			
Light meat (1 oz)	0.3	0.3	20
Dark meat (1 oz)	0.7	0.6	24
Cod (fillet) (1 oz)	0.1	0.1	35
Tuna (canned) (1 oz)	0.6	0.5	19
Shrimp (1 oz)	0.1	0.2	59
Navy beans (1 cup)	0.2	0.4	0
Canned beans (1 cup)	0.4	0.4	0
Egg (1 large)			
Whole	1.7	0.7	274
Yolk	1.7	0.7	274
White	0	0	0
Fats and oils			
Lard (1 tbsp)	12.8	5.0	12
Butter (1 tbsp)	11.5	7.2	31
Margarine (1 tbsp)			
Hard (stick)	11.4	2.1	0
Soft (tub)	11.4	1.8	0
Mayonnaise (1 tbsp)	11.0	1.6	8
Corn oil (1 tbsp)	13.6	1.7	0
Peanut oil (1 tbsp)	13.5	2.3	0
Safflower oil (1 tbsp)	13.6	1.2	0
Soybean oil (1 tbsp)	13.6	2.0	0
Sunflower oil (1 tbsp)	13.6	1.4	0
Olive oil (1 tbsp)	13.5	1.8	0
Palm oil (1 tbsp)	13.6	6.7	0
Coconut oil (1 tbsp)	13.6	11.8	0

TABLE 10.1   (continued)

Selected foods	Total fat (grams)	Saturated fat (grams)	Cholesterol (milligrams)
Snacks			
Potato chips (10)	8.0	2.0	0
Corn chips (1/2 cup)	6.1	1.3	0
Popcorn (1 cup)	0.3	trace	0
Pretzels (10 thin)	0.1	trace	0
Saltine crackers (4)	1.4	0.3	0
Wheat crackers (4)	2.2	0.5	0
Peanuts (1/4 cup)	17.9	3.9	0
Cookie (1)			
Ginger snap	0.6	0.2	3
Chocolate chip	2.2	0.7	4
Sandwich-type	2.3	0.6	4
Doughnut (1)			
Cake-type	6.0	1.5	19
Raised	11.2	2.8	10

Note. These figures are derived from data presented by the U.S. Department of Agriculture (1971).

"protect" against the development of atherosclerosis. Monounsaturated fats, such as olive and canola oils, on the other hand, seem to lower serum cholesterol and low-density lipoprotein (LDL) cholesterol without suppressing the level of HDL cholesterol. In addition, polyunsaturated fats have been linked to cancer in laboratory animals, while monounsaturated fats have not (Grundy, Florentin, Nix, & Whelan, 1988). Most vegetable oils are made up of unsaturated fats. Exceptions to this rule are palm and coconut oils, both of which are extremely high in saturated fats (see Table 10.1).

Although fats provide a potent source of calories, their satiety value is also high. This is an important characteristic for the clinician to keep in mind. When lipids reach the stomach, hormones that inhibit the discharge of food are released, thereby increasing and prolonging a sensation of fullness. Dietary fats also stimulate the release of cholecystokinin, a hormone with documented appetite-suppressing effects (Smith, 1984). Thus, in planning a diet for the management of obesity, the satiety potential of dietary fats must be balanced against their high caloric density. Diets that are too low in fat can leave a patient with chronic feelings of hunger. On the other hand, the high caloric density of fats, combined with their enhanced palatability, may lead to the consumption of a greater number of calories than desired.

Vitamins

Vitamins are organic compounds that are essential for tissue construction, for the control of specific metabolic functions, and for the prevention of disease. Vitamins differ from proteins, carbohydrates, and fats, in that they do not provide energy. Nonetheless, vitamins are essential nutrients that cannot be manufactured by the body and must be supplied by the diet.

Vitamins are traditionally classified based on their solubility. Vitamin C and all of the B vitamins are water soluble, whereas vitamins A, D, E, and K are fat soluble. The water-soluble vitamins are transported in the fluids of the tissues and cells. Because these nutrients cannot be stored, they must be consumed daily. Excessive amounts of water-soluble vitamins tend to be excreted in the urine. Ingesting more of these vitamins than recommended will be of limited or no benefit. The fat-soluble vitamins, on the other hand, tend to be retained within the body and stored in fat. They are not readily excreted and may be toxic in large doses. A nutritionally balanced diet provides the necessary amounts of all vitamins.

The issue of vitamin supplementation has been a topic of lively debate for many years (Krehl, 1985). Opponents of supplementation argue that a balanced intake provides an adequate supply of vitamins. Those who favor supplementation point out that individual diets often are nutritionally deficient. Moreover, they note that the tremendous growth of the fast food industry indicates that millions of people are consuming diets high in fat, sugar, and sodium, and low in important micronutrients (Cassell, 1989). Thus, proponents view vitamin supplementation as an important means of providing many people with essential nutrients that may be missing from their diet. Both critics and proponents of vitamin supplementation agree, however, that when caloric intake is low (i.e., less than 1000 calories per day), it is difficult to meet the RDAs for many micronutrients. Supplementation with a multivitamin plus minerals appears to be a reasonable means of ensuring adequate nutrition in individuals who are consuming low-calorie diets over extended periods of time.

Minerals

Minerals are inorganic elements that are required by the body to build tissues, to regulate bodily fluids, and to assist in the production of energy. Minerals originate in water and soil. Consumption of water and foods that have not been processed provides the dietary source of minerals. Minerals are often classified into two groups, based on the amount required by the body. The *macrominerals*, which are required in relatively large amounts, include calcium, phosphorous, magnesium, sodium, potassium, chlorine, and sulfur. Trace elements or *microminerals*, which are required only in very small amounts, include iron, copper, iodine, manganese, zinc, fluorine, cobalt, chromium, molybdenum, and selenium.

Mineral deficiencies can result in a variety of disease conditions, ranging from anemia (due to iron deficiency) to cardiac arrhythmias (due to potassium deficiency). However, as is the case with vitamins, a balanced diet will provide a healthy adult with all necessary minerals. Mineral supplements are generally unnecessary except in unusual circumstances. Moreover, consumption of concentrated sources of minerals over extended periods of time can produce toxicity, and an excessive intake of one mineral can produce a deficiency in another mineral.

Minerals that ionize in water (i.e., separate into electrically charged particles) are referred to as "electrolytes" and include sodium, potassium, and chloride. Sodium plays a critical role in regulating fluid balance in the body. For obese individuals, understanding the role of sodium is particularly important, both for planning a healthy diet and for understanding minor changes in weight.

High levels of sodium in the diet can cause excessive fluid retention and can result in increased blood pressure. Indeed, a significant relationship exists between the sodium content of the diet and the incidence of hypertension (e.g., Page, Damon, & Moellering, 1974). Moreover, because obese individuals are at increased risk of hypertension due to their adiposity (Bray, 1986), attention to the intake of sodium represents prudent dietary practice.

The primary source of sodium in the American diet is table salt (i.e., sodium chloride). Current estimates show that Americans typically consume 4000–6000 milligrams of sodium per day. About one third of this amount comes from naturally occurring food sources. Processed foods, which use sodium as a preservative and flavor enhancer, also contribute approximately one third of the sodium in the diet. The final third comes from additions by the individual. The American Heart Association guidelines (AHA, 1988) suggest that sodium intake be limited to less than 3000 milligrams per day.

One teaspoon of table salt contains approximately 2000 milligrams of sodium. Thus, control of the salt shaker often represents an obvious target for change. In addition, hidden sources of sodium can add significantly to an individual's daily intake. Many foods that might not be expected to contain sodium (such as breakfast cereals, diet drinks, canned vegetables, prepared soups, and low-calorie frozen dinners) use sodium to enhance sweetness and lengthen shelf life. Thus, the use of these sodium-enriched foods pose a special problem for obese individuals who may find that by selecting these low-calorie alternatives, they are consuming many high-sodium foods. An important starting point in limiting sodium intake is to educate patients about the sodium content of foods. Table 10.2 provides examples of foods that are low, moderate, or high in sodium content.

Although sodium has no direct impact on body fat, high levels can result in increased weight due to fluid retention. As a consequence, obese patients sometimes report a sensation of "being bloated." Unfortunately, many interpret this sensation in an inappropriate and negative way (i.e., as evidence that their diet is not working). As a result, they experience a variety of negative moods, including feelings of guilt and depression. Such feelings can have a negative impact on motivation to sustain the weight-

TABLE 10.2 SELECTED FOODS THAT ARE LOW, MODERATE, OR HIGH IN
SODIUM CONTENT

Low-sodium foods (less than 140 mg of sodium per 100 grams)
   Apples, apricots, asparagus (fresh not canned), avocados, beans (not canned),
   beef (retail cuts), berries, broccoli, cabbage, carrots, cauliflower, celery,
   cherries, chicken (roasted), corn, eggs, eggplant, flatfish (e.g., flounder, sole),
   grapefruit, grapes, jams, lamb (retail cuts), milk (not dry), mushrooms,
   oranges, peaches, perch, pears, peas (not canned), plums, popcorn (plain),
   pork (retail cuts), potatoes, puddings, raisins, spinach (not canned), squash,
   tomatoes, tuna (canned in water), turkey, turnips, veal (retail cuts), walnuts,
   yogurt.

Medium-sodium foods (140 to 500 mg of sodium per 100 grams)
   Beans (canned), beef liver, black-eyed peas, cakes, cottage cheese, coleslaw,
   cookies, farina (enriched), haddock (fried), lobster, macaroni and cheese,
   muffins, oatmeal (cooked), oysters (cooked), nuts (roasted and salted), peas
   (canned), pies, rice (cooked), scallops (cooked), soups (canned).

High-sodium foods (more than 500 mg of sodium per 100 grams)
   Bacon, barbecue sauce, beans and frankfurters (canned), corned beef, biscuits,
   bologna, bouillon, bran, bread, butter, caviar, cheeses (American, cheddar,
   parmesan, processed, Swiss), chocolate-flavored beverages, cod (dehydrated),
   corn cereals, cornbread, crab (canned), crackers, cream substitutes, doughnuts
   (cake-type), frankfurters, ham, hard rolls, herring (smoked), ketchup, margarine, milk (dry nonfat), mustard, oat cereals, olives, pancakes, peanut butter,
   pickles, pizza, pork (cured), pretzels, rice cereals, salad dressings, sardines,
   sauerkraut, sausage, soy sauce, tartar sauce, tuna (canned in oil), waffles.

loss effort. Understanding the effect of sodium on fluid retention and
weight change can often help patients to interpret the bloated sensation in
an appropriate and constructive manner.

Water

Water is also an essential nutrient. Indeed, people can live several
weeks without food, but they cannot live more than a few days without
water. Water functions as a component of all body tissue, serves as a
transport for nutrients and wastes, and plays a critical role in digestion,
metabolism, and temperature control. Water is supplied not only by
drinking, but also from the fluid content of foods. Approximately 42
ounces of water are required each day, directly from fluid intake. Greater
amounts may be needed in warm weather or when exercise levels are high
(Dunne, 1990). Patients frequently ask about water intake in dieting. Although water does not have a direct impact on weight, some diet programs
recommend drinking a minimum of 64 ounces per day. Except in protein-
sparing modified fasts, the rationale for this level of intake is related less
to its physiological benefits than to the indirect impact it may have on the

consumption of food. Drinking water increases feelings of fullness, particularly if it is consumed with meals. In addition, for the dieter, drinking water may satisfy an urge to eat, without adding calories.

IMPROVING THE NUTRITIONAL ADEQUACY OF THE DIET

Assessing Patients' Diets for Nutritional Soundness

After educating patients about the basics of nutrition and the guidelines for a healthy diet, the next task for the clinician is to assess how well the patient's intake matches the recommendations for a nutritionally sound diet. Several methods can be used for this purpose. If the patient has been keeping a food diary that includes the type and amounts of foods eaten, the records can be analyzed to determine the relative proportions of nutrients consumed. This process can be facilitated by the use of software programs that provide nutritional analyses, including detailed breakdowns of the amounts and percentages of nutrients consumed. If computer analysis is not available, then the clinician and patient can use reference tables (e.g., Dunne, 1990) containing the nutritional components of foods to analyze the food diary.

If the patient has not been keeping a food diary, a 24-hour recall procedure (using either a questionnaire or an interview format) can be used to record all food and drink consumed by the patient during the previous day. In using data from a 24-hour recall procedure, the clinician must assess the extent to which the foods consumed during the period sampled represent the patient's usual intake. Indeed, there is considerable within-person variability in food consumption from day to day. In general, the accuracy of food assessments is increased by sampling longer periods of time. However, limitations of memory generally preclude extending a dietary recall beyond 48 hours.

In analyzing data from a food diary or dietary recall, the clinician will want to derive the following information:

1. Total calories consumed
2. Percentage of calories consumed as protein
3. Percentage of calories consumed as carbohydrates
4. Percentage of calories consumed as simple carbohydrates
5. Percentage of calories consumed as complex carbohydrates
6. Percentage of calories consumed as fats
7. Percentage of calories consumed as saturated fats
8. Percentage of calories consumed as polyunsaturated fats
9. Percentage of calories consumed as monounsaturated fats
10. Milligrams of cholesterol consumed

11. Milligrams of sodium consumed
12. Amount of alcohol consumed

With this information in hand, the clinician can compare the patient's intake with the standards for an optimal diet, as detailed in the AHA (1988) recommendations. When major discrepancies are noted between the patient's actual intake and the recommended diet, the clinician must determine whether the mismatch is indeed a reflection of patient's dietary habits or whether the discrepancy might be due to an inaccurate sampling of the patient's typical intake. If discussion with the patient suggests a problem with sampling, then it may be wise for the clinician and patient to plan to use a food diary for 1 or 2 weeks, in order to obtain a more representative picture of the patient's typical pattern of food intake. If sampling is not a problem, then the clinician can use the problem-solving process outlined in Chapters 5 and 6 as a guide to help the patient solve the mismatch between actual and preferred dietary practices. It is important to note, however, that in working with obese patients who have known diseases, such as hypertension, hyperlipidemia, or diabetes mellitus, the clinician should consult a registered dietitian to provide the patient with a comprehensive nutritional assessment and treatment plan.

Ongoing Monitoring of Diet

Although this approach to assessing nutritional adequacy often yields a comprehensive picture of the patient's dietary intake, it is not without limitations. Because most patients do not have regular access to a computer and software for analysis of their diet, they must invest a fair amount of time and energy in calculating calories, grams, and milligrams of various nutrients. Few would be able or willing to continue such detailed calculations on an ongoing basis to allow long-term monitoring of changes in their diet. Two alternatives are available.

Narrowing the Focus.   The first option is for the clinician to limit the focus of dietary monitoring and to change no more than one or two target areas.

For example, our patient Ron (whom we described earlier in the chapter) was consuming a daily diet of 1800 calories, in which 50% of his intake was in the form of fats. The AHA guidelines indicate that fats should be limited to 30% of total intake. Thus, Ron's daily intake of fat should be limited to 540 calories (i.e., 30% of 1800 calories). Because a gram of fat has an energy value of 9 calories, dividing Ron's calorie allowance for fats (i.e., 540 calories) by 9 yields the number of grams of fat (i.e., 60 grams) that meet the target level for a total fat intake of 30%. Using this approach, the therapist worked with Ron to lower his daily consumption of fats from 100 grams per day (50% of intake) to 60 grams per day (30% of intake).

For 6 months, Ron had routinely monitored his caloric consumption. The therapist now asked him to monitor grams of fat that he consumed as well. This task was not exceedingly difficult because the calorie counting book that Ron used also listed the grams of protein, carbohydrates, and fats for each food item. Together, the therapist and Ron set an intermediate goal for Ron's fat intake. Specifically, for the first 2 weeks, Ron was to try to reduce his intake of fats from his previous average of 100 grams per day down to 90 grams per day. By *gradually* reducing the amounts of fat in his diet, the chances of Ron's succeeding at the task were increased. Also, by working on one aspect of dietary change, it is less likely that the patient will feel overwhelmed by the challenge of changing long-standing dietary practices.

Using Food-Exchange Lists. A second approach to assessing and modifying dietary behaviors involves the use of "exchange lists." Many patients find it tedious and time consuming to calculate grams of nutrient consumed. Thus, the American Diabetes Association and the American Dietetic Association (ADA, 1986) have jointly developed a system to simplify dietary planning. The exchange system is based on the concept of nutritional equivalency. Foods are grouped into six basic categories or lists, based on comparability in their composition of proteins, carbohydrates, fats, and caloric content. Foods within a particular group or subgroup are equivalent in their nutritional composition, thus allowing within-group substitutions or exchanges. The six categories are described next.

Starch/Bread List. One exchange from the starch and bread list contains about 80 calories and consists of approximately 15 grams of carbohydrate, 3 grams of protein, and a trace of fat. In general, 1 ounce (i.e., 1 slice) of bread is one exchange. For cereals, pasta, and starchy vegetables, such as corn, peas, and potatoes, $\frac{1}{2}$ cup is typically equivalent to one exchange.

Meat List. Foods on this list include not only beef, pork, and lamb, but also other items that are similar to meats in their nutritional composition, such as poultry, fish, cheese, and eggs. One exchange from the meat list consists of 7 grams of protein and a variable amount of fat and calories, depending on the type of food chosen. Thus, the list is subdivided into three groups: lean, medium-fat, and high-fat products. In general, 1 ounce of a product from the meat list is one exchange. One exchange of *lean* meat (e.g., chicken, fish, or lean cuts of beef or pork) consists of 7 grams of protein and 3 grams of fat, and contains 55 calories. One exchange of *medium-fat* meat (e.g., most cuts of beef and pork, egg, and skim or part-skim milk cheese) consists of 7 grams of protein and 5 grams of fat, and contains 75 calories. Finally, one exchange of *high-fat* meat (e.g., prime cuts of beef, luncheon meats, and most cheeses) consists of 7 grams of protein, and 8 grams of fat, and contains 100 calories. Patients are generally encouraged to select lean or medium-fat meats and to limit their use of high-fat meats.

Vegetable List.   One exchange from the vegetable list contains about 25 calories and consists of 5 grams of carbohydrate and 2 grams of protein. In general, 1 cup of raw vegetables, or ½ cup of cooked vegetables or vegetable juice, composes 1 vegetable exchange.

Fruit List.   One exchange from the fruit list contains 60 calories and consists of 15 grams of carbohydrate. In general, ½ cup of fresh fruit or fruit juice, or ¼ cup of dried fruit composes 1 fruit exchange.

Milk List.   One exchange from the milk list consists of 12 grams of carbohydrate, 8 grams of protein, and a variable amount of fat and calories, depending on the type of milk chosen. Thus, similar to the meat group, the milk list is subdivided into three groups: skim, low-fat, and whole milk products. In general, 1 cup of milk is one exchange, with the exception of evaporated milk, where ½ cup composes 1 exchange. One exchange of *skim* milk contains only a trace of fat and has 90 calories. One exchange of *low-fat* milk contains 5 grams of fat and 120 calories. Finally, one exchange of *whole* milk contains 8 grams of fat and 150 calories.

Fat List.   Foods on the fat list include avocados, bacon, butter, margarine, oils, olives, salad dressings, nuts, and seeds. One exchange from the fat list contains approximately 5 grams of fat and 45 calories. The amount of food that composes one exchange varies considerably. For example, 1 fat exchange may comprise 1 teaspoon of butter, margarine, or vegetable oil; 2 teaspoons of a mayonnaise-based salad dressing; or 1 tablespoon of an oil-based salad dressing.

Practical Applications of the Exchange Lists.   By reducing the universe of foods to six categories, the process of assessing and planning nutritional intake often becomes easier to manage. In terms of assessment, a patient can be asked to monitor his or her intake as the number of exchanges from each food list. Then, based on the patient's calorie goal, the actual distribution across the six groups can be compared with a nutritionally balanced distribution. Table 10.3 presents a nutritionally balanced distribution of exchanges at several different calorie levels. In comparing the patient's actual pattern with a balanced pattern, the clinician can determine which food groups have been inappropriately high or low in the patient's diet.

    In a similar fashion, the exchange lists can be used to assist patients in

TABLE 10.3 NUMBER OF EXCHANGES NEEDED TO OBTAIN A BALANCED INTAKE AT DIFFERENT CALORIE LEVELS

	Daily calorie level		
Food exchange groups	1200	1500	1800
Bread/starch	5	7	9
Meat	3	3	5
Vegetable	2	2	2
Fruit	4	5	5
Milk	2	2	2
Fat	3	4	4

Note. Assumes the use of medium-fat meat and skim milk.

planning an appropriate diet. For example, in helping our patient, Ron, to distribute his daily intake of 1800 calories in a nutritionally balanced fashion (i.e., 55% from carbohydrates, 15% from proteins, and 30% from fats), the therapist does not need to ask Ron to calculate grams of nutrient intake for each food that he consumes. Instead, the therapist can provide Ron with the numbers of exchanges per food group that would result in a balanced intake. Ron can select freely among equivalent foods within a particular list, so long as the number of exchanges for that list matches that required for a balanced intake.

SUMMARY

In this chapter, we considered nutritional principles and dietary intake in relation to weight control. In the long-term treatment of obesity, an appropriate diet must supply sufficient nutrients to maintain good health while providing an energy level that achieves an appropriate reduction or stabilization in weight. Obese patients need to know that successful long-term maintenance of a lower weight necessitates a lifelong commitment to lowered caloric intake.

In helping patients to determine an appropriate energy level for long-term weight control, the clinician's recommendations should be based on individualized assessment and treatment planning rather than on general guidelines that are uniformly applied to all patients. Expectations of weight change based on energy-balance equations should be made cautiously because obese individuals typically lose weight at a slower rate than would be predicted by such equations. When further weight loss continues as a goal during the secondary phase of treatment, caloric intake generally should be maintained at 1000 calories per day or greater, to decrease the potential of nutritional deficiencies or significant slowing of metabolic rate. When the clinician and patient agree that weight maintenance rather than weight loss is an appropriate goal, small and gradual increases in caloric intake should be made until stabilization of weight occurs.

Because most obese individuals must follow regimens of reduced caloric intake for extended periods of time, the adequacy of their nutritional intake takes on added importance. The dietary recommendations of the AHA represent an appropriate set of guidelines that can be used to judge the soundness of a patient's nutritional intake. The AHA recommendations suggest that patient's reduce their total intake of fats to 30%, that saturated fats and polyunsaturated fats each be limited to 10% of intake, and that dietary cholesterol not exceed 300 milligrams per day. The guidelines also recommend that carbohydrate intake should constitute 50% or more of calories (with an emphasis on complex carbohydrates), that sodium should not exceed 3 grams per day, and that alcohol consumption should not exceed 2 ounces of ethanol per day.

In order for patients to fully appreciate the dietary recommendations of the AHA, they need to have a good grasp of basic information about nutrition. Thus, it is often helpful for clinicians to provide patients with an overview of the dietary functions of proteins, carbohydrates, fats, vitamins, minerals, and water. Providing patients with an elementary understanding of nutrition serves as an essential first step toward their recognition of the need for changes in their dietary behavior.

After educating patients about the basics of nutrition and the guidelines for a healthy diet, the next task for the clinician is to assess how well the patient's intake matches the recommendations for a nutritionally sound diet. Using information derived from food diaries or dietary recalls, the clinician can compare the patient's typical intake with the standards for optimal diet. Exchange lists can sometimes be used to simplify the process of dietary assessment and nutritional planning. After identifying areas of the diet needing modification, the clinician can utilize the problem-solving model described in Chapters 5 and 6 to help the patient devise an eating-management plan that combines sound nutrition with a reduced calorie goal, without sacrificing flexibility, variety, or the inherent pleasure of food.

11

Social-Influence Strategies

For many individuals, successful long-term maintenance of weight loss will require help from others. In this chapter, we describe a variety of ways in which social-support and social-influence strategies can be used during the maintenance and follow-up phases of obesity management. These strategies include techniques that can be implemented in the context of group therapy, such as telephone networking, group contingency contracts, and competition among members, as well as procedures that can be used in conjunction with either group or individual therapy, including the involvement of partners or family members and the adjunctive use of self-help or commercial weight-loss programs.

RECEPTIVITY TO SOCIAL SUPPORT

An initial task for the clinician is to determine whether an individual is likely to benefit from social support during the maintenance phase. Some patients may prefer to work on managing their obesity independently of others. Often, such individuals believe that they work best in a solo mode. Table 11.1 presents a number of questions that can be explored to deter-

TABLE 11.1 ASSESSMENT OF THE PATIENT'S AVAILABILITY TO SOCIAL SUPPORT

1. In general, does the patient view himself or herself as
   - Friendly and outgoing or a loner?
   - Open to discussing difficult personal issues with others?
   - Comfortable with others commenting on their weight?
   - Preferring to exercise with others rather than alone?
2. In the context of group treatment, does the patient
   - Display a willingness to participate actively?
   - Discuss negative as well as positive behaviors?
   - Appear open to the suggestions of others?
   - Offer suggestions to others?
   - Engage in problem solving with the group?
   - Take the problems of other group members seriously?
   - Allow others equal time?
3. In the context of social relationships, does the patient
   - Have at least one or two close friends?
   - Discuss personal problems?
   - Report positive work relationships?
   - Have avocational social contacts?
4. In the context of family relationships, does the patient
   - Report significant stresses?
   - Describe a good marital relationship?
   - Indicate that weight is an issue in the marriage?
   - Report excessive parent-child conflict?

mine how amenable a patient is to utilizing social support. The clinician can consider, with the patient, the various pros and cons of incorporating social support, and together, they can decide whether it is reasonable to develop a maintenance plan that involves social support. In most cases, patients are receptive to the idea of "getting help from others." However, some individuals may have potential sources of support available to them but may not use them effectively. Such patients may be reluctant to risk rejection in asking for help from others, or they may be uncomfortable with the thought of appearing dependent on others. In these instances, the therapist and patient can use problem solving to overcome obstacles to initiating the use of social support.

GROUP-THERAPY TECHNIQUES

Support from Peers

In the maintenance phase of obesity management, a group-treatment format offers a variety of opportunities for social support that are not typically available in individual therapy (see Yalom, 1985). Often, the group approach can provide powerful motivational incentives to sustain the behavior changes needed to maintain weight loss. By discovering that they are not alone in battling to maintain weight-loss progress, patients feel more hopeful about their chances of success and consequently may be more likely to persist in treatment. Moreover, homogeneity within the group creates a sense of symmetry that both encourages empathy and promotes personal disclosure. Although most obese patients recognize that many people have problems with maintaining weight loss, they may feel that their particular weight problems are unique. Hearing others describe weight-related problems, such as self-disparaging thoughts about body image or a history of yo-yo dieting, may reduce the sense of isolation that obese patients frequently experience and may provide the assurance needed to deal with the more personal aspects of their weight problems. Moreover, if the patient's eating problem involves an element of secrecy, as it often does with binge eating, self-disclosure can be a first step toward behavior change.

In group treatment, a patient's exposure to group members who are coping effectively with weight problems can instill a sense of hope and optimism. Moreover, substantial benefits can be experienced by both the individual who is modeling appropriate behavior and by other group members who are exposed to the model. The individual who is coping effectively is likely to receive social reinforcement for demonstrating progress. The observers are likely to benefit from both the information imparted by the model's behavior and the motivational incentives offered by observing the progress achieved by someone coping with a similar problem. In some instances, the vicarious learning that takes place in the group context may be as effective as learning from direct experience.

Group treatment also provides a safe setting in which members can work to identify effective solutions to common problems. Patients frequently recognize that other group members have an emotional, as well as an intellectual, understanding of their problems—that they have indeed "walked a mile in their shoes." For this reason, advice from a peer sometimes can be more powerful than suggestions from a therapist. Peers can be particularly effective in confronting dysfunctional attitudes, countering feelings of discouragement, and promoting a rational, problem-solving approach to impediments in treatment. Moreover, the *process* of exchanging advice and suggestions may be as important as the actual content of what is learned because it provides a vehicle for the expression of interest and caring among members. The emotional support among members can help sustain their long-term efforts in managing their obesity.

Group treatment can be used during the maintenance phase in several different ways. In those situations where initial weight-loss treatment was provided to patients in a *closed-group format* (i.e., no new members added after treatment is begun), the group can be continued in the same format during the maintenance phase, provided that there are enough members continuing in treatment to provide support. Our experience suggests that at least five or six patients are needed to make optimal use of the group format. In some instances, it may make sense for clinicians to consider conducting open-format maintenance groups. This format can accommodate patients who have undergone initial weight-loss treatment in individual therapy, as well as patients who are in varying stages of continuing care following initial treatment.

Telephone Networking

During the maintenance phase, group meetings are typically scheduled at less frequent intervals than during initial weight-loss treatment. Our own preference is to conduct maintenance-group meetings biweekly. Group members initially may feel relieved to attend sessions less frequently, but even a 2-week interval can seem like a long time to a patient who is experiencing difficulties. One method of bridging the gap between maintenance meetings is to arrange a telephone network among the members of the group. The goal of networking is to create a buddy system that will allow individuals to obtain support on a regular basis and to ensure that they will not be left without support during difficult periods. During the weeks between meetings, each person is responsible for calling a fellow group member. In this way, every patient has at least two contacts with other members because each is scheduled to make one telephone call and to receive one call.

It is not important for individuals to have an established social relationship for these calls to be beneficial; those who have relationships that extend beyond the group will probably be in contact between meetings anyway. Networking is an attempt to augment social supports by encouraging patients to get to know as many others in the group as possible, thereby expanding the number of persons who can potentially be available to provide support when a group member is experiencing a problem.

We have found that initially it is helpful to establish a round-robin schedule for network calls. In this way, the telephone contacts are perceived as a routine component of the maintenance program, as well as a special means of getting help during a crisis. Initially, members are instructed to make their network calls during the week that the group is *not* meeting. It is often helpful to suggest that the calls be made at the same time and day of the week that the group usually meets. Thus, if a group usually meets every other Monday evening from 7:00 to 9:00 P.M., group members can use that time during the off week to make their network calls. In this way, group members, rather than the therapist, review each others' weight-loss progress at the time during the week when they are accustomed to addressing weight-loss issues.

Guidelines for Providing Social Support

Although each member of the group may have been through the same initial treatment, it cannot be assumed that they are equally equipped to provide support. Some patients may feel overwhelmed at the thought of being responsible for another person's problems, particularly if they feel that they cannot solve their own. Therefore, instructing group members in *how* to provide support is a critical part of the networking process. We recommend that prior to implementing the telephone contacts, the clinician should use modeling, role playing, and rehearsal to demonstrate how support can be provided through the telephone network. Patients can be instructed to keep three simple rules in mind: (1) Be positive, (2) be specific, and (3) be available.

Rule 1. Be Positive.   Instruct group members to provide positive reinforcement when their "telephone buddy" reports that he or she is making good progress (e.g., "It sounds like you are doing a great job in maintaining your exercise, Gena; I bet that you are really proud of yourself."). Similarly, the group members should also be instructed to maintain a positive attitude in the face of any difficulties the other person is having. It is important to acknowledge empathically the difficulties that a buddy is experiencing and to remind them that coping with problems is a normal part of the maintenance process. This can be followed by pointing out progress made in other areas to help the individual see things in a more balanced way. For example, "Connie, I understand what you're going through. I know how difficult it is to stay within a calorie goal when there are out-of-town relatives staying in your home. This is the kind of problem we are all learning how to deal with. But don't let yourself get down about it. You've made such great progress in managing your weight, and I'm sure that you are going to be able to find some ways of dealing with this situation too."

Rule 2. Be Specific.   Group members should be encouraged to help the other person develop specific strategies for dealing with a problem. Encourage the individuals in the "helping" role to think about what has worked for them in the past, and to share these experiences. For example, "Something that seems to work for me when I have out-of-town guests, Connie, is to tell them that I have been trying to cook low-fat meals for the entire family because of my concerns about problems such as high cholesterol. You might be surprised to find out that your guests wouldn't mind your preparing some "heart healthy" foods for them as well. The other thing that sometimes works for me is to suggest that we go out for a seafood dinner. I find that guests like seafood, and I can keep to my diet as well." Once potential strategies have been identified, the individual can be asked to make a commitment to taking the appropriate steps (e.g.,

"Connie, I wonder if either of these ideas might make sense for you to try?"). It is important to avoid nonspecific suggestions such as "try harder." The individual may already be trying as hard as possible, and such advice does not provide them with an alternative to an unsuccessful strategy.

Rule 3. Be Available.   At maintenance sessions, group members should be encouraged to determine in advance the best times to call the person whom they are responsible for contacting. In this way, the planned telephone contacts can be made at a time that is mutually convenient. It is important that both persons be free of distractions in order to make good use of the opportunity to provide and receive support. In addition, if an individual is experiencing a problem, it is a good idea to plan an additional telephone contact or to let them know about times when a networking buddy would be available to talk further. For example, "Connie, if you would like to talk more, I'd be happy to give you a call later in the week to see how things are going for you, or you can feel free to give me a call too. My kids are in bed by 9 o'clock every night. So you can give me a ring after 9 on any night."

Group Contingency Contract

The use of a group contingency contract can effectively capitalize on both the cooperative and the competitive elements of the peer group to further weight-loss progress during the maintenance period. At the outset of initial weight-loss treatment, we typically ask patients to post a refundable deposit, usually $100 to $150, that is returned to them contingent on their attendance at treatment sessions and adherence to key weight-loss behaviors, such as self-monitoring of food intake. Those refunds that are forfeited by patients who miss sessions, fail to complete eating diaries, or drop out of treatment are placed into a special fund that is used to provide monetary incentives (i.e., "bonus bucks") during the maintenance phase. One way in which group contingencies with monetary incentives can be used to reinforce weight-loss progress during the maintenance phase is described next.

At the outset, the therapist explains how each member of the maintenance group can earn up to 10 "bonus points" during the 2-week interval between maintenance sessions. Table 11.2 illustrates a "Bonus Points Worksheet," which can be used to tabulate how many points are earned by a group member. Each person in attendance will earn a total of between 1 and 10 bonus points. One point is awarded for each of five key behaviors. Simply showing up at the maintenance session earns a point, and additional points can be obtained for completion of the food diary, for meeting the goals for exercise or caloric intake, and for completing a network telephone call.

An additional 5 points are awarded for progress toward achieving or

TABLE 11.2 BONUS POINTS WORKSHEET

Name _____ Date _____ Goal Weight _____

Part A: Adherence

1. Attendance: You have earned 1 point for attending
   tonight's meeting.   _____
2. Did you complete your eating diary on each of the past 14 days?
   Yes = 1 point, No = 0 points   _____
3. Did you complete one network telephone call during the past
   two weeks? Yes = 1 point, No = 0 points   _____
4. Did you stay within 100 calories of your daily calorie goal on
   10 of the past 14 days? Yes = 1 point, No = 0 points   _____
5. Did you complete 30 minutes of exercise on 10 of the past
   14 days? Yes = 1 point, No = 0 points   _____

   Total points for Part A   _____

Part B - Weight Loss Progress

6. What weight-loss goal did you have for the period comprising
   the past 2 weeks?   _____ pounds
7. What was your weight at the session held 2 weeks ago?
                                              _____ pounds
8. What is your weight tonight?   _____ pounds
9. How much have you lost (or gained) during these past 2 weeks?
                                              _____ pounds
10. If you had a weight-loss goal other than 0, divide the amount
    that you have lost (answer to Item 9) by your weight-loss goal
    (answer to Item 6).   _____
11. Determine the points you have earned (0–5) for weight- loss progress
    according to the following schedule:
    • 5 points for reaching 100% or more of your weight-loss goal
    • 4 points for reaching 75–99% of your weight-loss goal
    • 3 points for reaching 50–74% of your weight-loss goal
    • 2 points for reaching 25–49% of your weight-loss goal
    • 1 point for maintaining your weight or reaching up to 24% of your
      weight-loss goal
    • 0 points for any weight gain

    Total points for Part B   _____

    Total score (A + B)   _____

maintaining goal weight. For each patient, a reasonable goal weight is
established by considering the lowest weight that they have been able to
maintain for 1 year during their past decade of life. We recommend that
patients not shoot for a goal weight that is lower than the top end of the
weight range for their height from Metropolitan Tables. Next, each group
member agrees to a weight-loss goal for the 2-week period between
maintenance sessions. These goals range from 0 to 2.0 pounds. For those
individuals who already are below their goal weights, their weight-loss

goal for the 2-week period is 0 (i.e., no weight gain). For all others, the 2-week weight-loss goal cannot exceed either 2.0 pounds or 1% of their total body weight (whichever is the smaller amount). The number of bonus points earned for weight-loss progress is determined by the percentage of their weight-loss goal achieved by the patient (see Table 11.2).

Thus, if Connie, who weighs 215 pounds, accomplishes her 2-week weight-loss goal of 2 pounds, she earns all 5 of the bonus points allocated for weight-loss progress. If she stayed the same weight over the 2 weeks, she would earn 1 point (see Table 11.2). Lydia, on the other hand, has lost 32 pounds and is now at her goal weight of 152 pounds. Her weight-loss goal for the 2-week period is 0, and she earns 5 points for not gaining weight during this interval.

The bonus points can be used as part of a group contingency contract in the following way: The therapist and group members collaborate to determine a group goal for a 2-week period. The goal is specified in terms of the total number of bonus points earned by all members. If the group meets or exceeds the group goal, then everyone in the group is rewarded with "bonus bucks," usually one or two dollars per person. For example, our Monday night maintenance group has 12 members, each of whom can earn up to 10 bonus points, for a maximum group total of 120 points. The therapist and group members decide that to kick off the bonus system, the first group contract will be based on a total group score of 60 points. If the group achieves 60 points or more at the next maintenance session, then every member will receive a one-dollar bonus. Members who are absent cannot contribute to the group's total, but if the group makes its goal, everyone, including those who are absent, receives a bonus buck. This procedure often encourages group cohesion and sparks in each member a sense of responsibility to the group. We have often heard individuals remark that they were thinking about skipping a maintenance session but decided to attend so as to contribute to their buddies' chances of earning bonus bucks.

At each maintenance session, the therapist and the group members can negotiate the terms of the bonus bucks contract for the next 2-week period. The contract should reflect reasonable expectations for continuing group progress in adherence and weight loss. During the later stages of the maintenance period, it may be important to plan a transition from group to individual contingencies, to taper reliance on the group and shift greater responsibility to the individual. The use of a "maintenance lottery" is one means of facilitating this transition.

The "Maintenance Lottery"

A lottery can stimulate healthy competition among peers and can be an effective technique to keep patients on track with important maintenance-phase goals. The maintenance lottery can be derived from the procedures used in the group contingencies. Each group member continues to earn bonus points, but there is no longer a group goal. Instead, for each point that an individual earns, he or she receives a ticket for a lottery that is conducted during the maintenance session. Thus, the more bonus points that an individual has achieved, the more tickets he or she earns for the lottery, and the greater the chances for winning. A simple way to conduct the lottery is to have a drawing of a name from a hat, with the number of slips of paper placed in the hat with particular patient's name equal to the number of bonus points that he or she has earned.

The prize for the maintenance lottery can be set at a fixed amount, such as ten dollars, or it can be made contingent on some aspect of *group* performance. For example, one dollar can be placed in the "pot" for each group member who is present at the maintenance meeting. Because everyone who attends the session earns a minimum of one bonus point (i.e., for simply showing up), each group member has a chance to win the lottery, regardless of whether they have done well on other aspects of the adherence and weight-loss goals. This procedure provides an incentive for each member to do well and to encourage peers to attend the session as well. Our experience shows that patients really enjoy the maintenance lottery. They perceive it as a fun way to encourage weight-loss progress, and they enjoy the chance of winning the prize.

Learning by Teaching

By the maintenance stage of treatment, patients have acquired a great deal of information about weight loss, diets, and exercise. As they have become better informed, they are able to discriminate between sound, factual information and compelling but unscientific fads. One of the best ways to learn a subject thoroughly is to teach it. Teaching can help the individual to consolidate relevant knowledge and can provide the group with relevant information. More important, assuming the role of a group leader often provides an experience of success that enhances the individual's personal sense of effectiveness and self-esteem.

During the maintenance phase, we incorporate learning by teaching as a routine component of group treatment sessions. Fifteen minutes of every session is allocated to a presentation by one of the group members. All patients are scheduled in a round-robin fashion to take their turns at preparing and presenting a weight-related topic to the group. Potential issues can pertain to eating, exercise, nutrition, health, motivation, or any topic that the presenter believes would in some way be relevant to the other group members. The actual presentation can be brief (e.g., 10 minutes) and can be extrapolated from material obtained from newspapers, magazines, books, audio- or videotapes, fitness programs, television news, or special reports. We have found that most patients take this role of teacher seriously, and many even prepare handouts or copies of articles to supplement their oral presentations. In some instances, a group member may be anxious about doing a presentation, and extra support, encouragement, and coaching by the clinician may be needed to help the patient successfully complete the teaching assignment.

Group Support Outside the Therapy Session

As an extension of therapy, the maintenance group can provide abundant opportunities for social support. Each member is a potential resource for others in the group. The development of social networking outside the group greatly extends the parameters of support that are available to each patient. Individuals who have been through treatment together can be a valuable resource during the follow-up period and well beyond the final stage of treatment.

In the treatment of alcoholism, self-help groups such as AA assist patients in a variety of different ways. One important method is the opportunity for social contact. The patient who is struggling to overcome an alcohol problem often finds that to achieve success in giving up drinking, they must change their former social network in order to avoid the risk of resuming drinking. AA provides an alternative to the isolation and alienation the individual might otherwise experience. Among patients in treatment for obesity, expanding contact may not be as critical as for the alcoholic patient, but it can also provide important benefits. If much of an individual's past social activities revolved around food, finding new outlets for interaction may help the individual to adhere to weight-loss goals. A natural point of interaction for individuals in treatment for obesity would be to develop relationships centered around exercise. In addition to allowing opportunities for socialization, exercise can provide physical and psychological benefits to reinforce the maintenance of weight loss.

In addition to exercising together, group members often want to get together over a meal. Eating in a restaurant situation can represent a significant high-risk situation for many patients. Thus, we often recommend, and initially orchestrate, potluck dinners as a means of having patients deal with eating together in an appropriate manner. Potluck dinners allow individuals who have become acquainted in a treatment setting to expand their social relationships. In addition, such dinners can offer the chance to exchange creative ideas about food. Group members can be encouraged to experiment with new tastes and combinations of ingredients. Consistent with the objectives of the maintenance group, the member who is hosting the dinner can suggest an appropriate theme for the get together, such as "low-calorie appetizers," "heart-healthy entrees," or "low-fat desserts." Each member can be asked to prepare and bring a dish that meets the theme of the dinner. Planned events of this kind can provide an opportunity for the positive expression of interest in food, rather than the sense of deprivation that characterizes much of the patient's struggle with weight.

INFORMAL SOURCES OF SOCIAL SUPPORT

Natural Support Groups

Families and friends are powerful sources of social influence in the obese patient's life. However, this influence can be negative as well as positive. It is important to recognize that negative aspects of the social environment can have deleterious effects on weight loss. Interpersonal conflict produces emotional states that are known predictors of relapse (Brownell et al., 1986). The task of the therapist in working with the social milieu involves (a) helping the patients to effectively utilize available support, (b) teaching them to resist the negative influences in their social environment, and (c) instructing significant others in ways in which they can support the patient's weight-control efforts.

Black and his colleagues (Black, Gleser, & Kooyers, 1990) described the ways in which partners can help in the treatment of obesity in terms of three types of assistance: esteem support, informational support, and instrumental support. *Esteem support* entails the ability to provide encouragement or praise without being directive. This type of support has greatest impact when it comes from a significant person in the patient's life. For example, when a spouse attends a weight-loss meeting, it communicates care and concern, and it conveys to the patient a message of positive regard. *Informational support* is similar to the support provided by an individual in a teaching or coaching role. Prompting, cuing, and modeling of appropriate behaviors, as well as providing feedback about performance are examples of informational support. Finally, *instrumental support* refers to a partner's making specific changes in his or her own actions that can assist the patient. Thus, a partner may agree to refrain from negative behaviors, such as nagging or criticizing the patient, or may initiate positive behaviors consistent with the patient's weight-loss effort, such as beginning a walking program together with the patient.

To determine who in the social environment can best provide support, and who may be a negative influence, Marcoux, Trenkner, and Rosenstock (1990) have recommended the following exercise. Patients create a list of those with whom they are in close contact, such as family members, friends, co-workers and neighbors. Next, each person on the list is evaluated along the dimensions of esteem, informational, and instrumental support by having patients address the following questions: (1) How often does he or she compliment you when you do something well? (2) How often does he or she praise you for following your diet? (3) To what extent would he or she be able to help you with tasks you need to do? (4) How often does he or she join in some physical activity with you? (5) How often does he or she hassle you or make too many demands on you? (6) To what extent does he or she encourage you to have snacks, desserts, and so forth?

In many cases, the patient will have a clear idea about who is likely to be helpful and who is not. However, when there is some doubt, rating individuals along these dimensions will enable patients to make the best use of available supports and to identify the specific areas that need further work.

There are a wide variety of ways in which family members and close friends can assist in the patient's weight-management endeavor. The types and amounts of support that can best help a particular patient need to be assessed idiographically. Some patients will value signs of esteem support from their spouses and will not need other types of assistance. Other individuals may benefit most from a combination of all three types of support. In developing a plan for partner support, the therapist must assess not only the needs of a particular patient, but also the willingness and ability of a spouse or significant other to provide such support.

Good communication is essential to the optimal utilization of supports. Too often, individuals may not get the support they would like simply because they have not let anyone know what they find helpful and what they do not. Even individuals who have lived together for a long time may not be able to predict how the other person feels in a particular situation.

For example, Evelyn, a 41-year old teacher who was moderately overweight would become upset with her husband Jack because each evening after dinner he would continuously watch TV and snack on junk foods until bedtime. Evelyn assumed that Jack was being insensitive to her needs, but rather than express these feelings directly, she reported that she would "clam up" and give her spouse the "silent treatment." Although her husband was aware something was wrong, he had no way of understanding what this was about. Until Evelyn was able to address this issue more directly, both she and her husband felt angry and misunderstood.

Patients can use three simple rules of good communication in asking others for assistance with problems related to their weight: (1) Tell others *how* you would like to be helped; (2) make *specific* requests of others; and (3) state your request *positively*.

Thus, in Evelyn's situation, Evelyn could be encouraged to approach her spouse directly about helping her out. The therapist might model and role play some of the alternatives available to the patient: "Jack, I would like your help with a problem. I find it really hard to stay with my calorie goal when there are so many snack foods around each evening. I would really appreciate it if you and I could talk about this problem and find a way to deal with it. I had a couple of ideas that I wanted to ask you about, and I thought you might have some good suggestions as well. One of my thoughts is that maybe you would like to join me when I go out for my walk after dinner. I would like your company, and it would be better than our just sitting around like a couple of couch potatoes. The other idea I had was maybe it would be helpful for us to try some healthier snacks rather than just having chips and peanuts all the time. Maybe we can come up with some other choices that are less fattening and still taste good."

How Others Can Help

Spouses, family members, and significant others can influence the patient's weight-loss progress through their attitudes and behavior. Cormillot (cited in Brownell, 1990) has described specific dos and don'ts for the family's interactions with the person who is trying to lose weight, such as:

Do keep the house and family relaxed.

Do ask the dieter how you can help.

Do learn to ignore and forgive lapses.

Do exercise with the dieter.

Do not hide food from the dieter.

Do not lecture, criticize, or reprimand.

Do not expect perfection or 100% recovery.

These recommendations are reasonable guidelines for spouses, family members, and significant others to use. For example, because dieting can become tedious and discouraging for both the patient and other members of the family, it is important for all involved to work at keeping a positive attitude and a relaxed atmosphere. The family should not get caught up with setbacks and lapses that the patient is likely to experience. In particular, it is helpful to avoid using guilt or shame as motivators. Encouragement and support are generally more effective influences on behavior. Finally, it is very important for family members to recognize that the person trying to lose weight deserves acceptance and respect (i.e., esteem support), independent of his or her successes or failings in weight management.

Potential Problems in Partner Support

A complex relationship exists between marital or family adjustment and the partner's ability to be supportive of weight-maintenance efforts. Thus, family members are often perceived as both the most and the least helpful to individuals attempting to control their weight (Marcoux et al., 1990). In some cases, a partner in a good relationship may not be able to be supportive with weight loss. In other instances, individuals in a somewhat troubled relationship may be able to provide support in a circumscribed area of the partner's life, such as weight control. However, spouses who are in relationships characterized by a high degree of discord are unlikely to be of much help in obesity treatment, and the patient's weight may simply become a new arena for conflict. For example, a disapproving spouse who views the partner as generally undisciplined or impulsive is also likely to perceive these same negative characteristics in the partner's management of his or her weight.

Weight loss can affect patients and their spouses in both positive and negative ways. While spouses are often quite pleased to see their partner lose weight, in some cases, such change can be experienced as threatening. Spouses sometimes fear that loss of weight will also result in personality or behavioral changes that will affect their relationship. For example, people who lose significant amounts of weight typically look more physically attractive than they did at their higher weights. Such changes may enhance feelings of self-esteem and lead to greater involvement by the patient in social activities. Some spouses may interpret such changes negatively, out of fear that their spouses are less interested in them. In working with couples, the clinician needs to evaluate the implications of weight loss for both the patient and the spouse. By addressing problems such as this, potential obstacles to long-term success can be overcome.

In a small number of cases, intractable problems with weight may reflect serious difficulties within a family system (Minuchin, Rosman, & Baker, 1978). If the overweight individual is the identified patient within the family system, attempting to treat that person alone is unlikely to succeed unless other problems within the family are handled as well. A signal that this may be happening is that the individual in treatment describes dysfunctional patterns of conflict within the family. Although the details of these conflicts may vary, the underlying issues tend to remain the same.

If the patient appears unable to resolve difficulties with the partner, the therapist should consider asking the spouse to come in so that these issues can be discussed together. These meetings should focus on major sources of conflict to help the couple develop a mutually agreeable solution. If these meetings are not effective in producing change, a more intensive couples treatment is probably indicated. The therapist needs to decide whether he or she feels qualified to provide this treatment or whether it would be best to refer the couple to someone specializing in marital or family therapy.

Dealing with Children's Eating

One recent study indicated that among those in the social environment, children were generally perceived as "least helpful" to weight-maintenance efforts (Marcoux et al., 1990). Although the specific reasons were not identified, several explanations come to mind. Young children often eat a number of small meals throughout the day, resulting in increased contact with food for the person responsible for preparing these meals. Also, parents of young children often get into the habit of finishing up food the child has left so that it does not "go to waste." These situations increase difficulty with stimulus control for the overweight individual. In addition, children demand a great deal of attention. It may be extremely difficult to find time for tasks related to weight control such as self-monitoring, preparation of special foods, or exercise when one has primary responsibility for the care of a child. Finally, child-rearing is a difficult task that occasionally may cause anxiety and frustration, mood states that can lead to relapse. Eating in response to emotional cues is more likely to occur under these circumstances.

If the therapist is aware that the care of children creates difficulties with stimulus control or that increased emotionality triggers eating, the therapist should take a problem-solving approach to help the patient with these issues. Definition of the problem is an important step in the process. The patient may be so caught up in the tribulations of everyday life that they do not recognize the degree to which they can achieve greater control over the situation. If lack of time seems be the most prominent issue, teaching the patient better time-management strategies and how to set priorities can be helpful.

Dealing with Negative Social Influences

There are many situations in which overweight individuals must be prepared to meet resistance to their efforts to diet. Both family members and friends may unwittingly sabotage weight-loss efforts. It is not uncommon for the host at a party to insist that a guest eat more than they had planned. "Oh, please, at least try one!" or "This is no time for a diet!" are difficult statements to resist, particularly when food is enticingly prepared, as it is likely to be for special events.

Overweight individuals often face pressure to eat when they are with their families. It is difficult to resist a favorite food when the individual anticipates that refusal may result in hurt, angry feelings. Breaking a diet may seem like the lesser of evils when the alternative is emotional conflict. This is a no-win situation: Individuals are likely to feel upset with themselves if they break their restraint or upset by the reactions of others if they do not.

External pressure to eat reinforces patients' underlying ambivalence and may weaken their resolve. Although some individuals may be assertive in most situations, those who are overweight will almost certainly have more difficulty when the issue is food. There are times when these pressures will inevitably occur. Identifying the elements of an assertive response and practicing these responses will make these situations more manageable. The following five recommendations can help patients to deal more assertively in social situations where they are offered food:

1. Use your tone of voice and facial expression to express sincere conviction about not wanting the food.
2. Maintain good eye contact throughout the interaction.
3. Make clear and simple statements of your preferences.
4. Compliment the efforts of the other person.
5. Suggest an appropriate alternative.

The first step in working with patients who have difficulty asserting themselves in food-related situations is to help them analyze their problem interactions.

Bob, a 42-year-old moderately overweight engineer reported having the most difficulty at social events when he felt that someone would be offended by his refusal to eat what they had prepared. As a guest, he found it difficult to say "no" to food when the person hosting a party would encourage him to eat, with statements such as "I'll be very upset if you don't try one of these; they're my specialty." Individuals who hesitate to express themselves clearly often confuse assertiveness with aggression and, like Bob, may be fearful of hurting others.

In addition to being clear and direct, the patients who are concerned about hurting people by their refusal should acknowledge the feelings of the other person.

Rita, a 32-year old nurse who is moderately overweight described her tendency to overeat when she visited her parents' home: "If I don't eat everything, Mom will feel I didn't enjoy the food. She might even think something is wrong, or that I was angry with her." An assertive response to this situation might encompass the aforementioned five elements. Rita was able to assert her own needs successfully by looking directly at her mother and saying in a firm and sincere manner, "Mom, no thank you. I just couldn't take a second helping. The food was great and I'm really full. It's so good to be home—your cooking is a treat. You work so hard to make everything perfect. If any of the casserole is left over, I'd love to take it for lunch tomorrow." The therapist can help the patient develop more assertive behaviors by role-playing typical problem situations and modeling assertive responses.

FORMAL SELF-HELP GROUPS

During the maintenance or follow-up phase of continuous care, it may be appropriate for the clinician to consider whether the patient might benefit from the additional support offered by self-help groups. OA (Overeaters Anonymous) is the most prominent of the weight-related self-help groups. This organization addresses the needs of the subgroup of overweight individuals for whom compulsive eating is a prominent problem. OA is a 12-step program based on the model of treatment used in AA. Thus, the 12 steps of OA have been adapted from AA and differ only in the reference to food rather than to alcohol or other drugs. For example, Step 1 of OA is "We admitted we were powerless over food—that our lives had become unmanageable."

The major premises of OA can be summarized as follows:

- The "disease" of compulsive eating is threefold: physical, emotional, and spiritual
- The individual must recognize the self-destructive behavior connected with obesity—namely, dieting, starving, overexercising, or purging
- Denial and attempts to split off problems related to eating from other parts of one's life must be confronted
- Food is used as an avoidance—to "sate the fears, anxieties, angers and disappointments of life"
- Control is an issue, not only in the realm of food, but also in many other areas of the individual's life
- The individual's life had been "out of balance"
- Compulsive eaters are "people of extremes" who overreact to small things while ignoring larger issues
- Compulsive eaters pursue short-term solutions to long-term problems
- Overeating has become less comforting over time
- The solution is in giving oneself over to a "Higher Power"
- Recovery comes through helping others with the same problem and living one day at a time

Although the conceptual model espoused by OA is not consistent with current biobehavioral perspectives on eating disorders, the help offered by OA groups may have practical value, particularly in terms of the support that some patients derive from their involvement in OA. OA attempts to help members through a process of self-awareness. A major objective is to have members acknowledge their eating problem and demonstrate a willingness to attempt to change. The emphasis on spirituality represents an effort to have the individual develop a more reflective approach to living.

The pervasive emphasis on spirituality in the writings of OA may make it difficult for individuals who are not religious to relate to this group. However, a distinction is generally made between spirituality and religion. For example, a higher power can be defined traditionally as God, or in terms that some individuals find personally meaningful (e.g., "the shared love of the group").

The various methods of OA include a commitment to what they call "abstinence," (i.e., from compulsive overeating), regular attendance at meetings, extensive reading and writing assignments, supportive telephone contacts, and the guidance of a sponsor. Each member has a sponsor who is the primary source of support, and who has successfully controlled his or her own "addiction" for a significant period of time, usually a minimum of 12 months. In addition to having a sponsor, members are encouraged to obtain the phone numbers of others in the group, and to have at least six people on whom they can call in a personal crisis. Members can "work the steps" with whomever they feel most comfortable, including their sponsor, other group members, or someone outside the group, such as a therapist.

OA groups vary significantly in their interpretation of spirituality and the degree to which the rule of abstinence is applied. In general, abstinence is espoused, not from food, but from compulsive eating. A rigid interpretation of the abstinence rule would prohibit foods that previously led to binging, while a more liberal interpretation would encourage controlled use of these foods. The more extreme application of the abstinence rule has been criticized for the same reasons as has the abstinence model of alcohol treatment. Abstinence creates dichotomous thinking in which the individual is either totally "in" or "out" of control of their "addiction." In some cases, this approach may unwittingly reinforce an overly restrictive approach to the management of eating problems.

There is little research available about the effectiveness of OA. However, anecdotal evidence suggests that this approach can be helpful for some individuals. Clinicians should consider OA as a potential resource for those individuals who need and desire an extensive network of support. If the circumstances warrant it, the clinician might encourage a patient to attend several OA groups to determine whether this approach might be a useful source of help and support in the long-term management of the patient's weight.

COMMERCIAL WEIGHT-LOSS PROGRAMS

Most patients are likely to have had experiences with commercial weight-loss programs. Although these programs may not have met the patient's needs during the initial phase of treatment, they may be important sources of support during maintenance or follow-up periods. For example, Weight Watchers, one of the first commercial weight-loss programs, and probably the most well-known, includes advice and recommendations that are consistent with a comprehensive, conservative approach to the management of obesity. In addition to advice on nutrition and exercise, Weight Watchers also encourages the use of behavioral techniques, such as self-monitoring, and provides an opportunity for social support. The weekly weigh-ins that are a central feature of the program can help an individual to monitor weight-loss progress and can encourage adherence through the effects of social influence. In addition, the program is low in cost and is available in most areas of the country. As noted in Chapter 3, one drawback of commercial programs is their high attrition rates. This problem is more salient when the commercial program is being used as an initial treatment for obesity; it is much less of an issue if a patient is using the program as a source of support during the maintenance or follow-up period. Indeed, the ease of access through which patients can enter and exit from a program such as Weight Watchers can make it an important resource in the patient's long-term effort at weight control.

SUMMARY

For most patients, the long-term management of obesity often means that they will need help and support from others. In this chapter, we described a number of ways in which social-support and social-influence strategies can be used in the continuous care of the obese patient. In a group-therapy context, a variety of social-influence techniques can be used, including telephone networking, group contingency contracts, and competition among members. Other social-support procedures can be implemented in conjunction with either group or individual therapy and include the involvement of partners or family members and the adjunctive use of self-help or commercial weight-loss programs. Through the use of the problem-solving model, the clinician can assess and plan how and when social-support and social-influence procedures can best be implemented to enhance the patient's success in the long-term management of obesity.

References

Abramson, E. E., & Wunderlich, R. A. (1972). Anxiety, fear, and eating: A test of the psychosomatic concept of obesity. *Journal of Abnormal Psychology, 79,* 317–321.

Agras, W. S. (1987). *Eating disorders: Management of obesity, bulimia, and anorexia nervosa.* New York: Pergamon Press.

American College of Sports Medicine. (1991). *Guidelines for exercise testing and exercise prescription* (4th ed.). Philadelphia: Lea & Febiger.

American Diabetes Association. (1986). *Exchange lists for meal planning.* Alexandria, VA: Author.

American Heart Association. (1988). Dietary guidelines for healthy American adults: A statement for physicians and health care professionals by the nutrition committee, American Heart Association. *Circulation, 77,* 721A–724A.

Andersen, T., Stockholm, K. H., Backer, O. G., & Quaade, F. (1988). Long–term (5-year) results after either horizontal gastroplasty or very-low-calorie diet for morbid obesity. *International Journal of Obesity, 12,* 277–284.

Andres, R., Elahi, D., Tobin, J. D., Muller, D. C., & Brant, L. (1985). Impact of age on weight goals. *Annals of Internal Medicine, 103,* 1030–1033.

Ashby, W. A., & Wilson, G. T. (1977). Behavior therapy for obesity: Booster sessions and long-term maintenance of weight. *Behaviour Research and Therapy, 14,* 451–464.

Ashley, F. W., & Kannel, W. B. (1974). Relation of weight change to changes in atherogenic traits: The Framingham study. *Journal of Chronic Diseases, 27,* 103–114.

Ashwell, M. (1978). Commercial weight loss groups. In G. Bray (Ed.), *Recent advances in obesity research: Proceedings of the Second International Congress on Obesity* (Vol. 2; pp. 266–272). London: Newman Publishing.

Ashwell, M. A., & Garrow, J. S. (1975). A survey of three slimming and weight control organisations in the UK. *Nutrition, 29*, 347–356.

Atkinson, R. L. (1989). Low and very low calorie diets. *Medical Clinics of North America, 73*, 203–215.

Ballor, B., Katch, V. L., Becque, M. D., & Marks, C. R. (1988). Resistance weight training during caloric restriction enhances lean body weight maintenance. *American Journal of Clinical Nutrition, 47*, 19–25.

Bannister, E. W., & Brown, S. R. (1968). The relative energy requirements of physical activity. In H. B. Falls (Ed.), *Exercise physiology* (pp. 268–322). New York: Academic Press.

Barrows, K., & Snook, J. T. (1987). Effects of a high-protein, very-low-calorie diet on resting metabolism, thyroid hormones, and energy expenditure of obese middle-aged women. *American Journal of Clinical Nutrition, 45*, 391–398.

Baucom, D. H., & Aiken, P. A. (1981). Effect of depressed mood on eating among obese and nonobese dieting and nondieting persons. *Journal of Personality and Social Psychology, 41*, 577–585.

Beck, A. T., Ward, C. H., Mendelsohn, M., Mock, J., & Erbaugh, J. (1961). An inventory for measuring depression. *Archives of General Psychiatry, 5*, 561–571.

Bellack, A. S., Hersen, M., & Kazdin, A. E. (Eds.). (1990). *International handbook of behavior modification and therapy* (2nd ed.). New York: Plenum.

Beneke, W. M., & Paulsen, B. K. (1979). Long-term efficacy of behavior modification weight loss programs: A comparison of two follow-up maintenance strategies. *Behavior Therapy, 10*, 8–13.

Benn, R. T. (1970). Indices of height and weight as measures of obesity. *British Journal of Preventive and Social Medicine, 24*, 64.

Bennett, G. A. (1986). Behavior therapy for obesity: A quantitative review of selected treatment characteristics on outcome. *Behavior Therapy, 17*, 554–562.

Bernstein, R. A., Giefer, E. E., Vieira, J. J., Werner, L. H., & Rimm, A. A. (1977). Gallbladder disease. II. Utilization of the life table method in obtaining clinically useful information: A study of 62,739 weight conscious women. *Journal of Chronic Diseases, 30*, 529–541.

Billings, A. G., & Moos, R. H. (1981). The role of coping resources and social resources in attenuating the impact of stressful life events. *Journal of Behavioral Medicine, 4*, 139–157.

Bjorntorp, P. (1978). Physical training in the treatment of obesity. *International Journal of Obesity, 2*, 149–156.

Bjorntorp, P. (1985). Regional patterns of fat distribution: Health implications. *Annals of Internal Medicine, 103*, 994–995.

Bjorntorp, P. (1986). Fat cells and obesity. In K. D. Brownell & J. P. Foreyt, (Eds.), *Handbook of eating disorders: Physiology, psychology, and treatment of obesity, anorexia, and bulimia* (pp. 88–98). New York: Basic Books.

Bjorntorp, P., Holm, G., Jacobsson, B., Schiller-de Jounge, K., Lundberg, P., Sjostrom, L., Smith, U., & Sullivan, L. (1977). Physical training in human hyperplastic obesity: Effects on the hormonal status. *Metabolism, 26*, 319–328.

Bjorntorp, P., & Yang, M. (1982). Refeeding after fasting in the rat: Effects on body composition and food efficiency. *American Journal of Clinical Nutrition, 36*, 444–449.

Bjorvell, H., & Rossner, S. (1985). Long-term treatment of severe obesity: Four year follow-up of results of combined behavioural modification programme. *British Medical Journal, 291*, 379–382.

Bjorvell, H., & Rossner, S. (1990). A ten year follow-up of weight change in severely obese subjects treated in a behavioural modification programme. *International Journal of Obesity, 14*(Suppl. 2), 88.

Black, D. R. (1987). A minimal intervention program and a problem-solving program for weight control. *Cognitive Therapy and Research, 11*, 107–120.

Black, D. R., Coe, W. C., Friesen, J. G., & Wurzmann, A. G. (1984). A minimal intervention for weight control: A cost-effective alternative. *Addictive Behaviors, 9*, 279–285.

Black, D. R., Gleser, L. J., & Kooyers, K. J. (1990). A meta-analytic evaluation of couples weight-loss programs. *Health Psychology, 9*, 330–347.

Black, D. R., & Threlfall, W. E. (1986). A stepped approach to weight control: A minimal intervention and a bibliotherapy problem-solving program. *Behavior Therapy, 17*, 144–157.

Black, D. R., & Threlfall, W. E. (1989). Partner weight status and subject weight loss: Implications for cost-effective programs and public health. *Addictive Behaviors, 14*, 279–289.

Blackburn, G. L., Bistrian, B. R., & Flatt, J. P. (1975). Role of protein-sparing modified fast in a comprehensive weight reduction program. In A. N. Howard (Ed.), *Recent advances in obesity research* (pp. 279–281). London: Newman.

Blackburn, G. L., Lynch, M. E., & Wong, S. L. (1986). The very-low-calorie diet: A weight reduction technique. In K. D. Brownell & J. P. Foreyt (Eds.), *Handbook of eating disorders: Physiology, psychology, and treatment of obesity, anorexia, and bulimia* (pp. 198–213). New York: Basic Books.

Blackburn, G. L., Phinney, S. D., & Moldawer, L. I. (1981). Mechanisms of nitrogen sparing with severe calorie restricted diets. *International Journal of Obesity, 5*, 215–216.

Blackburn, G. L., Wilson, G. T., Kanders, B. S., Stein, L. J., Lavin, P. T., Adler, J., & Brownell, K. D. (1989). Weight cycling: The experience of human dieters. *American Journal of Clinical Nutrition, 49*, 1105–1109.

Block, J. (1985). Sleep apnea and related disorders. *Disease-a-Month, 31*, 1–56.

Bogardus, C., Lillioja, S., Ravussin, E., Abbott, J. K., Zawadzk, A., Young, W. C., Knowler, R., Jacobowitz, R., & Moll, P. P. (1986). Familial dependence of the resting metabolic rate. *New England Journal of Medicine, 315*, 96–100.

Bouchard, C. (1989). Genetic factors in obesity. *Medical Clinics of North America, 73*, 67–81.

Bouchard, C. (1991). Heredity and the path to overweight and obesity. *Medicine and Science in Sports and Exercise, 23*, 285–291.

Bouchard, C., Perusse, L., Leblanc, C., Tremblay, A., & Theriault, G. (1988). Inheritance of the amount and distribution of human body fat. *International Journal of Obesity, 12*, 205–215.

Bouchard, C., Tremblay, A., Despres, J., Nadeau, A., Lupien, P. J., Theriault, G.,

Dussault, J., Moorjani, S., Pinault, S., & Fournier, G. (1990). The response to long-term overfeeding in identical twins. *New England Journal of Medicine, 322,* 1477–1482.

Braitman, L. E., Adlin, E. V., & Stanton, J. L. (1985). Obesity and caloric intake: The National Health and Nutrition Examination Survey of 1971–1975 (HANES I). *Journal of Chronic Diseases, 38,* 727–732.

Bray, G. A. (1969). Effects of caloric restriction on energy expenditure in obese patients. *Lancet, 2,* 397–398.

Bray, G. A. (1985). Complications of obesity. *Annals of Internal Medicine, 103,* 1052–1062.

Bray, G. A. (1986). Effects of obesity on health and happiness. In K. D. Brownell & J. P. Foreyt (Eds.), *Handbook of eating disorders: Physiology, psychology, and treatment of obesity, anorexia, and bulimia.* (pp. 3–44), New York: Basic Books.

Bray, G. A. (1990). Exercise and obesity. In C. Bouchard, R. J. Shepherd, T. Stephens, J. R. Sutton, & B. D. McPherson (Eds.), *Exercise, fitness, and health: A consensus of current knowledge* (pp. 497–509). Champaign, IL: Human Kinetics Press.

Bray, G. A., Glennon, J. A., Ruedi, B., Cheifetz, P., & Cassidy, C. E. (1969). Triiodothyronine and mercurial diuretics: Effects on excretion of a water load and on plasma free fatty acids in obese patients. *American Journal of Clinical Nutrition, 22,* 1420–1422.

Bray, G. A., & Gray, D. S. (1988). Obesity: II. Treatment. *Western Journal of Medicine, 149,* 555–571.

Brehm, S., & McAllister, D. A. (1980). Social psychological perspectives on the maintenance of therapeutic change. In P. Karoly & J. J. Steffen (Eds.), *Improving the long-term effects of psychotherapy* (pp. 381–406). New York: Gardner Press.

Brolin, R. E. (1987). Results of obesity surgery. *Gastroenterology Clinics of North America, 16,* 317.

Brownell, K. D. (1982). Obesity: Understanding and treating a serious, prevalent, and refractory disorder. *Journal of Clinical and Counseling Psychology, 50,* 820–840.

Brownell, K. D. (1990). *The LEARN program for weight control.* Dallas, TX: Brownell & Hager.

Brownell, K. D. (1991). Dieting and the search for the perfect body: Where physiology and culture collide. *Behavior Therapy, 22,* 1–12.

Brownell, K. D., & Foreyt, J. P. (1985). Obesity. In D. H. Barlow (Ed.), *Clinical handbook of psychological disorders* (pp. 299–345). New York: Guilford.

Brownell, K. D., Greenwood, M. R. C., Stellar, E., & Shrager, E. E. (1986). The effects of repeated cycles of weight loss and regain in rats. *Physiology and Behavior, 38,* 459–464.

Brownell, K. D., & Jeffery, R. W. (1987). Improving long-term weight loss: Pushing the limits of treatment. *Behavior Therapy, 18,* 353–374.

Brownell, K. D., Marlatt, G. A., Lichtenstein, E., & Wilson, G. T. (1986). Understanding and preventing relapse. *American Psychologist, 41,* 765–782.

Brownell, K. D., & Rodin, J. (1990). *The weight maintenance survival guide.* Dallas, TX: Brownell & Hagar.

Brownell, K. D., & Stunkard, A. J. (1980). Physical activity in the development and control of obesity. In A. J. Stunkard (Ed.), *Obesity* (pp. 300–324). Philadelphia: W. B. Saunders.

Brownell, K. D., Stunkard, A. J., & Albaum, J. M. (1980). Evaluation and modification of exercise patterns in the natural environment. *American Journal of Psychiatry, 137,* 1540–1545.

Brownell, K. D., & Wadden, T. A. (1986). Behavior therapy for obesity: Modern approaches and better results. In K. D. Brownell & J. P. Foreyt (Eds.), *Handbook of eating disorders: Physiology, psychology, and treatment of obesity, anorexia, and bulimia* (pp. 180–197). New York: Basic Books.

Brownell, K. D., & Wadden, T. A. (1991). The heterogeneity of obesity: Fitting treatments to individuals. *Behavior Therapy, 22,* 153–177.

Bruch, H. (1981). Developmental considerations of anorexia nervosa and obesity. *Canadian Journal of Psychiatry, 26,* 212–217.

Cassell, J. A. (1989). Commentary: American food habits in the 1980s. *Topics in Clinical Nutrition, 4,* 47–58.

Centers for Disease Control. (1990, June). CDC surveillance summaries. *Morbidity and Mortality Weekly Report, 39* (SS-2), 8.

Clark, M. M., Abrams, D. B., Niaura, R. S., Eaton, C. A., & Rossi, J. S. (1991). Self-efficacy in weight management. *Journal of Consulting and Clinical Psychology, 59,* 739–744.

Clarys, J. P., Martin, A. D., & Drinkwater, D. T. (1984). Gross tissue weight in the human body by cadaver dissection. *Human Biology, 56,* 459–473.

Cleary, M. P. (1986). Consequences of restricted feeding/refeeding cycles in lean and obese female Zucker rats. *Journal of Nutrition, 116,* 290–303.

Cohn, C., & Joseph, D. (1962). Influence of body weight and body fat on appetite of "normal" lean and obese rats. *Yale Journal of Biology, 34,* 598–607.

Colvin, R. H., & Olson, S. B. (1983). A descriptive analysis of men and women who have lost weight and are highly successful at maintaining the loss. *Addictive Behaviors, 8,* 287–296.

Cook, T. D. (1985). Post-positivist critical multiplism. In L. Shotland & M. M. Marks (Eds.), *Social science and social policy* (pp. 21–62). Beverly Hills, CA: Sage.

Craighead, L. W. (1987). Behavior therapy and pharmocotherapy in the treatment of obesity. In W. G. Johnson (Ed.), *Advances in eating disorders: Vol. 1. Treating and preventing obesity* (pp. 65–86). Greenwich, CT: JAI.

Craighead, L. W., & Blum, M. D. (1989). Supervised exercise in behavioral treatment for moderate obesity. *Behavior Therapy, 20,* 49–59.

Craighead, L. W., Stunkard, A. J., & O'Brien, R. (1981). Behavior therapy and pharmacotherapy for obesity. *Archives of General Psychiatry, 38,* 763–768.

Craighead, W. E. (1980). Away from a unitary model of depression. *Behavior Therapy, 11,* 112–118.

Dahlkoetter, J., Callahan, E. J., & Linton, J. (1979). Obesity and the unbalanced energy equation. *Journal of Consulting and Clinical Psychology, 47,* 898–905.

Derogatis, L. R., Lipman, R. S., & Covi, L. (1975). SCL-90: An outpatient psychiatric rating scale—Preliminary report. *Psychopharmacology Bulletin, 9,* 13–27.

deVries, H. A., & Adams, G. M. (1972). Electromyographic comparison of single dose of exercise and meprobamate as to effects on muscular relaxation. *American Journal of Physical Medicine, 51,* 130–141.

Dishman, R. K. (1988). *Exercise adherence: Its impact on public health.* Champaign, IL: Human Kinetics.

Dishman, R. K., Sallis, J. F., & Orenstein, D. (1985). The determinants of physical activity and exercise. *Public Health Reports, 100,* 158–171.

Doherty, J. U., Wadden, T. A., Zuk, L., Letizia, K. A., Foster, G. D., & Day, S. C. (1991). Long-term evaluation of cardiac function in obese patients treated with a very-low-calorie diet: A controlled clinical study of patients without underlying cardiac disease. *American Journal of Nutrition, 53,* 854–858.

Donahoe, C. P., Lin, D. H., Kirschenbaum, D. S., & Keesey, R. E. (1984). Metabolic consequences of dieting and exercise in the behavioral treatment of obesity. *Journal of Consulting and Clinical Psychology, 52,* 827–836.

Doyne, E. J., Chambless, D. L., & Beutler, L. E. (1983). Aerobic exercise as a treatment for depression in women. *Behavior Therapy, 14,* 434–440.

Doyne, E. J., Ossip-Klein, D. J., Bowman, E. D., Osborn, K. M., McDougall-Wilson, I. B., & Neimeyer, R. A. (1987). Running versus weight lifting in the treatment of depression. *Journal of Consulting and Clinical Psychology, 55,* 748–754.

Drenick, E. J., & Smith, R. (1964). Weight reduction by starvation. *Postgraduate Medicine,* A-95 through A-100.

Dreon, D. M., Frey-Hewitt, B., Ellsworth, N., Williams, P. T., Terry, R. B., & Wood, P. D. (1988). Dietary fat: Carbohydrate ratio and obesity in middle-aged men. *American Journal of Clinical Nutrition, 47,* 995–1000.

Ducimetiere, P., Avons, P., Cambien, F., & Richard, J. L. (1983). Corpulence history and fat distribution in CHD etiology—The Paris Prospective Study. *European Heart Journal, 4,* 8.

Dunne, L. J. (1990). *Nutrition almanac* (3rd ed.). New York: McGraw-Hill.

Durnin, J., & Womersley, J. (1974). Body fat assessed from total body density and its estimation from skinfold thickness: Measurements on 481 men and women aged from 16 to 72 years. *British Journal of Nutrition, 32,* 77–97.

D'Zurilla, T. J., & Goldfried, M. R. (1971). Problem solving and behavior modification. *Journal of Abnormal Psychology, 78,* 107–126.

D'Zurilla, T. J., & Nezu, A. M. (1982). Social problem solving in adults. In P. C. Kendall (Ed.), *Advances in cognitive-behavioral research and therapy* (Vol. 1, pp. 202–274). New York: Academic Press.

D'Zurilla, T. J., & Nezu, A. M. (1990). Development and preliminary evaluation of the Social Problem-Solving Inventory (SPSI). *Psychological Assessment: A Journal of Consulting and Clinical Psychology, 2,* 156–163.

Eaton, S. B., & Konner, M. (1985). Paleolithic nutrition: A consideration of its nature and current implications. *New England Journal of Medicine, 312,* 283–289.

Epstein, L. H., & Wing, R. R. (1980). Aerobic exercise and weight. *Addictive Behaviors, 5,* 371–388.

Falls, H. B., Baylor, A. M., & Dishman, R. K. (1980). *Essentials of fitness.* Philadelphia: Saunders.

Faust, I. M., Johnson, P. R., Stern, J. S., & Hirsch, J. (1978). Diet-induced adipocyte number increase in adult rats: A new model of obesity. *American Journal of Physiology, 235,* E279–E286.

References   265

Ferguson, J. M., & Feighner, J. P. (1987). Fluoxetine-induced weight loss in over-weight non-depressed humans. *International Journal of Obesity, 11*(Suppl. 3), 163–170.

Ferster, C. B., Nurnberger, J. I., & Levitt, E. E. (1962). The control of eating. *Journal of Mathetics, 1*, 87–109.

Feurer, I. D., & Mullen, J. L. (1986). Measurement of energy expenditure. In J. Rombeau & M. Caldwell (Eds.), *Clinical nutrition* (Vol. 2, pp. 224–236). Philadelphia: Saunders.

Flatt, J. P. (1987). The difference in the storage capacities for carbohydrate and for fat, and its implications in the regulation of body weight. In R. J. Wurtman & J. J. Wurtman (Eds.), *Human obesity* (pp. 104–123). New York: New York Academy of Sciences.

Folkins, C. H., & Sime, W. E. (1981). Physical fitness training and mental health. *American Psychologist, 36*, 373–389.

Fontaine, E., Savard, R., Tremblay, A., Despres, J. P., Poehlman, E. T., & Bouchard, C. (1985). Resting metabolic rate in monozygotic and dizygotic twins. *Acta Geneticae Medicae et Gemellologiae, 34*, 41–47.

Foreyt, J. P. (1987a). The addictive disorders. In C. M. Franks, G. T. Wilson, P. C. Kendall, & J. P. Foreyt (Eds.), *Review of behavior therapy: Theory and practice* (Vol. 11, pp. 187–233). New York: Guilford.

Foreyt, J. P. (1987b). Issues in the assessment and treatment of obesity. *Journal of Consulting and Clinical Psychology, 55*, 677–684.

Foreyt, J. P. (1990). The addictive disorders. In C. M. Franks, G. T. Wilson, P. C. Kendall, & J. P. Foreyt (Eds.), *Review of behavior therapy: Theory and practice* (Vol. 12, pp. 178–224). New York: Guilford Press.

Foreyt, J. P., & Goodrick, G. K. (1991). Factors common to successful therapy for the obese patient. *Medicine and Science in Sports and Exercise, 23*, 292–297.

Foster, G. D., Wadden, T. A., Feurer, I. D., Jennings, A. S., Stunkard, A. J., Crosby, L. O., Ship, J., & Mullen, J. L. (1990). Controlled trial of the metabolic effects of a very-low-calorie diet: Short- and long-term effects. *American Journal of Clinical Nutrition, 51*, 167–172.

Foster, G. D., Wadden, T. A., Mullen, J. L., Stunkard, A. J., Wang, J., Feurer, I. D., Pierson, R. N., Yang, M. U., Presta, E., Van Itallie, T. B., Lemberg, P. S., & Gold, J. (1988). Resting energy expenditure, body composition, and excess weight in the obese. *Metabolism, 37*, 467–472.

Frey-Hewitt, B., Vranizan, K. M., Dreon, D. M., & Wood, P. D. (1990). The effect of weight loss by dieting or exercise on resting metabolic rate in overweight men. *International Journal of Obesity, 14*, 323–330.

Friedman G. D., Kannel, W. B., & Dawber, T. R. (1966). The epidemiology of gall bladder disease: Observations in the Framingham study. *Journal of Chronic Diseases, 19*, 273–292.

Garb, J. R., & Stunkard, A. J. (1974). Effectiveness of a self-help group in obesity control: A further assessment. *Archives of Internal Medicine, 134*, 716–720.

Garfield, S. L., & Bergin, A. E. (1986). *Handbook of psychotherapy and behavior change* (3rd ed.). New York: Wiley.

Garn, S. M., Leonard, W. R., & Hawthorne, V. M. (1986). Three limitations of the body-mass index. *American Journal of Clinical Nutrition, 44*, 996.

Garner, D. M., & Garfinkel, P. (1979). The Eating Attitudes Test: An index of the symptoms of anorexia nervosa. *Psychological Medicine, 13,* 821–828.

Garner, D. M., & Olmsted, M. P. (1984). *The Eating Disorder Inventory manual.* Odessa, FL: Psychological Assessment Resources.

Garnett, E. S., Bernard, D. L., Ford, J., Goodbody, R. A., & Woodhouse, M. A. (1969). Gross fragmentation of starvation for obesity. *Lancet, 1,* 14–16.

Garrow, J. S. (1974). *Energy balance and obesity in man.* New York: Elsevier.

Garrow, J. S. (1978). *Energy balance and obesity in man* (2nd ed.). New York: Elsevier.

Garrow, J. S. (1981). *Treat obesity seriously.* London: Churchill Livingstone.

Garrow, J. S. (1986). Physiological aspects of obesity. In K. D. Brownell & J. P. Foreyt (Eds.), *Handbook of eating disorders: Physiology, psychology, and treatment of obesity, anorexia, and bulimia* (pp. 45–62). New York: Basic Books.

Geissler, C. A., Miller, D. S., & Shah, M. (1987). The daily metabolic rate of the post-obese and the lean. *American Journal of Clinical Nutrition, 45,* 914–920.

Gentry, K., Halverson, J. D., & Heisler, S. (1984). Psychologic assessment of morbidly obese patients undergoing gastric bypass: A comparison of preoperative and postoperative adjustment. *Surgery, 95,* 215–220.

Gibson, G. S., Gerberich, S. G., & Leon, A. S. (1983). Writing the exercise prescription: An individualized approach. *Physical Sports Medicine, 11,* 87–110.

Goldstein, A. P. (1975). Relationship-enhancement methods. In F. H. Kanfer & A. P. Goldstein (Eds.), *Helping people change.* New York: Pergamon.

Gormally, J., Black, S., Daston, S., & Rardin, D. (1982). The assessment of binge eating severity among obese persons. *Addictive Behaviors, 7,* 47–55.

Gormally, J., & Rardin, D. (1981). Weight loss and maintenance and changes in diet and exercise for behavioral counseling and nutrition education. *Journal of Counseling Psychology, 28,* 295–304.

Gortmaker, S. L., Dietz, W. H., & Cheung, L. W. Y. (1990). Inactivity, dieting, and the fattening of America. *Journal of the American Dietetic Association, 90,* 1247–1252.

Gortmaker, S. L., Dietz, W. H., Sobol, A. M., & Wehler, C. A. (1987). Increasing pediatric obesity in the United States. *American Journal of Diseases of Childhood, 141,* 535.

Gotestam, K. G., & Hauge, L. S. (1987). Drug treatment of obesity. In W. G. Johnson (Ed.), *Advances in eating disorders: Vol. 1. Treating and preventing obesity* (pp. 39–64). Greenwich, CT: JAI.

Gray, D. S., Fisler, J. S., & Bray, G. A. (1988). Effects of repeated weight loss and regain on body composition in obese rats. *American Journal of Clinical Nutrition, 47,* 393–399.

Grilo, C. M., Shiffman, S., & Wing, R. R. (1989). Relapse crises and coping among dieters. *Journal of Consulting and Clinical Psychology, 57,* 488–495.

Grundy, S. M., Florentin, L., Nix, D., & Whelan, M. F. (1988). Comparison of monounsaturated fatty acids and carbohydrates for reducing raised levels of plasma cholesterol in man. *American Journal of Clinical Nutrition, 47,* 966–969.

Guy-Grand, B. J. P. (1987). A new approach to the treatment of obesity. In R. J. Wurtman & J. J. Wurtman (Eds.), *Human obesity* (pp. 313–317). New York: New York Academy of Sciences.

Guy-Grand, B., Apfelbaum, M., Crepalki, G., Gries, A., Lefebvre, P., & Turner, P. (1989). International trial of long-term dexfenfluramine in obesity. *Lancet, 2,* 1142–1145.

Hagberg, J. M. (1990). Exercise, fitness, and hypertension. In C. Bouchard, R. J. Shepherd, T. Stephens, J. R. Sutton, & B. D. McPherson (Eds.), *Exercise, fitness, and health: A consensus of current knowledge* (pp. 455–466). Champaign, IL: Human Kinetics Books.

Hall, S. M., Bass, A., & Monroe, J. (1978). Continued contact and monitoring as follow-up strategies: A long-term study of obesity treatment. *Addictive Behaviors, 3,* 139–147.

Hall, S. M., Hall, R. G., Borden, B. L., & Hanson, R. W. (1975). Follow-up strategies in the behavioral treatment of overweight. *Behaviour Research and Therapy, 13,* 167–172.

Halmi, K. A., Long, M., & Stunkard, A. J. (1980). Psychiatric diagnosis of morbidly obese gastric bypass patients. *American Journal of Psychiatry, 137,* 470–472.

Halmi, K. A., Stunkard, A. J., & Mason, E. E. (1980). Emotional responses to weight reduction by three methods: Diet, jejunoileal bypass, and gastric bypass. *American Journal of Clinical Nutrition, 33,* 351–357.

Halverson, J. D., Wise, L., Wazna, R. F., & Ballinger, W. F. (1978). Jejunoileal bypass for morbid obesity: A critical appraisal. *American Jounal of Medicine, 64,* 461–475.

Hamm, P., Shekelle, R. B., & Stamler, J. (1989). Large fluctuations in body weight during young adulthood and twenty-five-year risk of coronary death in men. *American Journal of Epidemiology, 129,* 312–318.

Harris, M. B., & Hallbauer, E. S. (1973). Self-directed weight control through eating and exercise modification. *Behaviour Research and Therapy, 11,* 523–529.

Harrison, G. G. (1984). Purposes and types of classification. *International Journal of Obesity, 8,* 481–490.

Hartz, A. J., & Rimm, A. A. (1980). Natural history of obesity in 6,946 women between 50 and 59 years of age. *American Journal of Public Health, 70,* 385–388.

Hartz, A. J., Rupley, D. C., & Rimm, A. A. (1984). The association of girth measurements with disease in 32,856 women. *Journal of Epidemiology, 119,* 71–80.

Herman, C. P., & Mack, D. (1975). Restrained and unrestrained eating. *Journal of Personality, 43,* 647–660.

Herman, C. P., & Polivy, J. (1975). Anxiety, restraint, and eating behavior. *Journal of Abnormal Psychology, 84,* 666–672.

Herman, C. P., & Polivy, J. (1980). Restrained eating. In A. J. Stunkard (Ed.), *Obesity* (pp. 208–225). Philadelphia: Saunders.

Hersen, M. (1981). Complex problems require complex solutions. *Behavior Therapy, 12,* 15–29.

Hill, J. O., Sparling, P. B., Shields, T. W., & Heller, P. A. (1987). Exercise and food restriction: Effects on body composition and metabolic rate in obese women. *American Journal of Clinical Nutrition, 46,* 622–630.

Hill, S., & McCutcheon, N. (1975). Eating responses of obese and nonobese humans during dinner meals. *Psychological Medicine, 37,* 395–401.

Hirsch, J., & Batchelor, B. (1976). Adipose tissue cellularity in human obesity. *Clinical Endocrinology and Metabolism, 5,* 299–311.

Hirsch, J., Fried, S. K., Edens, N. K., & Leibel, R. L. (1989). The fat cell. *Medical Clinics of North America, 73,* 83–96.

Hocking, M. P., Kelly, K. A., & Callaway, C. W. (1986). Vertical gastroplasty for morbid obesity: Clinical experience. *Mayo Clinic Procedures, 61,* 287–291.

Hoiberg, A., Berard, S., Watten, R. H., & Caine, C. (1984). Correlates of weight loss in treatment and at follow-up. *International Journal of Obesity, 8,* 457–465.

Hovell, M. F., Koch, A., Hofstetter, C. R., Sipan, C., Faucher, P., Dellinger, A., Borok, G., Forsyther, A., & Felitti, V. J. (1988). Long-term weight loss maintenance: Assessment of a behavioral and supplemented fasting regimen. *American Journal of Public Health, 78,* 663–666.

Howard, A. N., Grant, A., Edwards, O., Littlewood, E. R., & McLean Baird, I. (1978). The treatment of obesity with a very-low-calorie liquid-formula diet: An inpatient/outpatient comparison using skimmed milk as the chief protein source. *International Journal of Obesity, 2,* 321–332.

Howley, E. T., & Glover, M. E. (1974). The caloric costs of running and walking one mile for men and women. *Medicine and Science in Sports, 6,* 235.

Hoyt, M. F., & Janis, I. L. (1975). Increasing adherence to a stressful decision via a motivational balance-sheet procedure: A field experiment. *Journal of Personality and Social Psychology, 31,* 833–839.

Hubert, H. B., Feinleib, M., McNamara, P. M., & Castelli, W. P. (1983). Obesity as an independent risk factor for cardiovascular disease: A 26-year follow-up of participants in Framingham heart study. *Circulation, 67,* 968–977.

Hughes, J. R. (1984). Psychological effects of exercise. *Preventive Medicine, 13,* 66–78.

Jeffery, R. W. (1987). Behavioral treatment of obesity. *Annals of Behavioral Medicine, 9,* 20–24.

Jen, K.-L. C. (1988). Effects of diet composition on food intake and carcass composition in rats. *Physiology and Behavior, 42,* 551–556.

Jequier, E. (1987). Energy, obesity, and body weight standards. *American Journal of Clinical Nutrition, 45,* 1035–1047.

Johnson, W. G., & Stalonas, P. M. (1981). *Weight no longer.* Gretna, LA: Pelican.

Kanfer, F. H. (1985). Target selection for clinical change programs. *Behavioral Assessment, 7,* 7–20.

Kanfer, F. H., & Goldstein, A. P. (Eds.). (1991). *Helping people change: A textbook of methods* (4th ed.). New York: Pergamon.

Kanfer, F. H., & Phillips, J. S. (1970). *Learning foundations of behavior therapy.* New York: Wiley.

Kanner, A. D., Coyne, J. C., Schaefer, C., & Lazarus, R. S. (1981). Comparison of two modes of stress measurement: Daily hassles and uplifts versus major life events. *Journal of Behavioral Medicine, 4,* 1–39.

Kaplan, K. K., & Wadden, T. A. (1986). Childhood obesity and self-esteem. *Journal of Pediatrics, 109,* 367–370.

Katahn, M., Pleas, J., Thackrey, M., & Wallston, K. A. (1982). Relationship of eating and activity reports to follow-up weight maintenance in the massively obese. *Behavior Therapy, 13,* 521–528.

Katzeff, H. L. (1988). Energy metabolism and thermogenesis in obesity. In R. Frankle & M.-U. Yang (Eds.), *Obesity and weight control* (pp. 55–70). Rockville, MD: Aspen.

Katzeff, H. L., O'Connell, M., Horton, E. S., Danforth, E., Young, J. B., & Landsberg, L. (1986). Metabolic studies in human obesity during overnutrition and undernutrition: Thermogenic and hormonal responses to norepinephrine. *Metabolism*, *35*, 166–175.

Kayman, S., Bruvold, W., & Stern, J. S. (1990). Maintenance and relapse after weight loss in women: Behavioral aspects. *American Journal of Clinical Nutrition*, *52*, 800–807.

Keesey, R. E. (1980). The regulation of body weight: A set-point analysis. In A. J. Stunkard (Ed.), *Obesity* (pp. 144–165). Philadelphia: Saunders.

Keesey, R. E. (1986). A set-point theory of obesity. In K. D. Brownell & J. P. Foreyt (Eds.), *Handbook of eating disorders: Physiology, psychology, and treatment of obesity, anorexia, and bulimia* (pp. 63–87). New York: Basic Books.

Keesey, R. E. (1989). Physiological regulation of body weight and the issue of obesity. *Medical Clinics of North America*, *73*, 15–28.

Kern, P. A., Ong, J. M., Saffari, B., & Carty, J. (1990). The effects of weight loss on the activity and expression of adipose-tissue lipoprotein lipase in very obese humans. *New England Journal of Medicine*, *322*, 1053–1059.

Keys, A. (1979). Dietary survey methods. In R. Levy, B. Rifkind, & B. Dennis (Eds.), *Nutrition, lipids, and coronary heart disease* (pp. 1–23). New York: Raven Press.

Keys, A., Brozek, J., Henschel, A., Mickelsen, O., & Taylor, H. L. (1950). *The biology of human starvation*. Minneapolis: University of Minnesota Press.

Keys, A., Fidanza, F., Karvonen, M. J., Kimura, N., & Taylor, H. (1972). Indices of relative weight and obesity. *Journal of Chronic Diseases*, *25*, 329–343.

King, A. C., Frey-Hewitt, B., Dreon, D. M., & Wood, P. D. (1989). Diet vs. exercise in weight management: The effects of minimal intervention strategies on long-term outcomes in men. *Archives of Internal Medicine*, *149*, 2741–2746.

King, A. C., & Tribble, D. C. (1991). The role of exercise in weight reduction in nonathletes. *Sports Medicine*, *11*, 331–349.

Kingsley, R. G., & Wilson, G. T. (1977). Behavior therapy for obesity: A comparative investigation of long-term efficacy. *Journal of Consulting and Clinical Psychology*, *45*, 288–298.

Kinsell, L. W., Gunning, B., Michaels, G. D., Richardson, J., Cox, C. B., & Lemon, C. (1964). Calories do count. *Metabolism*, *13*, 195–203.

Kirby, R., Anderson, J., & Sieling, B. (1981). Oat-bran intake selectively lowers serum low-density lipoprotein cholesterol concentrations of hypercholesterolemic men. *American Journal of Clinical Nutrition*, *34*, 824–829.

Kirschenbaum, D. S. (1987). Self-regulatory failures: A review with clinical implications. *Clinical Psychology Review*, *7*, 77–104.

Kissebah, A. H., Pieris, A., & Evans, D. J. (1986). Mechanisms associating body fat distribution with abnormal metabolic profiles in obesity. In E. Berry (Ed.), *Recent advances in obesity research*. London: John Libbey.

Kissebah, A. H., Vydelingum, N., Murray, R., Evans, D. J., Hartz, A. J., Kalkoff, R. K., & Adams, P. W. (1982). Relationship of body fat distribution to metabolic complications of obesity. *Journal of Clinical Endocrinology and Metabolism, 54,* 254–260.

Kisseleff, H. R., Klingsberg, G., & Van Itallie, T. B. (1980). Universal eating monitor for continuous recording of solid or liquid consumption in man. *American Journal of Physiology, 238,* 14–22.

Klajner, F., Herman, C. P., Polivy, J., & Chhabra, R. (1981). Human obesity, dieting, and anticipatory salivation to food. *Physiology and Behavior, 27,* 195–198.

Klein, M. H., Greist, J. H., Gurman, A. S., Neimeyer, R. A., Lesser, D. P., Bushnell, N. J., & Smith, R. E. (1985). A comparative outcome study of group psychotherapy vs. exercise treatments for depression. *International Journal of Mental Health, 13,* 148–175.

Knittle, J. L., Timmens, K., Ginsberg-Fellner, F., Brown, R. E., & Katz, D. P. (1979). The growth of adipose tissue in children and adolescents. *Journal of Clinical Investigation, 63,* 239–246.

Kolterman, O. G., Olefsky, J. M., Kurahara, C., & Taylor, K. (1982). A defect in cell-mediated immune function in insulin-resistant diabetic and obese subjects. *Journal of Laboratory and Clinical Medicine, 96,* 535–543.

Kral, J. (1988). Surgery for obesity. In R. T. Frankle & M.-U. Yang (Eds.), *Obesity and weight control* (pp. 297–313). Rockville, MD: Aspen.

Kral, J. G. (1989). Surgical treatment of obesity. *Medical Clinics of North America, 73,* 251–269.

Kramer, F. M., Jeffery, R. W., Forster, J. L., & Snell, M. K. (1989). Long-term follow-up of behavioral treatment for obesity: Patterns of weight gain among men and women. *International Journal of Obesity, 13,* 123–136.

Kramer, F. M., Jeffery, R. W., Snell, M. K., & Forster, J. L. (1986). Maintenance of successful weight loss over 1 year: Effects of financial contracts for weight maintenance or participation in skills training. *Behavior Therapy, 17,* 295–301.

Krehl, W. A. (1985). Vitamin supplementation: A practical view. In R. H. Garrison & E. Somer (Eds.), *The nutrition desk reference* (pp. 121–123). New Canaan, CT: Keats Publishing.

Krotkiewski, M., Bjorntorp, P., Sjostrom, L., & Smith, U. (1983). Impact of obesity on metabolism in men and women: Importance of regional adipose tissue distribution. *Journal of Clinical Investigations, 72,* 1150–1162.

Lantingua, R. A., Amatruda, J. A., Biddle, T. L., Forbes, G. B., & Lockwood, D. H. (1980). Cardiac arrhythmias associated with a liquid protein diet for the treatment of obesity. *New England Journal of Medicine, 303,* 735–738.

Lapidus, L., & Bengtsson, C. (1988). Regional adiposity as a health hazard in women: A prospective study. *Acta Medica Scandinavia 723*(Suppl.), 53.

Lapidus, L., Bengtsson, C., Larsson, B., Pennert, K., Rybo, E., & Sjostrom, L. (1984). Adipose tissue distribution and risk of cardiovascular disease and death: A 12-year follow-up of participants in the population study of women in Gothenburg, Sweden. *British Medical Journal, 289,* 1257–1261.

Larsson, B., Svardsuud, K., Welin, L., Wilhelmsen, L., Bjorntorp, P., & Tibblin, G. (1984). Abdominal adipose tissue distribution, obesity, and risk of cardiovascular disease and death: 13 year follow-up of participants in the study of men born in 1913. *British Medical Journal, 288,* 1401–1404.

Lebow, M. D., Goldberg, P., & Collins, A. (1977). A methodology for investigating differences in eating between obese and nonobese persons. *Behavior Therapy, 5,* 707–709.

Leibel, R. L., Berry, E. M., & Hirsch, J. (1983). Biochemistry and development of adipose tissue in man. In H. L. Conn, E. A. De Felice, & P. Huo (Eds.), *Health and obesity* (pp. 21–48). New York: Raven Press.

Leibel, R. L., & Hirsch, J. (1984). Diminished energy requirements in reduced-obese patients. *Metabolism, 33,* 164–179.

Lennon, D., Nagle, F., Stratman, F., Shrago, E., & Dennis, S. (1984). Diet and exercise training effects on resting metabolic rate. *International Journal of Obesity, 9,* 39–47.

Leon, A. S., & Blackburn, H. (1983). Physical inactivity. In N. M. Kaplan & J. Stamler (Eds.), *Prevention of coronary heart disease* (pp. 86–97). Philadelphia: Saunders.

Levin, B. E., Triscari, J., & Sullivan, A. C. (1986). Metabolic features of diet-induced obesity without hyperphagia in young rats. *American Journal of Physiology, 251,* R433–R440.

Levine, A. S., Tallman, J. A. R., Grace, M. K., Parker, S. A., Billington, C. B., & Levitt, M. D. (1989). Effect of breakfast cereals on short-term food intake. *American Journal of Clinical Nutrition, 50,* 1303–1307.

Levine, L. R., Rosenblatt, S., & Bosomworth, J. (1987). Use of a serotonin re-uptake inhibitor, fluoxetine, in the treatment of obesity. *International Journal of Obesity, 11*(Suppl. 3), 185–190.

Levitsky, D. A. (1970). Feeding patterns of rats in response to fasts and changes in environmental conditions. *Physiology and Behavior, 5,* 291–300.

Lew, E. A., & Garfinkel, L. (1979). Variations in mortality by weight among 750,000 men and women. *Journal of Chronic Diseases, 32,* 563–576.

Linn, R., & Stuart, S. L. (1976). *The last chance diet.* Secaucus, NJ: Lyle Stuart.

Lissner, L., Andres, R., Muller, D. C., & Shimokata, H. (1990). Body weight variability in men: Metabolic rate, health and longevity. *International Journal of Obesity, 14,* 373–383.

Lissner, L., Bengtsson, C., Lapidus, L., Bengtsson, B., & Brownell, K. D., (1989). Body weight variability and mortality in the Gothenburg prospective studies of men and women. In P. Bjorntorp & S. Rossner (Eds.), *Obesity in Europe 88: Proceedings of the First European Congress on Obesity* (pp. 55–60). London: Libbey.

Lissner, L., Levitsky, D. A., Strupp, B. J., Kalkwarf, H. J., & Roe, D. A. (1987). Dietary fat and the regulation of energy intake in human subjects. *American Journal of Clinical Nutrition, 46,* 886–892.

Lissner, L., Odell, P. M., D'Agostino, R. B., Stokes, J., III, Kreger, B. E., Belanger, A. J., & Brownell, K. D. (1991). Variability of body weight and health outcomes in the Framingham population. *New England Journal of Medicine, 324,* 1839–1844.

MacLean, L. D., Rhode, B. M., & Shizgal, H. M. (1983). Nutrition following gastric operations for morbid obesity. *Annals of Surgery, 198,* 347–355.

MacMahon, S. W., Wilcken, D. E. L., & Macdonald, G. J. (1986). The effect of weight reduction on left ventricular mass. *New England Journal of Medicine, 314,* 334–339.

Mahoney, M. J. (1975). The obese eating style: Bites, beliefs, and behavior modification. *Addictive Behaviors, 1,* 47–53.

Mahoney, M. J., & Mahoney, K. (1976). *Permanent weight control*. New York: Norton.

Makarewicz, P. A., Freeman, J. B., Burchett, H., & Brazeau, P. (1985). Vertical banded gastroplasty: Assessment of efficacy. *Surgery, 98*, 700–707.

Manson, J. E., Colditz, G. A., Stampfer, M. J., Willett, W. C., Rosner, B., Monson, R. R., Speizer, F. E., & Hennekens, C. H. (1990). A prospective study of obesity and risk of coronary heart disease in women. *New England Journal of Medicine, 322*, 882–889.

Marcoux, B. C., Trenkner, L. L., & Rosenstock, I. M. (1990). Social networks and social support in weight loss. *Patient Education and Counseling, 15*, 229–238.

Marcus, M. D., & Wing, R. R. (1987). Binge eating among the obese. *Annals of Behavioral Medicine, 9*, 23–27.

Marcus, M. D., Wing, R. R., & Hopkins, J. (1988). Obese binge eaters: Affect, cognitions, and responses to behavioral weight control. *Journal of Consulting and Clinical Psychology, 56*, 433–439.

Marlatt, G. A. (1985). Relapse prevention: Theoretical rationale and overview of the model. In G. A. Marlatt & J. R. Gordon (Eds.), *Relapse prevention: Maintenance strategies in the treatment of addictive behaviors* (pp. 3–70). New York: Guilford.

Marlatt, G. A. (1988). Matching clients to treatment: Treatment models and stages of change. In D. M. Donovan & G. A. Marlatt (Eds.), *Assessment of addictive behaviors* (pp. 474–484). New York: Guilford.

Marlatt, G. A., & Gordon, J. R. (Eds.). (1985). *Relapse prevention: Maintenance strategies in the treatment of addictive behaviors*. New York: Guilford.

Marshall, J. D., Hazlett, C. B., Spady, D. W., & Quinney, H. A. (1990). Comparison of convenient indicators of obesity. *American Journal of Clinical Nutrition, 51*, 22–28.

Marston, A. R., & Criss, J. (1984). Maintenance of successful weight loss: Incidence and prediction. *International Journal of Obesity, 8*, 435–439.

Martin, J. E., & Dubbert, P. M. (1982). Exercise applications and promotion in behavioral medicine: Current status and future directions. *Journal of Consulting and Clinical Psychology, 50*, 1004–1017.

Mason, E. E., Doherty, C., Maher, J. W., Scott, D. H., Rodriguez, E. M., & Blommers, T. J. (1987). Super obesity and gastric reduction procedures. *Gastroenterology Clinics of North America, 16*, 495–502.

Mayer, J., & Goldberg, J. P. (1990). *Dr. Jean Mayer's diet and nutrition guide*. New York: Pharos Books.

McArdle, W. D., Katch F. I., & Katch V. L. (1986). *Exercise physiology: Energy, nutrition, and human performance* (2nd ed.). Philadelphia: Lea & Febiger.

McArdle, W. D., & Toner, M. M. (1988). Application of exercise for weight control. In R. T. Frankle & M.-U. Yang (Eds.), *Obesity and weight control* (pp. 257–274). Rockville, MD: Aspen.

McCann, K. L., Perri, M. G., Nezu, A. M., & Lowe, M. R. (1992). Dietary restraint in obese clinic attenders. *International Journal of Eating Disorders*.

McKenna, R. J. (1972). Some effects of anxiety level and food cues in the behavior of obese and normal subjects. *Journal of Personality and Social Psychology, 22*, 311–316.

McReynolds, W. T. (1982). Toward a psychology of obesity: Review of research on the role of personality and level of adjustment. *International Journal of Eating Disorders, 2*, 37–57.

Melby, C. L., Schmidt, W. D., & Corrigan, D. (1990). Resting metabolic rate in weight-cycling collegiate wrestlers compared with physically active noncycling control subjects. *American Journal of Clinical Nutrition, 52*, 409–414.

Metropolitan Life Insurance Company. (1984). 1983 Metropolitan height and weight tables. *Statistical Bulletin of the Metropolitan Life Insurance Company, 64*, 2–9.

Miller, P. M., & Sims, K. L. (1981). Evaluation and component analysis of a comprehensive weight control program. *International Journal of Obesity, 5*, 57–65.

Miller, W. C. (1991). Obesity: Diet composition, energy expenditure, and treatment of the obese patient. *Medicine and Science in Sports and Exercise, 23*, 273–274.

Miller, W. C., Lindeman, A. K., Wallace, J., & Niederpruem, M. (1990). Diet composition, energy intake, and exercise in relation to body fatness in men and women. *American Journal of Clinical Nutrition, 52*, 426–430.

Minuchin, S., Rosman, B. L., & Baker, L. (1978). *Psychosomatic families: Anorexia nervosa in context*. Cambridge, MA: Harvard University Press.

Mole, P. A., Stern, J. S., Schultz, C. L., Bernauer, E. M., & Holcomb, B. J. (1989). Exercise reverses depressed metabolic rate produced by severe metabolic restriction. *Medicine and Science in Sports and Exercise, 21*, 29–33.

Moore, M. E., Stunkard, A. J., & Srole, L. (1962). Obesity, social class, and mental illness. *Journal of the American Medical Association, 181*, 962–966.

Morgan, W. P., & Horstman, O. H. (1976). Anxiety reduction following acute physical activity. *Medicine and Science in Sports, 8*, 62.

Munro, J. F., & Ford, M. J. (1982). Drug treatment of obesity. In T. Silverstone (Ed.), *Drugs and appetite* (pp. 125–157). London: Academic Press.

Nash, J. D. (1977). *Curbing drop-out from treatment for obesity*. Unpublished doctoral dissertation, Stanford University, Palo Alto, CA.

National Center for Health Statistics. (1966). *Weight by height and age of adults, United States, 1960–1962*. (Vital and Health Statistics, Series 11, No. 14). Hyattsville, MD: Author.

National Center for Health Statistics. (1979). *Weight and height of adults 18–74 years of age, United States, 1971–1974* (DHEW Publication No. [PHS] 79-1659, Vital and Health Statistics, Series 11, No. 211). Hyattsville, MD: Author.

National Center for Health Statistics. (1981). *Plan and operation of the National Health and Nutrition Examination Survey, 1976–1980* (DHHS Publication No. [PHS] 81-1317, Vital and Health Statistics, Series 1, No. 15). Hyattsville, MD: Author.

National Center for Health Statistics. (1986). Prevalence and impact of known diabetes in the United States. In *Advance data from vital health statistics* (DHHS Publication No. [PHS] 86-1250, pp. XXII, 469–479). Hyattsville, MD: U.S. Public Health Service.

National Diabetes Data Group (1979). Classification and diagnosis of diabetes mellitus and other categories of glucose intolerance. *Diabetes, 28*, 1039–1059.

National Institutes of Health Consensus Development Panel on the Health Implications of Obesity. (1985). Health implications of obesity. *Annals of Internal Medicine, 103*, 147–151.

National Research Council. (1989). *Diet and health: Implications for reducing chronic disease risk.* Washington, DC: National Academy Press.

Nezu, A. M., & D'Zurilla, T. J. (1981a). Effects of problem definition and formulation on decision making in the social problem-solving process. *Behavior Therapy, 12,* 100–106.

Nezu, A. M., & D'Zurilla, T. J. (1981b). Effects of problem definition and formulation on the generation of alternatives in the social problem-solving process. *Cognitive Therapy and Research, 5,* 265–271.

Nezu, A. M., & D'Zurilla, T. J. (1989). Social problem solving and negative affective states. In P. C. Kendall & D. Watson (Eds.), *Anxiety and depression: Distinctive and overlapping features* (pp. 285–315). New York: Academic Press.

Nezu, A. M., & Nezu, C. M. (Eds.). (1989). *Clinical decision making in behavior therapy: A problem-solving perspective.* Champaign, IL: Research Press.

Nezu, A. M., Nezu, C. M., & Perri, M. G. (1989). *Problem-solving therapy for depression: Theory, research, and clinical guidelines.* New York: Wiley.

Nicholas, P., & Dwyer, J. (1986). Diets for weight reduction: nutritional considerations. In K. D. Brownell & J. P. Foreyt (Eds.), *Handbook of eating disorders: Physiology, psychology, and treatment of obesity, anorexia, and bulimia* (pp. 122–145). New York: Basic Books.

Nisbett, R. E. (1968). Determinants of food intake in obesity. *Science, 159,* 1254–1255.

Ohlson, L. O., Larsson, B., Svardsudd, K., Welin, L., Eriksson, H., & Wilhelmsen, L., (1985). The influence of body fat distribution on the incidence of diabetes: 13.5 years of follow-up of the participants in the study of men born in 1913. *Diabetes, 34,* 1055–1058.

Orme, C. M., & Binik, Y. M. (1987). Recidivism and self-cure of obesity: A test of Schacter's hypothesis in diabetic patients. *Health Psychology, 6,* 467–475.

Oscai, L. B., Brown, M. M., & Miller, W. C. (1984). Effect of dietary fat on food intake, growth and body composition in rats. *Growth, 48,* 415–424.

Oscai, L. B., Miller, W. C., & Arnall, D. A. (1987). Effect of dietary sugar and of dietary fat on food intake and body fat content in rats. *Growth, 51,* 64–73.

Page, L. B., Damon, A., & Moellering, R. C. (1974). Antecedents of cardiovascular disease in six Solomon Islands societies. *Circulation, 49,* 1132–1146.

Passmore, R., & Durnin, J. V. G. A. (1955). Human energy expenditure. *Physiological Reviews, 35,* 801.

Paul, G. L. (1969). Behavior modification research: Design and tactics. In C. M. Franks (Ed.), *Behavior therapy: Appraisal and status* (pp. 29–62). New York: McGraw-Hill.

Pavlou, K. N., Krey, S., & Steffee, W. P. (1989). Exercise as an adjunct to weight loss and maintenance in moderately obese subjects. *American Journal of Clinical Nutrition, 49*(Suppl.), 1115–1123.

Pepper, S. C. (1942). *World hypotheses.* Berkeley: University of California Press.

Perri, M. G. (1985). Self-change strategies for smoking, obesity, and problem drinking. In S. Shiffman & T. A. Wills (Eds.), *Coping and substance use* (pp. 295–317). Orlando, FL: Academic Press.

Perri, M. G. (1987). Maintenance strategies for the management of obesity. In W. G.

Johnson (Ed.), *Advances in eating disorders: Vol. 1. Treating and preventing obesity* (pp. 177–194). Greenwich, CT: JAI.

Perri, M. G. (1989). Obesity. In A. M. Nezu & C. M. Nezu (Eds.), *Clinical decision making in behavior therapy: A problem-solving perspective* (pp. 193–226). Champaign, IL: Research Press.

Perri, M. G., McAdoo, W. G., McAllister, D. A., Lauer, J. B., Jordan, R. C., Yancey, D. Z., & Nezu, A. M. (1987). Effects of peer support and therapist contact on long-term weight loss. *Journal of Consulting and Clinical Psychology, 55,* 615–617.

Perri, M. G., McAdoo, W. G., McAllister, D. A., Lauer, J. B., & Yancey, D. Z. (1986). Enhancing the efficacy of behavior therapy for obesity: Effects of aerobic exercise and a multicomponent maintenance program. *Journal of Consulting and Clinical Psychology, 54,* 670–675.

Perri, M. G., McAdoo, W. G., Spevak, P. A., & Newlin, D. B. (1984). Effect of a multicomponent maintenance program on long-term weight loss. *Journal of Consulting and Clinical Psychology, 52,* 480–481.

Perri, M. G., McAllister, D. A., Gange, J. J., Jordan, R. C., McAdoo, W. G., & Nezu, A. M. (1988). Effects of four maintenance programs on the long-term management of obesity. *Journal of Consulting and Clinical Psychology, 56,* 529–534.

Perri, M. G., McKelvey, W. F., Schein, R. L., Renjilian, D. A., Viegener, B. J., & Nezu, A. M. (1990, November). *Relapse prevention training versus frequent therapist contacts as weight-loss maintenance strategies.* Paper presented at the annual meeting of the Association for Advancement of Behavior Therapy, San Francisco.

Perri, M. G., Nezu, A. M., Patti, E. T., & McCann, K. L. (1989). Effect of length of treatment on weight loss. *Journal of Consulting and Clinical Psychology, 57,* 450–452.

Perri, M. G., & Richards, C. S. (1977). An investigation of naturally occurring episodes of self-controlled behavior. *Journal of Counseling Psychology, 25,* 178–183.

Perri, M. G., Shapiro, R. M., Ludwig, W. W., Twentyman, C. T., & McAdoo, W. G. (1984). Maintenance strategies for the treatment of obesity: An evaluation of relapse prevention training and posttreatment contact by mail and telephone. *Journal of Consulting and Clinical Psychology, 52,* 404–413.

Perusse, L., Tremblay, A., Leblanc, C., & Bouchard, C. (1989). Genetic and environmental influences on level of habitual physical activity and exercise participation. *American Journal of Epidemiology, 129,* 1012–1022.

Phinney, S. D., LaGrange, B. M., O'Connell, M., & Danforth, E. (1988). Effects of aerobic exercise on energy expenditure and nitrogen balance during very-low-calorie dieting. *Metabolism, 37,* 758–765.

Pi-Sunyer, F. X. (1988). Exercise in the treatment of obesity. In R. T. Frankle & M.-U. Yang (Eds.), *Obesity and weight control* (pp. 241–255). Rockville, MD: Aspen.

Poehlman, E. T., Melby, C. L., & Badylak, S. F. (1988). Resting metabolic rate and postprandial thermogenesis in highly trained and untrained males. *American Journal of Clinical Nutrition, 47,* 793–798.

Polivy, J. (1976). Perception of calories and regulation of intake in restrained and unrestrained subjects. *Addictive Behaviors, 1,* 237–243.

Polivy, J., & Herman, C. P. (1976). Effects of alcohol on eating behavior: Influences of mood and perceived intoxication. *Journal of Abnormal Psychology, 85,* 601–606.

Polivy, J., & Herman, C. P. (1985). Dieting and binging: A causal analysis. *American Psychologist, 40,* 193–201.

Price, R. A. (1987). Genetics of human obesity. *Annals of Behavioral Medicine, 9,* 9–14.

Price, R. A., Cadoret, R. J., Stunkard, A. J., & Troughton, E. (1987). Genetic contributions to human fatness: An adoption study. *American Journal of Psychiatry, 144,* 1003–1008.

Prior, I. A. (1971). The price of civilization. *Nutrition Today, 6,* 2–11.

Prochaska, J. O., & DiClemente, C. C. (1982). Transtheoretical therapy: Toward a more integrative model of change. *Psychotherapy: Theory, Research, and Practice, 19,* 276–288.

Prochaska, J. O., & DiClemente, C. C. (1984). *The transtheoretical approach: Crossing traditional boundaries of therapy.* Homewood, IL: Dow Jones–Irwin.

Rathus, S. A. (1973). A 30-item schedule for assessing assertive behavior. *Behavior Therapy, 4,* 398–406.

Ravussin, E., Acheson, K., Vernet, O., Danforth, E., & Jequier, E. (1985). Evidence that insulin resistance is responsible for decreased thermic effect of glucose in human obesity. *Journal of Clinical Investigations, 76,* 1268–1273.

Ravussin, E., Lillioja, S., Anderson, T. E., Christin, L., & Bogardus, C. (1986). Determinants of 24-hour energy expenditure in man: Methods and results using a respiratory chamber. *Journal of Clinical Investigations, 78,* 1568–1578.

Ravussin, E., Lillioja, S., Knowler, W. C., Christin, L., Freymond, D., Abbott, W. G. H., Boyce, V., Howard, B. V., & Bogardus, C. (1988). Reduced rate of energy expenditure as a risk factor for body-weight gain. *New England Journal of Medicine, 318,* 462–472.

Rifkind, H. (Ed.). (1984). *The physician's guide to type II diabetes (NIDDM): Diagnosis and treatment.* New York: American Diabetes Association.

Roberts, S. B., Savage, J., Coward, W. E., Chew, B., & Lucas, A. (1988). Energy expenditure and intake in infants born to lean and overweight mothers. *New England Journal of Medicine, 318,* 461–466.

Rodin, J. (1981). The current status of the internal–external obesity hypothesis: What went wrong? *American Psychologist, 36,* 361–372.

Rodin, J. (1985). Insulin levels, hunger and food intake: An example of feedback loops in body weight regulation. *Health Psychology, 4,* 1–18.

Rodin, J., Radke-Sharpe, N., Rebuffe-Scrive, M., & Greenwood, M. R. C. (1990). Weight cycling and fat distribution. *International Journal of Obesity, 14,* 303–310.

Rodin, J., Schank, D., & Striegel-Moore, R. (1989). Psychological features of obesity. *Medical Clinics of North America, 73,* 47–66.

Rodin, J., Wack, J., Ferrannini, E., & DeFronzo, E. (1985). Effects of insulin and glucose on feeding behavior. *Metabolism, 34,* 826–831.

Romieu, I., Willett, W. C., Stampfer, M. J., Colditz, G. A., Sampson, L., Rosner, B., Hennekens, C. H., & Speizer, F. E. (1988). Energy intake and other determinants of relative weight. *American Journal of Clinical Nutrition, 47,* 406–412.

Ruderman, A. J. (1983). Obesity, anxiety, and food consumption. *Addictive Behaviors, 8,* 235–242.

Ruggerio, L., Williamson, D., Davis, C. J., Schlundt, D. G., & Carey, M. P. (1988).

Forbidden Foods Survey: Measure of bulimics anticipated reactions to specific foods. *Addictive Behavior, 13,* 267–274.

Salans, L. B., Knittle, J. L., & Hirsch, J. (1983). Obesity, glucose intolerance, and diabetes mellitus. In M. Ellenberg & M. Rifkind (Eds.), *Diabetes mellitus: Theory and practice* (3rd ed., pp. 469–480). New Hyde Park, NY: Medical Examination Publishing.

Sallis, J. F., Hovell, M. F., Hofstetter, C. R., Elder, J. P., Faucher, P., Spry, V. M., Barrington, E., & Hackley, M. (1990). Lifetime history of relapse from exercise. *Addictive Behaviors, 15,* 573–579.

Sarason, I. G., Johnson, J. H., & Siegel, J. M. (1978). Assessing the impact of life changes: Development of the Life Experiences Survey. *Journal of Consulting and Clinical Psychology, 46,* 932–946.

Schachter, S. (1982). Recidivism and self-cure of smoking and obesity. *American Psychologist, 37,* 436–444.

Schachter, S., Goldman, R., & Gordon, A. (1968). Effects of fear, food deprivation, and obesity on eating. *Journal of Personality and Social Psychology, 10,* 91–97.

Schachter, S., & Rodin, J. (1974). *Obese humans and rats.* Washington, DC: Erlbaum/Halsted.

Schlundt, D. G., & Johnson, W. G. (1990). *Eating disorders: Assessment and treatment.* Needham Heights, MA: Allyn & Bacon.

Schlundt, D. G., Johnson, W. G., & Jarrell, M. P. (1985). A naturalistic functional analysis of eating behavior in bulimia and obesity. *Advances in Behaviour Research and Therapy, 7,* 149–162.

Schutz, Y., Flatt, J. P., & Jequier, E. (1989). Failure of dietary fat intake to promote fat oxidation: A factor favoring the development of obesity. *American Journal of Clinical Nutrition, 50,* 307–314.

Scoville, B. (1975). Review of amphetamine-like drugs by the Food and Drug Administration. In G. A. Bray (Ed.), *Obesity in perspective* (Vol. 2, pp. 441–460). Washington, DC: U.S. Government Printing Office.

Segal, K. R., Gutin, B., Albu, J., & Pi-Sunyer, F. X. (1987). Thermic effects of food and exercise in lean and obese men of similar lean body mass. *American Journal of Physiology, 252,* E110–E117.

Segal, K. R., Gutin, B., Nyman, A. M., & Pi-Sunyer, F. X. (1985). Thermic effect of food at rest, during exercise, and after exercise in lean and obese men of similar body weight. *Journal of Clinical Investigations, 76,* 1107–1112.

Segal, K. R., & Pi-Sunyer, F. X. (1989). Exercise and obesity. *Medical Clinics of North America, 73,* 217–236.

Shadish, W. R. (1986). Planned critical multiplism: Some elaborations. *Behavioral Assessment, 8,* 75–103.

Shapiro, L., Koehl, C., Springen, K., Manley, H., Pyrillis, R., Hager, M., & Starr, M. (1991, May 27). Feeding frenzy. *Newsweek,* pp. 46–53.

Sharp, J. T., Barrocas, M., & Chokroverty, S. (1983). The cardiorespiratory effects of obesity. *Clinics in Chest Medicine, 1,* 103–118.

Sikand, G., Kondo, A., Foreyt, J. P., Jones, P. H., & Gotto, A. M. (1988). Two-year follow-up of patients treated with a very-low-calorie diet and exercise training. *Journal of the American Dietetic Association, 88,* 487–488.

Silverstone, T. (1987). Appetite-suppressant drugs in the management of obesity: The current view. *International Journal of Obesity, 11*(Suppl. 3), 135–139.

Sims, E. A. H. (1974). Studies in human hyperphagia. In G. Bray & J. Bethune (Eds.), *Treatment and management of obesity* (pp. 29–46). New York: Harper & Row.

Sjostrom, L. (1980). Fat cells and body weight. In A. J. Stunkard (Ed.), *Obesity* (pp. 72–100). Philadelphia: Saunders.

Smith, D. E., & Wing, R. R. (1991). Diminished weight loss and behavioral compliance using repeated diets in obese women with Type II diabetes. *Health Psychology, 10*, 378–383.

Smith, G. P. (1984). Gut hormone hypothesis of postprandial satiety. In A. J. Stunkard & E. Stellar (Eds.), *Eating and its disorders* (pp. 67–75). New York: Raven Press.

Smith, U. (1985). Regional differences in adipocyte metabolism and possible consequences in vivo. In J. Hirsch & T. B. Van Itallie (Eds.), *Recent advances in obesity research* (Vol. 4, pp. 33–36). London: John Libbey.

Smoller, J. W., Wadden, T. A., & Stunkard, A. J. (1987). Dieting and depression: A critical review. *Journal of Psychosomatic Research, 31*(4), 429–440.

Snyder, D. K. (1979). *Marital satisfaction inventory*. Los Angeles: Western Psychological Services.

Society of Actuaries and Association of Life Insurance Medical Directors of America. (1980). *Build study of 1979*. Chicago, IL: Author.

Solow, C., Silberfarb, P. M., & Swift, K. (1974). Psychosocial effects of intestinal bypass surgery for severe obesity. *New England Journal of Medicine, 290*, 300–304.

Sorensen, T. I. A., Price, R. A., Stunkard, A. J., & Schulsinger, F. (1989). Genetics of obesity in adult adoptees and their biological siblings. *British Medical Journal, 298*, 87–90.

Southard, D. R., Winett, R. A., Walberg-Rankin, J. L., Neubauer, T. E., Donckers-Roseveare, K., Burkett, P. A., Gould, R., & Moore, J. F. (in press). Increasing the effectiveness of the National Cholesterol Education Program: Dietary and behavioral strategies. *Annals of Behavioral Medicine*.

Spencer, I. O. B. (1968). Death during therapeutic starvation for obesity. *Lancet, 1*, 1288–1290.

Society of Actuaries and Association of Life Insurance Medical Directors of merica. (1980). *Build study of 1979*. Chicago, IL: Author.

Spevak, P. A. (1981). Maintenance of therapy gains: Strategies, problems, and progress. *JSAS Catalog of Selected Documents in Psychology, 11*(Ms. No. 2255), 35.

Spiegel, T. A., Wadden, T. A., & Foster, G. D. (1991). Objective measurement of eating rate during behavioral treatment of obesity. *Behavior Therapy, 22*, 61–67.

Spielberger, C. D., Gorsuch, R. L., & Luschene, R. E. (1979). *Manual for the State-Trait Anxiety Inventory*. Palo Alto, CA: Consulting Psychologists Press.

Spitzer, R. L., Devlin, M., Walsh, B. T., Hasin, D., Wing, R., Marcus, M., Stunkard, A., Wadden, T., Yanovski, S., Agras, S., Mitchell, J., & Nonas, C. (in press). Binge eating disorder: A multisite field trial of the diagnostic criteria. *International Journal of Eating Disorders*.

Stalonas, P. M., Johnson, W. G., & Christ, M. (1978). Behavior modification for obesity: The evaluation of exercise, contingency management, and program adherence. *Journal of Consulting and Clinical Psychology, 46*, 463–469.

Stalonas, P. M., & Kirschenbaum, D. S. (1985). Behavioral treatment for obesity: Eating habits revisited. *Behavior Therapy, 16,* 1–14.

Stalonas, P. M., Perri, M. G., & Kerzner, A. B. (1984). Do behavioral treatments of obesity last? A five-year follow-up investigation. *Addictive Behaviors, 9,* 175–184.

Stanton, A. L., Garcia, M. E., & Green, S. B. (1990). Development and validation of the Situation Appetite Measures. *Addictive Behaviors, 15,* 460–472.

Steen, S. N., Opplinger, R. A., & Brownell, K. D. (1988). Metabolic effects of repeated weight loss and regain in adolescent wrestlers. *Journal of the American Medical Association, 260,* 47–50.

Stephen, A. M., & Wald, N. J. (1990). Trends in individual consumption of dietary fat in the United States, 1920–1984. *American Journal of Clinical Nutrition, 52,* 457–469.

Stern, J. S., & Lowney, P. (1986). Obesity: The role of physical activity. In K. D. Brownell & J. P. Foreyt (Eds.), *Handbook of eating disorders: Physiology, psychology, and treatment of obesity, anorexia, and bulimia* (pp. 145–158). New York: Basic Books.

Stevens, J., & Lissner, L. (1990). Body weight variability and mortality in the Charleston Heart Study. *International Journal of Obesity, 14,* 385–386.

Stewart, A. L., & Brook, R. H. (1983). Effects of being overweight. *American Journal of Public Health, 73,* 171–178.

Stillman, I. M., & Baker, S. (1977). *The doctor's quick weight loss diet.* New York: Dell.

Straw, M. K., Straw, M. B., Mahoney, M. J., Rogers, T., Mahoney, B. K., Craighead, L. W., & Stunkard, A. J. (1984). The Master Questionnaire: Preliminary report of an obesity assessment device. *Addictive Behaviors, 9,* 1–10.

Stuart, R. B. (1980). Weight loss and beyond: Are they taking it off and keeping it off? In P. O. Davidson & S. M. Davidson (Eds.), *Behavioral Medicine: Changing health lifestyles* (pp. 151–192). New York: Brunner/Mazel.

Stunkard, A. J. (1957). The dieting depression: Untoward responses to weight reduction. *American Journal of Medicine, 23,* 77–86.

Stunkard, A. J. (1976). *The pain of obesity.* Palo Alto, CA: Bull Publishing.

Stunkard, A. J. (1984). The current status of treatment for obesity in adults. In A. J. Stunkard & E. Stellar (Eds.), *Eating and its disorders* (pp. 157–174). New York: Raven Press.

Stunkard, A. J. (1987). Conservative treatments for obesity. *American Journal of Clinical Nutrition, 45,* 1142–1154.

Stunkard, A. J. (1989). Perspectives on human obesity. In A. J. Stunkard & A. Baum (Eds.) *Perspectives in behavioral medicine: Eating, sleeping, and sex* (pp. 9–30). Hillsdale, NJ: Erlbaum.

Stunkard, A. J., Harris, J. R., Pedersen, N. I., & McClearn, G. E. (1990). The body-mass index of twins who have been reared apart. *New England Journal of Medicine, 322,* 1483–1487.

Stunkard, A. J., Levine, H., & Fox, S. (1970). The management of obesity: Patient self-help and medical treatment. *Archives of Internal Medicine, 125,* 1067–1072.

Stunkard, A. J., & Messick, S. (1988). *Eating Inventory manual.* San Antonio, TX: Psychological Corporation.

Stunkard, A. J., & Rush, A. J. (1974). Dieting and depression reexamined: A critical review of reports of untoward responses during weight reduction for obesity. *Annals of Internal Medicine, 81,* 526–533.

Stunkard, A. J., Sorensen, T. I. A., Hanis, C., Teasdale, T. W., Chakraborty, R., Schull, W. J., & Schlusinger, F. (1986). An adoption study of human obesity. *New England Journal of Medicine, 314,* 193–198.

Stunkard, A. J., Stinnett, J. L., & Smoller, J. W. (1986). Psychological and social aspects of the surgical treatment of obesity. *American Journal of Psychiatry, 143,* 417–429.

Sturdevant, R. A. L., Pearce, M. L., & Dayton, S. (1973). Increased prevalence of cholelithiasis in men ingesting a serum cholesterol-lowering diet. *New England Journal of Medicine, 288,* 24–27.

Sugerman, H. J., Londrey, G., Kellum, J. M., Wolf, L., Liszka, T., Engle, K. M., Birkenhauer, R., & Starkey, J. V. (1989). Weight loss with vertical banded gastroplasty and Roux-Y gastric bypass for morbid obesity with selective versus random assignment. *American Journal of Surgery, 157,* 93–102.

Sugerman, H. J., Starkey, J. V., & Birkenhauer, R. (1987). A randomized prospective trial of gastric bypass versus vertical banded gastroplasty for morbid obesity and their effects on sweets versus non-sweets eaters. *Annals of Surgery, 205,* 613–624.

Sullivan, A. C., & Comai, K. (1978). Pharmacological treatment of obesity. *International Journal of Obesity, 2,* 167–189.

Tarnower, H., & Baker, S. S. (1978). *The complete Scarsdale medical diet.* New York: Bantam Books.

Task Force of the American Society for Clinical Nutrition. (1985). Guidelines for surgery for morbid obesity. *American Journal of Clinical Nutrition, 42,* 904–905.

Telch, C. F., Agras, W. S., & Rossiter, E. M. (1988). Binge eating increases with increasing adiposity. *International Journal of Eating Disorders, 7,* 115–119.

Thompson, J. K., Jarvie, G. J., Lahey, B. B., & Cureton, K. H. (1982). Exercise and obesity: Etiology, physiology, and intervention. *Psychological Bulletin, 91,* 55–79.

Tremblay, A., Plourde, G., Despres, J. P., & Bouchard, C. (1989). Impact of dietary fat content and fat oxidation on energy intake in humans. *American Journal of Clinical Nutrition, 49,* 799–805.

Trowell, H. C., & Burkitt, D. P. (1981). *Western diseases: Their emergence and prevention.* Cambridge, MA: Harvard University Press.

U.S. Department of Agriculture. (1971). *Nutritive value of foods* (Home and Garden Bulletin No. 72, rev.). Washington, DC: Author.

U.S. Department of Agriculture. (1984). *Nationwide food consumption survey: Nutrient intakes—Individuals in 48 states, years 1977–1978* (Report No. 1-2; Consumer Nutrition Division, Human Nutrition Information Service). Hyattsville, MD: Author.

Van Dale, D., & Saris, W. H. M. (1989). Repetitive weight loss and weight regain: Effects on weight reduction, resting metabolic rate, and lipolytic activity before and after exercise and/or diet treatment. *American Journal of Clinical Nutrition, 49,* 409–416.

Van Itallie, T. B. (1978). Liquid protein mayhem [Editorial]. *Journal of the American Medical Association, 240,* 140–145.

Van Itallie, T. B. (1980). Dietary approaches to the treatment of obesity. In A. J. Stunkard (Ed.), *Obesity* (pp. 249–261). Philadelphia: Saunders.

Van Itallie, T. B. (1985). Health implications of overweight and obesity in the United States. *Annals of Internal Medicine, 103,* 983–988.

Van Itallie, T. B., & Hadley, L. (1988). *The best spas.* New York: Harper & Row.

Viegener, B. J., Perri, M. G., Nezu, A. M., Renjilian, D. A., McKelvey, W. F., & Schein, R. L. (1990). Effects of an intermittent, low-fat, low-calorie diet in the behavioral treatment of obesity. *Behavior Therapy, 21,* 499–509.

Volkmar, F. R., Stunkard, A. J., Woolston, J., & Bailey, B. A. (1981). High attrition rates in commercial weight reduction programs. *Archives of Internal Medicine, 141,* 426–428.

Wadden, T. A., Bartlett, S., Letizia, K. A., Foster, G. D., Stunkard, A. J., & Conill, A. (in press). Relationship of dieting history to resting metabolic rate, body composition, eating behavior and subsequent weight loss. *American Journal of Clinical Nutrition.*

Wadden, T. A., & Bell, S. T. (1990). Obesity. In A. S. Bellack, M. Hersen, & A. E. Kazdin (Eds.), *International handbook of behavior modification and therapy* (Vol. 2, pp. 449–473). New York: Plenum.

Wadden, T. A., Foster, G. D., Brownell, K. D., & Finley, B. (1984). Self-concepts in obese and normal weight children. *Journal of Consulting and Clinical Psychology, 52,* 1104–1105.

Wadden, T. A., Sternberg, J. A., Letizia, K. A., Stunkard, A. J., & Foster, G. A. (1989). Treatment of obesity by very low calorie diet, behavior therapy, and their combination: A five-year perspective. *International Journal of Obesity, 13,* 39–46.

Wadden, T. A., & Stunkard, A. J. (1985). Social and psychological consequences of obesity. *Annals of Internal Medicine, 103,* 1062–1067.

Wadden, T. A., & Stunkard, A. J. (1986). Controlled trial of very-low-calorie diet, behavior therapy, and their combination in the treatment of obesity. *Journal of Consulting and Clinical Psychology, 54,* 482–488.

Wadden, T. A., & Stunkard, A. J. (1987). Psychopathology and obesity. In R. J. Wurtman & J. J. Wurtman (Eds.), *Human obesity* (pp. 55–65). New York: New York Academy of Sciences.

Wadden, T. A., Stunkard, A. J., & Brownell, K. D. (1983). Very low calorie diets: Their efficacy, safety, and future. *Annals of Internal Medicine, 99,* 675–684.

Wadden, T. A., Stunkard, A. J., Brownell, K. D., & Day, S. C. (1985). A comparison of two very-low-calorie diets: Protein-sparing-modified fast versus protein-formula-liquid diet. *American Journal of Clinical Nutrition, 41,* 533–539.

Wadden, T. A., Stunkard, A. J., & Liebschutz, J. (1988). Three year follow-up of the treatment of obesity by very-low-calorie diet, behavior therapy and their combination. *Journal of Consulting and Clinical Psychology, 56,* 925–928.

Wadden, T. A., Stunkard, A. J., Rich, L., Rubin, C. J., Sweidel, G., & McKinney, S. (1990). Obesity in black adolescent girls: A controlled trial of treatment by diet, behavior modification and parental support. *Pediatrics, 85,* 345–352.

Waxman, M., & Stunkard, A. J. (1980). Caloric intake and expenditure of obese boys. *Journal of Pediatrics, 96,* 187–193.

Webster, J. D., & Garrow, J. S. (1989). Weight loss in 108 obese women on a diet supplying 800 kcal/d for 21 d. *American Journal of Clinical Nutrition, 50,* 41–45.

282   References

Weintraub, M., & Bray, G. A. (1989). Drug treatment of obesity. *Medical Clinics of North America, 73,* 237–249.

Westlund, K., & Nicholaysen, R. (1972). Ten year mortality and morbidity related to serum cholesterol: A follow–up of 3,751 men aged 40–49. *Scandinavian Journal of Clinical and Laboratory Medicine, 127*(Suppl.), 1–24.

Whiting, M. G. (1958). *A cross-cultural nutrition survey.* Unpublished doctoral dissertation, Harvard School of Public Health, Cambridge, MA.

Williamson, D. A., Kelley, M. L., Davis, C. J., Ruggerio, L., & Blouin, D. (1985). Psychopathology of eating disorders: A controlled comparison of bulimic, obese, and normal subjects. *Journal of Consulting and Clinical Psychology, 53,* 161–

& Kupfer, D. J. (1984). Mood changes ...nal of Psychosomatic Research, 28, 189–

...les, M., Kriska, A., Nowalk, M. P., & ...ioural weight control programme for ...dependent) diabetes. *Diabetologia, 31,*

...nt treatments of obesity: A comparison ...rnational Journal of Obesity, 3, 261–279.

...valk, M. P., Gooding, W., & Becker, D. ...ight loss in Type II diabetic patients. ...753.

Woo, R., Garrow, J. S., & Pi-Sunyer, F. X. (1982). Effect of exercise on spontaneous caloric intake in obesity. *American Journal of Clinical Nutrition, 36,* 470–477.

Woo, R., & Pi-Sunyer, F. X. (1985). Effect of increased physical activity on voluntary intake in lean women. *Metabolism, 34,* 836–841.

Wood, P. D., Stefanick, M. L., & Haskell, W. L. (1985). Exercise offsets adverse lipoprotein effects of a "heart healthy" diet for weight loss. *Arteriosclerosis, 9,* 773a.

Wooley, S. C., Wooley, O. W., & Dyrenforth, S. (1979). Theoretical, practical, and social issues in behavioral treatment of obesity. *Journal of Applied Behavioral Analysis, 12,* 3–25.

Yalom, I. D. (1985). *The theory and practice of group psychotherapy.* New York: Basic Books.

Zerbe, R. L. (1987). Safety of fluoxetine in the treatment of obesity. *International Journal of Obesity, 11*(Suppl. 3), 191–199.

Author Index

Subject Index

Date Due

JAN - 5 1998	
NO- 9 '98	
NOV 3 0 1999	
APR 0 6 2000	
AUG 2 4 2000	
JAN 0 2 2001	
NOV 3 0 2002	

PRINTED IN U.S.A.   CAT. NO. 24 161

Date Due

JAN - 5 1998			
NO- 9 '98			
NOV 3 0 1999			
APR 0 8 2000			
AUG 2 4 2000			
JAN 0 2 01			
NOV 3 0 2002			

PRINTED IN U.S.A.   CAT. NO. 24 161   BRO DART